HOSPITAL EXTENSION SERVICES

(Encyclopaedia of Hospital Management—11)

DR. S.L. GOEL
Professor of Public Administration (Retd.),
Panjab University, Chandigarh
Editor, Indian Journal of Public Administration, IIPA, New Delhi
Former Member, UGC, Former Member Distance Education Council
Former Member All India Board of Management, AICTE
Member, Executive Council, IIPA, New Delhi.
Former Vice-President, IIPA, New Delhi.
Emeritus Fellow, University Grants Commission
Former Director, State Bank of India (Local Board) Chandigarh
Former Director, National Horticulture Board, Ministry of Agriculture,
Government of India, New Delhi.

and

DR. R. KUMAR
MBBS, MS, Ex. PGI
President, Chandigarh Ophthalmological Society, 2000-01,
Columnist on Health Education and Management,
Advisor on Health Care and Medical Tourism,
Member Tourism Advisory Forum,
Chandigarh Administration, Chandigarh

DEEP & DEEP PUBLICATIONS PVT. LTD.
F-159, Rajouri Garden, New Delhi-110027

HOSPITAL EXTENSION SERVICES
(Encyclopaedia of Hospital Management—11)

ISBN 978-81-8450-226-8

Typeset by S.S. COMPOSERS
3190, Mohindra Park, Shakur Basti, Delhi-110034.

Printed in India at MAYUR ENTERPRISES
WZ Plot No. 3, Gujjar Market, Tihar Village, New Delhi-110018.

Published by DEEP & DEEP PUBLICATIONS PVT. LTD.
F-159, Rajouri Garden, New Delhi-110027.
Phones: 25435369, 25440916
E-mail: ddpbooks@yahoo.co.in • ddpubs@gmail.com
Showroom:
2/13, Ansari Road, Daryaganj, New Delhi-110002 • Telefax: 23245122

Contents

Preface

While hospitals may touch someone once in a lifetime kind situation, extension services have a wide reach/horizon and need to touch a large population on a continuing basis, from birth to death, viz. delivery huts in the remote areas to funeral services organised by an agency like Red-Cross. In fact in many situations, the extension services are the hospital services provided by the hospitals at the door steps of the beneficiaries. China's concept of barefoot doctors or India's National rural health mission encompassing immunisation, nutrition services and implementation of reproductive and child health services and national health programmes are the living examples of extension services of hospital duties.

In India, where the hospitals are over-crowded, the doctor-patient ratio is low and the resources are limited, the need for providing satisfactory outreach services is all the more. Now with the rise of longevity and increase in the graying population the need to look after the chronically ill and terminally ill is also rising. Hospitals are not the best places for such clients. Such patients can be looked after better in a domestic set-up or another home-like set-up, which is not a part of the hospitals. Similarly, hospitals are not the best places to give well baby services or care to maternity cases, since they are not patients in a real sense. They are normal beings requiring medical supervision; why to expose them to the stresses and strains and infections of the hospitals. More so such services outside the hospitals can be provided at a much lower cost to the nation and the beneficiary persons. The benefits of such a care are tremendous, since the child has a long way to go in life. Similarly, why to burden a hospital bed with a cancer patient or a complicated diabetic, since the chances of cure are minimal and the costs to all concerned is very high. Such cases may be better dealt and more cost effective outside the hospitals.

Holding of free eye camps and medical camps, family planning operation camps, de-addiction services, services to homeless and those in jails, mentally ill patients, administration of vaccines, mobile trauma and critical care teams, specialised clinics of physiotherapy/imaging, advanced services in various branches of medicine and clinics thereof, prevention and treatment of lifestyle diseases, HIV/sexually transmitted diseases and other infections, supplements for malnutrition containment viz. vitamin and iron deficiency, iodine deficiency diseases, delivery huts for safe and hygienic childbirth, school health programmes, etc. are only some of the examples of ever expanding extension services meant for non-admitted patients and the community at large. It also entails services like sending nurses or care-givers for the chronically ill at home or services like hospice for the terminally ill. Often it may mean providing medical services or wellness services at the door steps of the patient/person.

Non-admitted Patients (NAPs)

NAPs are those who receive care from a hospital but who do not undergo the hospital's formal admission process. The categories of **non-admitted patient services** offered by hospitals are: emergency department; outpatient; others viz. community, domiciliary and other **outreach services**. This concept is well known in Australia. Accurate detailed information is required on the **outpatient services** provided by hospitals to the Outpatient Care Data Collection (OPCDC). The data are used to quantify activity and inform planning and resourcing decisions. An Outpatient Department in the context of this reporting is an outpatient setting in a specialty unit or under an organisational arrangement administered by a hospital, excluding emergency department and **services** provided through community health settings such as community or child health centers. **Patients** meeting the criteria for **non-admitted** outpatient may receive treatment in a designated outpatient department or clinic within a hospital. Currently the required measures of recording scheduled visits to outpatient clinics are an 'occasion of service'.

Group Sessions (Group Occasions of Service)

An occasion of service is defined as any examination, consultation, treatment or other service provided to a patient, or a group of **patients**, in each functional unit of a health service or hospital on each occasion that such a service was provided. Other occasions of service to be recorded for counting include **outreach** clinic **services**, **services** delivered in a multidisciplinary mode and services delivered in group sessions.

For example if a patient has been **admitted** for orthopedic surgery but has an outpatient appointment for the diabetes clinic, the appointment at the diabetes clinic is a valid outpatient occasion of service even though the patient was **admitted** at the time of the appointment. Where the hospital provides a component of a service, i.e. a private specialist provides a service at a rural site but uses that hospital's staff, the hospital staff activity can be included in reporting.

Outreach Services for the Community

Setting-up of Outreach teams to provide regular services to a section of community on a continuing basis is a new and evolving concept. It is imperative that there are nationally agreed standards and minimum levels of competence, both within existing and recently developed teams. These may take the form of advanced assessment skills. All of these should, however, draw on the existing skills of allied health professions such as physiotherapy, acute pain teams and dietetics. To offer some minimum basic medical facilities at or near the doorsteps of the population in the area of trauma and critical care is essential in any situation, but is a stupendous task and may be even risky for the reputation of the providers and health of the beneficiaries. The need for incorporating such facilities in the mobile vans; with the necessary technology and trained manpower is all the more being felt. As of now the ambulances are being used only transport vehicles, devoid of any critical care services on the way. In fact in many cases the ambulance services should obviate the need to take the patient to the hospital, by administering the vital treatment in the van itself. This can reduce load on the hospital emergency services and provide patient friendly care at the door steps of the patient.

The authors have described the extension and outreach services in the following chapters:

1. Extension and Outreach Services in Health Care
2. Non-communicable, Lifestyle and Lifetime Diseases: Role of Hospitals
3. Immunisation in Hospitals: Extension Services Essential
4. Overview of Blindness and Ophthalmic Services
5. Hepatitis Clinic in a Hospital
6. Specialised Services of Radiotherapy and Oncology in a Hospital
7. Management of Mid-life Clinic for Women
8. Rehabilitation Centre: Essential in Every Hospital
9. Physiotherapy in a Hospital: Immense Scope
10. Hospital Library Services: Great Resource

Chandigarh

S.L. GOEL
R. KUMAR

1

Extension and Outreach Services in Health Care

Extension services in health care are not a new concept, though it is evolving on a continuing basis for the welfare of the community in general and the economically weaker and other less privileged beings in particular. While hospitals may touch somebody once in a lifetime kind situation, extension services have a wide horizon and need to touch us on a continuing basis, from birth to death viz. delivery huts in the remote areas to funeral services organised by an agency like red-cross. In fact extension services are the hospital services provided by the hospitals at the door steps of the beneficiaries. Subsection 5D(1) of the National Health Act, 1953 Australia provides that the Minister may, by written determination, specify services provided by, or on behalf of, a specified hospital or day hospital facility for the purposes of the definition of outreach service in subsection

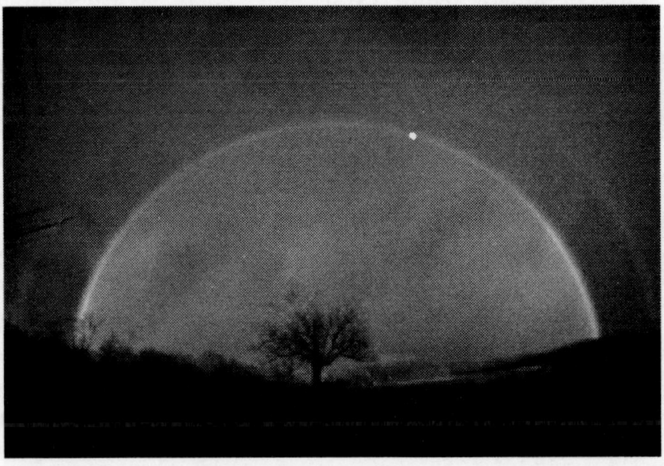

4(1) of the Act. Once a service is determined to be an outreach service then it is deemed to be hospital treatment (section 5C of the Act). Health funds can then pay benefits for those services (and associated professional services) under applicable benefits arrangements (hospital cover policies), provided that the services are provided as a direct substitute for hospital treatment that would otherwise be provided in a hospital or day hospital facility.

Holding of free eye camps and medical camps, family planning operation camps, de-addiction services, services to homeless and those in jails, mentally ill patients, administration of vaccines, mobile trauma and critical care teams, specialised clinics of physiotherapy/imaging, advanced services in various branches of medicine and clinics thereof, prevention and treatment of lifestyle diseases, HIV/sexually transmitted diseases and other infections, supplements for malnutrition containment viz. Vitamin and iron deficiency, iodine deficiency diseases, delivery huts for safe and hygienic childbirth, school health programmes, etc. are only some of the examples of ever expanding extension services meant for non-admitted patients and the community at large. It also entails services like sending nurses or care-givers for the chronically ill at home or services like hospice for the terminally ill. Often it may mean providing medical services or wellness services at the door steps of the patient/person.

DEFINITION

Dictionary definition of Outreach is 'the extending of services beyond current or usual limits' of the hospital premises. Setting up of Outreach teams to provide regular services to a section of community on a continuing basis is a new and evolving concept. It is imperative that there are nationally agreed standards and minimum levels of competence, both within existing and recently developed teams. These may take the form of advanced assessment skills. All of these should, however, draw on the existing skills of allied health professions such as physiotherapy, acute pain teams and dietetics. To offer some minimum basic medical facilities at or near the doorsteps of the population is a stupendous task and may be even risky for the reputation of the providers and health of the beneficiaries.

VISION 2020, a time honored approach in extension services

It is established that the magnitude of cataract-related blindness is high and it is not possible to treat all these cases in the available hospital resources. It is well known that they need to go out into communities to make services available to the patients, rather than wait for patients to come to them. This is usually done through outreach services. Aravind Eye hospital in Madurai, India is one such example in the voluntary sector. Eye units in Africa currently use a variety of outreach service approaches. A popular strategy is one in which a team goes out to examine large groups in the community, provides basic ocular medical services, makes definitive selection of patients who will benefit from surgery, then bring those selected back to the base hospital for surgery. This is sometimes referred to as the "Aravind model" and it has several advantages:

- It does not take the surgeon and team from their base station for too long (as compared to sending a team to do surgery outside the hospital)
- The quality of surgery provided at the base hospital is likely to be superior to that provided at a makeshift outreach clinic
- A team with skills enough to diagnose early operable cataract accurately should encourage patients to have surgery before they become blind and avoid the common testimony—"I was told to wait and come back when my vision was worse."
- A team with skills enough to diagnose and treat a number of causes of visual impairment as well as basic eye diseases brings the service into the community. This avoids needless trips to the hospital by patients who are merely "screened" by low level health workers. One concern of any approach that transports patients to the hospital is the cost.

Calculation of costs

It includes the costs of pre-outreach (promotional) activities, costs on the day of outreach, and costs of community follow up. They omitted all costs incurred during the hospitalisation. They considered salaries of personnel involved in outreach (pro-rata for % of time spent on the activity), special allowances, fuel costs, advertising costs, stationery, consumables including medicines given for free, and meals provided for staff or patients. Programmes that used their own vehicles included some depreciation for this. Four programmes provided services from community level to hospital in defined catchment areas. Two other programmes worked together, with one providing the community outreach and the other picking up patients from these outreaches and transporting them back for surgery. Data from these latter two were not included although, interestingly, when added the cost per patient operated from each of these, they arrived at a number very close to the average cost of the other programmes. All programmes provided similar services including registration, examination (including IOP measurement and funduscopy as indicated), consultation, medical treatment at the site if necessary, and return transport for cataract patients. Most programmes sold presbyopic spectacles and some provided more complete refractive services. One programme had an extensive community educational programme and rehabilitation for the blind integrated in its outreach activities.

- Number patients examined per outreach visit 85-191 (Range), 108 (Average).
- Cataract surgery acceptance rate 51%-93% (Range), 76% (Average).

- Cost per outreach visit $234-674 (Range), $421 (Average).
- Operable cataract per outreach visit 9-30 (Range), 14.75 (Average).
- Cost per cataract patient detected $23-46 (Range), $32 (Average)
- Cost per patient transported to hospital $33-56 (Range), $43 (Average).
- Cost per patient examined on outreach $1.8-4.8 (Range).

They estimated that it will cost outreach programmes in eastern Africa $35-45 per cataract patient transported. It is important to note that these figures include providing medical consultative (not just screening) and basic refractive services to the catchment populations as well. These costs are higher than those expected in Asian regions. Greater distances and sparse population density in eastern Africa are expected to result in higher costs for getting services to people. We recommend eye care institutions track and report their outreach programme cost per cataract patient brought for surgery, and the strategies they use to improve these results. Further we recommend that donor agencies become aware that the full cost of providing a cataract surgery is the community outreach. Using VISION 2020 targets of 2,000 cataract operations per million population in Africa, these programmes ought to be able to provide basic services for a population of 1 million for 5 years for about 1 million $US ($100 x 2000 x 5 years).

World Health Organisation (WHO) study in outreach services

In recent years developing countries, influenced heavily by findings in developed countries, have become increasingly interested in assessing the quality of their extension health care. Quality assessment studies usually measure one of three types of outcomes: medical outcomes, costs, and client satisfaction. For the last mentioned, clients are asked to assess not only their own health status after receiving care but their satisfaction with the services delivered.

The efforts of Bangladesh to improve its health care delivery system have increasingly emphasized quality of care. In accordance with the suggestions of the World Bank, the new Health and Population Programme of the Ministry of Health and Family Welfare (MOHFW), which began operating in July 1998, is recommending a thorough organisational restructuring of the entire sector with the aim of establishing health care services that are more sustainable, cost-effective, and responsive to client needs.

A study of 42 outreach services in Bangladesh

All 55 fixed services (services offered at an established physical structure) were studied, and simple random sampling was used to select 42 outreach services (services offered by a mobile health team at the house of a community member). These services are usually provided by two nurses.

Services sought by clients were divided into five categories: family planning, maternal care, female care, child care, common diseases. Clients were asked to supply the following information about themselves: age, sex, family size, marital status, occupation, level of education, distance between their houses and the health services, means of transport, care-seeking preferences, and expectations and level of satisfaction related to waiting and consultation time and to the behavior of providers. Clients were also asked about various aspects related to provider's technical competence during consultations. Level of satisfaction was assessed in two steps. First, users were asked whether or not they were satisfied with the care received, and then they were asked about their level of satisfaction or dissatisfaction. A total of 1913 persons were successfully interviewed. When children were the patients, their careers were interviewed. Approximately 88% of users were female, who were in general significantly younger than men. Most of the users were married, and 18% were children under 5 years of age. About 61% of respondents had never attended school, reflecting roughly the national educational pattern.

The same health worker provided services to people, irrespective of the condition they presented with. On average, 40 patients used the facilities daily, with the average waiting time at those facilities being 30 ± 2.5 min. Sufficient consultation time is of particular importance for provider–patient interrelations and for appropriate medical management of patients.

FIG. I

Boxplot Showing Client Waiting Times according to Services Received

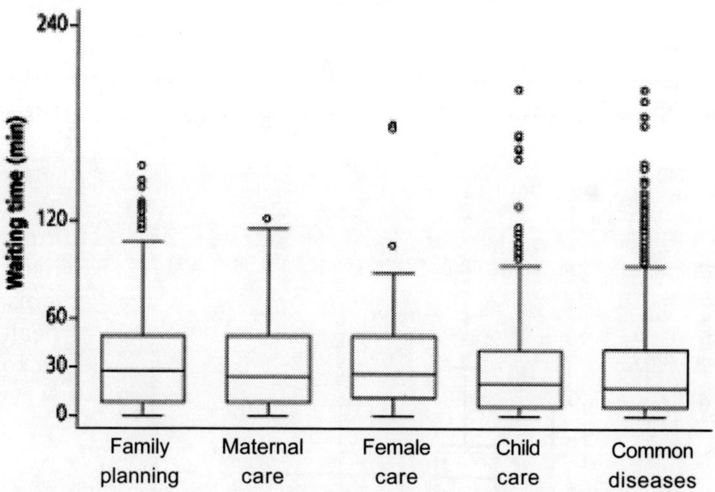

Boxes show the 95% distribution limits and bars the 97.5% distribution limits. Horizontal lines within the boxes show the median values. Widths of boxes correlate with the sample size in the various sub-categories.

FIG. 2

Boxplot Showing Consultation Times according to Services Received

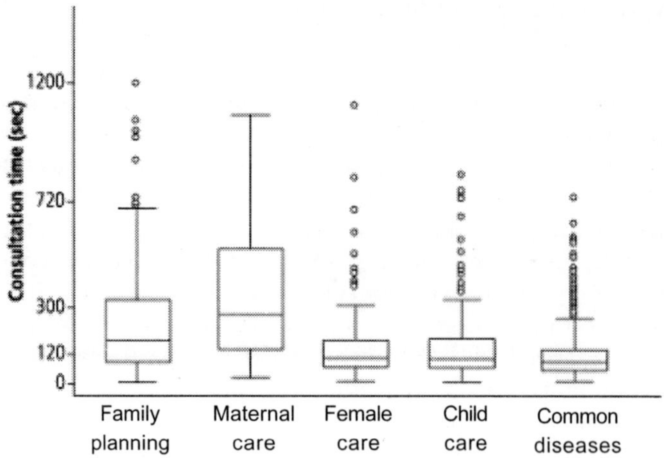

See legend to Fig. 1 for explanation of symbols.

The proportion of providers willing to ask patients their reasons for attending was relatively high (82.3%), but providers gave advice to only 53.5% of clients, and they gave some sort of explanation about the nature of their health problem only to 48.9%. A physical examination was performed on only 29% of all patients. No significant difference was found among health facilities, but providers performed physical examinations on 81.3% of patients for maternal care services, as opposed to 25.8% and 16.6% of clients coming for family planning and female care, respectively.

FIG. 3

Boxplot Showing Waiting Times according to Level of Satisfaction

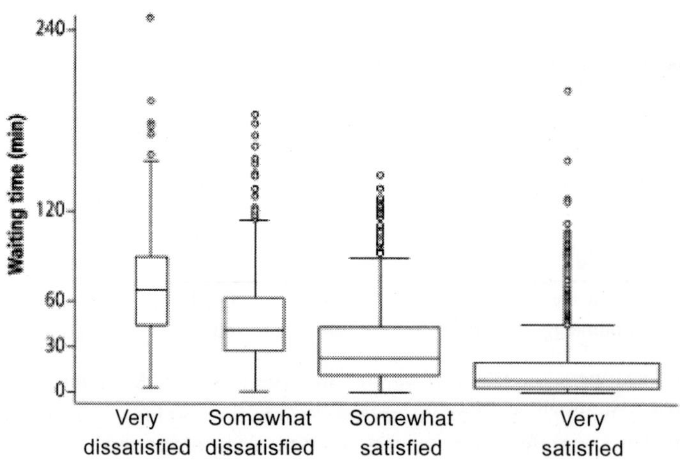

FIG. 4

Boxplot Showing Consultation Times according to Level of Satisfaction

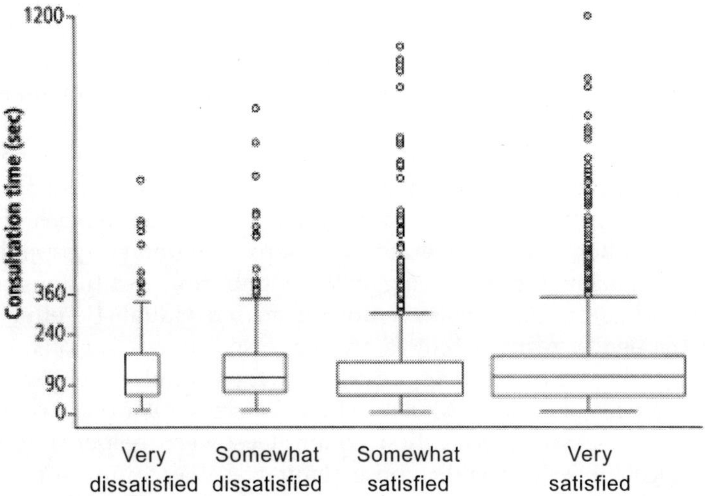

A total of 68% of patients expressed satisfaction with the services usually rendered, but almost half (45%) the clients presenting for female care were not satisfied at all. Satisfaction with the politeness of the provider was the most powerful predictor variable, followed by satisfaction with the providers respect for privacy, waiting time, and consultation time. The efficacy of medical treatment is enhanced by greater patient satisfaction.

The results of this study confirm findings in developed and some other developing countries that the perception and judgment of quality are highly individualistic and dynamic, in the sense that the criteria or elements used for judging quality at one moment may not be the same for the next, and that consequently client satisfaction reflects only part of the quality of the entire health care process. This aspect should not be misunderstood or overestimated, nor should it replace the notion of quality care. Although optimally care should meet both medical and psychosocial needs, in reality care that meets all medical needs may fail to meet client's emotional or social needs. Conversely, care that meets psychosocial needs may leave clients medically at risk. The results of research will enable policy-makers and decision-makers to improve the quality of health care effectively, keeping a balance between providers and patients ideas of what quality of health care means.

Many players in outreach services of health care; Co-ordination essential

One of the animating beliefs of health service reformers is that delivery would improve if greater co-ordination was imposed over disparate health care providers in the hospitals and outreach services. The fundamental divisions are between the voluntary, public and private sectors. Voluntary provision predominantly means some first aid kind of services and acute care hospitals, but also includes a range of other therapeutic and clinical services. The public sector delivered general practitioner (GP) and specialised services to the community through the state-run hospitals/dispensaries. The Government schemes also cover environmental health, isolation and general hospitals and a wide range of personal services addressing tuberculosis, venereal diseases, mental illness, and maternity and child welfare. Finally, the private sector provides nursing homes and GP attendance at commercial rates. The corporate hospitals provide world class services to the high end patients and foreign medical tourists. Within each area there were tendencies towards independent rather than co-operative working. Voluntary hospitals often lack any mechanism for conferring with neighboring institutions and the competitive logic of fund-raising enforced an individualistic ethic. In the public sector health responsibilities are dispersed across various agencies: local authority health committees, advised by the central/state governments or Medical Officer of Health (MOH), who oversees sanitation, hospitals and personal health services; education committees were responsible for the School Medical Service (SMS), whose remit was the compulsory medical inspection and treatment of elementary schoolchildren. Private practice co-exists with government services (though not allowed under the rules) and doctors tend to prioritize fee-paying rather than ordinary patients.

History of U.K. outreach Health Care systems

In U.K. the Dawson Report of 1920 responded to its remit from government to consider "the systematical provision of ... medical and allied services", by proposing a scheme for primary health centers affiliated to secondary centers, which in turn were attached to teaching hospitals. The Cave Committee of 1921 also attacked the "lack of organisation and co-operation among the voluntary hospitals", recommending local committees which would liaise with the Poor Law infirmaries to relieve waiting lists. Co-ordination within the public sector was central to the Local Government Act which sought to bring erstwhile Poor Law medical facilities under the control of health committees, while Section 13 of the Act called for joint voluntary/municipal hospital committees, giving statutory sanction to the collaboration which had failed to occur spontaneously. Shortly afterwards the non-governmental Sankey Report (1937) proposed regional co-ordination of voluntary hospitals "to bring their services into harmonious relationship" through joint fund-raising and planning.

The PEP report (1937) described Britain's health services as "a mass of separate expedients ... a bewildering variety of agencies, official and unofficial ... created during the past two or three generations", whose "general co-ordination ... is still fragmentary." The Cave and Sankey recommendations had not been met and the wartime hospital surveys of the Nuffield Provincial Hospitals Trust concluded bluntly: "there is no hospital system now." And the 1944 White Paper on the planned National Health Service (NHS), commenced with the observation that:

Many services are rendered by local authorities and others in special clinics and similar organisations ... These are, for the most part, thoroughly good in themselves ... But, owing to the way in which they have grown up piecemeal at different stages of history and under different statutory powers, they are usually conducted as quite separate and independent services.... There has to be somewhere a new responsibility to relate them, if a service for health is to be given in future which will be not only comprehensive and reliable but also easy to obtain.

The period saw the advance of expertise closely linked to academic medicine, for example, specialisation in fields such as eyes, orthopedics, skin, ear, nose and throat, facilities for laboratory analysis, departments of public health medicine and so on. Given the tendency for geographical concentration of such expertise in large towns it was in the interests of both practitioners and public to ensure that an area's health services worked together to establish referral mechanisms and rationalize patient flows to appropriate institutions: "hierarchical regionalism" in Fox's phrase. The banner of "co-ordination" was raised by different interest groups seeking to advance their positions. The "co-ordination" to achieve a comprehensive and universal service was not just more efficient, it was profoundly ideological.

The Gloucestershire Extension Medical Services

This was a local experiment in service organisation begun by Gloucestershire County Council in 1920, which sought in a novel way to integrate the work of GPs, the tax-funded public health services and the voluntary hospitals. Known as the Gloucestershire Extension of Medical Services Scheme (GEMSS), it was the brainchild of the County MOH, John Middleton Martin, and its innovative feature was the provision of "out-stations" in the rural parts of the county. These were small-scale health centers, either purpose built or situated in existing cottage hospitals or tuberculosis dispensaries, and staffed by GPs paid on a contractual basis. Gloucestershire was divided into administrative areas (Bristol, Gloucester and Cheltenham), each with its general hospital, to which the out-stations were affiliated for patient referrals, and with its specialist institutions such as tuberculosis sanatoria.

The GEMSS differed from other municipal health services in several ways. First, it utilised independent GPs and consultants rather than local government medical officers. Second, its out-stations were all-purpose treatment centers, as opposed to clinics targeted at a particular population or ailment. Third, it imposed a referral network upon existing institutions—public and voluntary—to fulfil public health duties, rather than building a separate municipal network. Finally, it was managed, at least at its inception, by a committee consisting of local authority and voluntary hospital representatives. Here, apparently, was a concrete expression of the reformers' vision of service co-ordination, both between the municipal, private and voluntary sectors, and within the municipal sector, which proved so elusive nationally. Indeed, the scheme was recognized both nationally and internationally, periodically attracting praise as a template that might be more widely applied. When the Ministry of Health conducted its public health surveys of local government in the early 1930s it too lauded the GEMSS's innovatory features, observing that it "deserves to be considered as a serious contribution to the theory and practice of public health in rural counties." There was also American interest, in the visit of Professor Winslow of Yale University to study the out-stations, and the GEMSS's inclusion in a major study of British health insurance. The PEP report also detailed the arrangements, arguing that it demonstrated how "to bridge the gulf between official and unofficial health services which is so frequent and so unsatisfactory a feature of the present situation." This then was an arrangement with more than just local interest, though as yet one which has attracted only passing mention from historians.

The over-arching goal was to knit together the different health providers—voluntary, public and private—in a coherent hierarchical network for referrals and treatment. Health services would therefore reach groups in rural areas where distance, or, for children, parental commitments, meant that even where early diagnosis was made, follow-up treatment was lacking.

Where did the idea for the GEMSS come from?

Given their apparently simultaneous gestation, it might be supposed that the Dawson Report provided the inspiration. The standard design included waiting, consulting and dressing rooms, and lavatories; equipment was limited to cabinets for medicines and filing, weighing machines and eye test posters. In the mid-1930s some additional coverage was achieved by subsidiary out-stations, based in a room in the house of the district nurse. Two types of session were run. First, there were regular weekly openings at which the medical officer and district nurse examined and treated patients for minor ailments, typically referrals from the nurse or the School Medical Service. Second, hospital consultants attended for intermediate sessions to treat patients for ophthalmic, ENT, orthopedic and tuberculosis complaints and rheumatic heart disease; surgical work performed at the out-stations was principally tonsils and adenoids operations. Two orthopedic nurses also visited the stations as necessary to offer treatment such as massage, and oversee more routine work conducted by district nurses. The main activity from the outset was dealing with schoolchildren.

The fundamental achievement of the GEMSS was therefore the provision of a systematic referral system which ensured that the diagnostic work of school medical inspections was followed up by treatment, a situation which did not obtain in many areas. Tuberculosis work remained a fairly minor aspect of the scheme, and continued to be dealt with principally through the county's public health administration, overseen by the deputy MOH. In practice, the scheme supplemented existing machinery by ensuring that country patients without easy access to urban dispensaries were seen regularly by the TB Officer. The same was true of maternity and child welfare work, where doctors acting as out-station medical officers were often also contracted by the MCW committee to run ante-natal and infant welfare clinics in isolated areas. Referrals were made where necessary to voluntary hospital consultants who made home visits in cases of puerperal pyrexia and difficult obstetrical cases, in 1932 five out-stations were equipped for dental work for expectant and nursing mothers. Finally, venereal disease work was a key area of growth in the 1930s, with some out-stations used as "VD sub-centres" at which the medical officer gave drug treatment, supervised by a Bristol VD specialist. GEMSS acted as a modest integrating force. The GEMSS was an imaginative plan which illustrates the scope for innovation afforded by the devolved health system of inter-war Britain. It was genuinely distinctive in four respects: the concept of general purpose out-stations went against the more typical practice of single-service clinics; its systematic outreach arrangements for rural areas were unusual; its reliance on private sector contracting contrasted with the standard municipal preference for public medical officers; and it offered a coherent and unique model of joint working premised on a hierarchical referral network. However, its ambitious conception was never realised. Despite the publicity which it generated, its practical achievement was very modest, and limited principally to the effective integration of the School Medical Service into the health system. Finally, what does the relative failure of the GEMSS experiment reveal of the barriers to service integration within the mixed economy of inter-war medicine? If the doctors were no barrier, the same could not be said for local or central government. The Gloucestershire scheme was an innovative project akin to the joint hospitals councils founded in major provincial cities.

Can outpatient treatment may mean 'hospital treatment' for insurance

"Hospital treatment" is defined by reference to its meaning in S. 67 (4) of the National Health Act 1953. Section 67 of that Act addresses the definition of hospital treatment for the purposes of identifying when a health insurance business must be registered. The operative part of subsection 67(4) is as follows: "hospital treatment" means accommodation and nursing care, whether provided for the purpose of permitting the provision of professional attention or, in the case of a nursing-home type patient, as an end in itself, and includes: (a) the provision at, or on behalf of, a hospital of relevant health services to a patient of the hospital; and (b) the provision at a hospital of a facility for a patient of the hospital. The definition of "hospital treatment" appears limited to "a patient of the hospital." Thus it is important to identify whether an outpatient is a patient of the hospital for the purposes of this definition. However, neither the National Health Act or the Parliamentary reading speeches provide any guidance on whether outpatients were intended to be covered under the category of "hospital treatment", or alternatively under the category of "ancillary health benefits."

Under the National Health Act, hospital treatment "means" accommodation and nursing care, and includes health services and hospital facilities provided to hospital patients. The words "means" and "and" must in this case be taken to support the presumption that where either accommodation or nursing care are not present, the supply will not constitute "hospital treatment." In the case of an outpatient who is not accommodated by a hospital, this would invite the conclusion that their treatment is not "hospital treatment." Much will therefore turn on the interpretation of "accommodation" and "nursing care", and whether the short-term care provided to, for instance, an emergency department patient, satisfies this test.

The inclusive aspects of the definition, relating to health services and facilities provided to patients of a hospital, in our view should be read in the context that they are part of hospital treatment where they are provided along with accommodation and nursing care. In a sense this would allow all supplies to patients of a hospital to be bundled under the single GST-free category of hospital treatment, rather than relying on separate categories of GST-free supplies.

An outpatient is one of the three categories of non-admitted patient as defined in the National Health Data Dictionary (together with emergency department and community/outreach patients). A non-admitted patient is a patient who does not undergo a hospital's formal admission process. This definition seems to mean that an outpatient is not formally a "patient of the hospital." If this formal classification is considered to be the intention of subsection 67(4) of the National Health Act, 1953 in referring to a "patient of a hospital" then it will be difficult to have outpatient treatment considered hospital treatment under the inclusive aspects of that definition (i.e. facilities and health services provided to a patient of the hospital). Further assistance regarding the definition of "outpatient" can be found in the Health Insurance Act, 1973. There an "outpatient service", in relation to a hospital, means a health service or procedure provided by the hospital to an eligible person other than a patient of the hospital. This reinforces the conclusion that an outpatient is not a patient of a hospital.

By contrast, an admitted patient, or "inpatient", is defined in the National Health Data Dictionary as a patient who undergoes a hospital's admission process to receive treatment or care, which can occur in hospital or in the person's home. A patient may be admitted if the patient's condition requires any of the following:

- clinical management not available in their usual residential environment;
- observation in order to be diagnosed or assessed;
- daily assessment of medication needs; or
- Procedures not able to be performed in a stand-alone facility.

While much of the concept of an admitted patient turns on accommodation during a period in which medical services are being provided, it is also clear that the category may include non-accommodated patients. On the definition of hospital treatment above, there may thus be "admitted patients" of a hospital who are not strictly receiving "hospital treatment."

However as a non-admitted patient is, by deduction, a person whose condition does not require the accommodation and nursing-based management and facilities described above, there appears to be a strong correlation between the test of "hospital treatment" and "admitted patients."

"Hospital in the home services" and "hospital outreach services" are not defined in any relevant legislation, however they tend to imply that it is not necessary for a patient to be a "formally admitted" patient of the hospital at the time of the hospital treatment taking place. Indeed "outreach services" are one of the categories of non-admitted patients in the National Health Data Dictionary, where patients are treated by hospital employees off the hospital site. As the very nature of "hospital in the home" and "hospital outreach" services do not include an accommodation element, there is a contradiction between the intention of the GST Act and the definition relied upon from the National Health Act, 1953.

GST-free supplies to outpatients

While it appears likely that supplies of goods and services by a hospital to outpatients will not be GST-free under the category of "hospital treatment", these supplies are likely to fall within one of a number of other categories of GST-free supplies. Medical services and a range of health services described in section 38-15 and the table in subsection (1) of section 38-10 of the GST Act are GST-free. It is possible that this range of services would encompass all services supplied by a hospital to outpatients.In addition to such services, the following supplies of goods to outpatients will also be GST-free; (a) a supply of goods made in the course of supplying a GST-free medical service (section 38-7(3)); (b) a supply of goods made in the course of supplying a GST-free health service described in the table in subsection (1) of section 38-10 of the GST Act (other than optical or pharmaceutical services), which is made at the premises at which the service is supplied (section 38-10(3)); (c) other GST-free health goods determined by the Health Minister (section 38-47); (d) prescription drugs and medicines (section 38-50).

Health Care for the Homeless

- o Lives on the streets or in a shelter.
- o Lives with a family member or friend due to an emergency situation.
- o Is incarcerated or have just been released without any stable home plan.

o Has been homeless before entering a drug and alcohol treatment center and will be going to a shelter or transitional living programme after completion.

Services Provided:

- Health Care
- Prescriptions
- Dental
- Optometry
- Case management
- Therapy
- Substance Abuse

Community Health Project

To help provide access to care and education, prevent infant mortality, reduce low-birth weight babies and premature delivery among high risk women and teens in the urban core of Jackson County.

Eligibility:

Pregnant mothers residing in the Jackson County area that receive prenatal care from safety-net providers such as Truman Medical Center, Cabot Westside Clinic, Swope Health Services and Samuel U. Rodgers Health Center.

Services Provided:

- Case management
- Prenatal and parenting workshops
- One on one labor and delivery, education, coaching and facilitation classes
- Prenatal/Infant Nutritional counseling
- Breastfeeding counseling
- Baby supplies (clothes, diapers, formula, etc. after child's birth)
- Transportation to and from prenatal exams, postpartum, well child checkups and follow up exams.
- Prenatal and parenting workshops

One on one labor and delivery, education, coaching and facilitation classes

Outreach services to homeless people with mental illness

During the 1980s, outreach services to homeless people with mental illness were identified as a unique component of the continuum of care for this growing population. The literature on outreach identified various strategies for engagement in street and shelter locations, including mobile units, intensive case management, shelter-based contact, and drop-in centers. Over the past decade, mental health programmes gradually have expanded their outreach to people with mental illness to include jailed populations.

The observed relationship between incarceration and the challenges of community re-entry suggests that the time of release from jail may be an especially auspicious one for reaching out to offenders and providing support for the transition back to community life. Health care professionals have developed models for clinical outreach in jails that are designed to link individuals who are arrested to community treatment programmes designed to facilitate reentry into the community and that can address medical, substance use, psychiatric, and social problems. Because outreach is designed to enroll difficult-to-engage clients in a continuum of care, its primary objective should be to link clients with the health and social welfare service systems.

Since 1987, the VA has provided outreach services to homeless veterans nationally through the Health Care for Homeless Veterans (HCHV) programme. HCHV is focused on delivering three kinds of service: outreach and case management in community locations, linkage with medical and psychiatric services available at VA medical centers, and community contract residential rehabilitation treatment services.

The outreach workers collected demographic, clinical, and social adjustment information by using a standard assessment form. This intake form records socio-demographic characteristics; homelessness status; financial and employment status; medical, psychiatric, and substance dependence problems; and assessment and referral information provided by the outreach worker. Veterans who spent the previous night in a shelter or on the streets or who had no residence and were staying with family or friends were considered to be homeless.

The outreach workers who completed the assessments were master's-level social work staff, paraprofessional social work staff, and nursing staff. The outreach workers recorded veterans' responses to questions about their psychiatric symptoms. The clinical assessments of the outreach workers were reviewed by licensed social workers, who determined whether the veterans had any psychiatric diagnoses. Clients were considered to have serious mental illness if a mood disorder, post-traumatic stress disorder, or schizophrenia or other psychotic disorder was documented. The presence of alcohol or drug abuse or dependence and any of the serious psychiatric disorders indicated dual diagnosis.

Costs for inpatient, residential, and outpatient services were estimated by using the VA's fiscal year 2000 cost distribution report. The cost distribution report uses standardized accounting procedures to assign direct costs, such as clinical salaries and supplies, and indirect costs, such as administration, building maintenance, engineering services, equipment, and depreciation, to each health care programme at each facility.

Sample characteristics

Of the 8,236 veterans who were assessed by outreach workers, 1,676 (20 percent) were assessed in jail. Both groups of veterans were, on average, middle-aged, and most were men. The ethnic distribution of the sample reflected the ethnic diversity of veterans in the Los Angeles area. Numerous statistically significant differences in social and clinical characteristics were observed. The veterans who were contacted in jail had higher scores on several measures of social stability than did the homeless veterans who were contacted in the community: they were more likely to be married and less likely either to be homeless over the long-term or to have relied on public support. However, the jailed veterans also had higher rates of unemployment over the previous three years.

The incarcerated veterans had fewer medical problems but higher rates of mental illness and substance use problems than the community homeless veterans. They were also more likely to have a diagnosis of alcohol or drug abuse, even though their current alcohol and drug use scores were lower, which probably reflects a lack of access to alcohol and drugs during incarceration. Except for posttraumatic stress disorder, higher rates of specific mental illnesses were observed among the veterans who were contacted in jail than among those who were contacted in the community, and the jailed veterans were twice as likely to have dual diagnoses.

This study sought to identify distinctive socio-demographic and clinical characteristics of veterans who received outreach contact in jail or in community settings and to test the hypothesis that veterans contacted through a jail outreach programme would have higher service use and costs than homeless veterans who were contacted through outreach in community settings. At the time of the intake assessment, the veterans who were contacted in jail were more likely to have been unemployed over the previous three years and to have higher levels of both substance abuse and mental illness. Although the veterans who were contacted in jail were better off as a group in terms of marital status and homelessness, they had very high rates of unemployment over the previous three years, even compared with a group of veterans who would be expected to have much higher unemployment rates than those in the general population. When veterans who were not available for work—for example, those who were disabled or retired—were removed from both samples, the unemployment rates were even higher: 83 percent for veterans contacted in jail and 64 percent for homeless veterans contacted in the community.

In the case of veterans who had been incarcerated previously, stigma associated with having been in jail may have prevented employment, an explanation consistent with O'Flaherty's hypothesis on attenuation of community ties. Alternatively, these very high unemployment rates may have been due in part to substance abuse or individual skill deficits. Still another possibility is that the jailed veterans had a high rate of long-term incarceration that would explain their high unemployment rate. However, data on the duration of incarceration were not available to enable this possibility to be evaluated.

The high levels of psychiatric and substance use problems among the jailed outreach clients were as serious as the high unemployment levels. One in three had a diagnosis of a serious mental illness, and one in two reported current drug abuse. Although these levels are not dramatically higher than rates found in other studies of homeless populations, these findings—coupled with the three-year unemployment pattern—demonstrate the seriousness of the challenges faced by jailed outreach clients as they reenter the community as well as by the community providers who attempt to assist them.

One area of hope is the fact that the rate of current alcohol and drug use was lower in the jailed group, which suggests that jailed veterans may be more open to engagement in treatment at the time of outreach contact. Even though the jailed veterans in this study had had shorter periods of homelessness than the veterans from the community, it has been shown that jailed veterans with substance use problems frequently lack stable housing and are likely to require substance abuse services with a residential component.

The lower use of medical services in the incarcerated group is consistent with this group's lower level of self-reported medical problems. However, given the high levels of need for mental health services among the jailed veterans, it might be expected that access to and use of VA services by this group would be higher than in the community homeless group. But this was not the case. The jailed group was only a quarter as likely to obtain services, even after adjustment for many other potentially confounding variables.

Another possibility is that the observed differences in use were due to differences in VA service eligibility between the two groups. To evaluate this possibility, we assessed eligibility in a random sample of 100 veterans from each of the two groups. No significant differences in eligibility rates were found (78 percent in the community group and 80 percent the incarcerated group). In addition, there were no significant differences in whether the veterans had service-connected disabilities, which is an indicator of service access priority; 8.3 percent in the community homeless group and 7.5 percent in the incarcerated group had service-connected disabilities. A third possible explanation for differences in service use is that the jailed veterans had a higher rate of drug abuse or dependence and were more treatment resistant. As noted above, differences in service use remained after adjustment for this clinical difference.

Still another possibility is that outreach workers planned more frequently to refer jailed veterans to non-VA community treatment providers. When such plans were included in regression models predicting service use and costs, there was no change in the service use odds ratio and only a small decrease in total costs explained by outreach group (R^2 change=.002, p<.001). Outreach workers' intentions to refer veterans to non-VA services thus did not explain differences in VA service use or costs.

Several other service and institutional variables could also explain lower levels of access to post-release services. Services that inmates receive while incarcerated may reduce their need for community services. Jail staff may be unwilling or unable to inform case managers of when inmates are to be released from jail, thus preventing linkages with community services. Transportation may not be available. Community service providers may not be enthusiastic about serving former inmates. Data were not available to assess differences in rates of access that might arise from these factors. A final important variable is that some veterans might have had lower levels of service use and cost a year after assessment because they were still incarcerated. We did not have access to jail release dates, so it is unclear how large a role this factor may play.

Cost differences between the two groups of veterans are more likely to be explained by differences in access to services than by differences in need. Although intake data suggest that the veterans who were contacted in jail had lower levels of need for medical services—corresponding to lower medical and surgical costs—these veterans had higher levels of need for mental health services yet lower mental health costs. Lower population costs for the jailed group across all cost categories could reflect indifference or fear on the part of the receiving programmes or service providers.

Incarceration and release dates in criminal justice records are necessary for determining more clearly the relationship of long-term incarceration to both the long-term unemployment and the lower levels of service use observed in our sample. A second limitation is that we studied male veterans—many of whom were homeless—who were receiving VA outreach services in one large city. This limits the generalizability of the study findings to the larger population of homeless or incarcerated people, although previous studies have shown few differences between homeless veterans and other homeless men.

Outreach can provide social bridging or support that O'Flaherty suggests may be especially lacking for inmates who are reentering community life. From a policy perspective, the findings of this study are a mixture of "good news and bad news." From one perspective, providing outreach services seems to connect some members of the jail population with needed services, and the resulting service use and increased cost burden are not likely to overwhelm health care system resources. Medical center administrators could thus comfortably support this kind of initiative.

From another perspective, among veterans who received outreach services in jail, a relatively small proportion actually followed through with VA services. Developing more effective methods of service linkage and more thorough evaluation of the impact of these services on clinical, functional, and criminal justice outcomes are important next steps in enhancing community treatment for offenders with mental illness.

Outreach services and the critical care facility

Early Identification of the critically ill is the key to preventing admission or readmission to the critical care facility. Outreach Services should have the following objectives:

1. Avert admissions to critical care.
2. Facilitate timely admission to critical care and discharge back to the wards.
3. Share critical care skills and expertise through an educational partnership.
4. Promote continuity of care.
5. Ensure thorough audit and evaluation of Outreach Services.

The primary role of Outreach Services is to ensure that patients receive appropriate and timely treatment in a suitable area. Adequate resources must be made available for outreach in addition to adequate ward provision. There should be particular emphasis on hospital trainees in acute specialties.

'The Critical Care Outreach Service is a multidisciplinary approach to the identification of patients, at risk of developing critical illness, and those patients recovering from a period of critical illness, to enable early intervention or transfer to an area suitable to care for that patient's individual needs. Outreach should be a collaboration and partnership between the critical care department and other departments to ensure a continuum of care for patients regardless of location, and should enhance the skills and understanding of all staff in the delivery of critical care. Thus, outreach care is a partnership aimed at prevention by education and action. A Critical Care Outreach Service is not a remedy for inadequate resources:

1. too few critical care beds,
2. inadequate ward facilities to care for lower dependency patients,
3. decreased ward nursing numbers or inappropriate skills mix, and
4. inexperienced trainee or lack of supervision.

The outreach team should be prepared to take over or at least direct the care of critically ill patients whose admission to a critical care facility is delayed and are deemed inappropriate for transfer. These patients may be being cared for in areas such as the general ward. The outreach concept requires investment to enable it to set-up a satellite service. The physical and psychological consequences of critical illness may extend beyond ward follow-up and outreach does not replace the requirement for formal and long-term post-intensive care follow-up clinics and rehabilitation services. 'Guidance for Admission and Discharge of Patients from Intensive Care High Dependency Units' gives clear guidance on the system failures which require patients to be cared for in the critical care environment. The skills and education necessary for their management should be the foundation of the educational base of both doctors and nurses.

In a complex system such as health care delivery, there are a large number of factors and individuals involved that may influence outcome and inadvertently contribute to sub-optimal care. These conditions are often deep rooted in the organisation but can usually be identified and prevented. The ability to be honest and to learn from mistakes will enable an organisation to address the wider causes of failure.

Respiratory rate, heart rate and adequacy of oxygenation are the indicators of critically ill patients in the general ward:

- Unfortunately the monitoring and charting of physiologic variables, especially respiratory rate, is often erratic. Sub-optimal care has been demonstrated inpatients prior to ICU admission and this may lead to increased morbidity and mortality. Inexperienced medical staff may not respond appropriately to patients with critical illness.
- Inadequate nursing provision may lead to failure to focus on groups of patients at risk of developing critical illness and on occasions nurses may be unsure when to call for assistance
- The patient population has become older and sicker as surgical, anesthetic and critical care techniques have improved, leading to higher risk patients being offered surgical intervention.
- Services are becoming increasingly specialised and this can lead to a de-skilling or lack of experience in the general wards. As a consequence of bed shortages patients may be cared for on inappropriate wards resulting in unfamiliarity with a patient's condition.
- The demands made on the health system particularly over busy periods can lead to patients being cared for in inappropriate areas. This may lead to unfamiliarity with treatment protocols amongst staff and difficulty for medical teams to keep track of their patients.

Critical Care Aspects

Level 0

Patient whose needs can be met through normal ward care in an acute hospital.

Level I

Patients at risk of their condition deteriorating, or those relocated from higher levels of care, whose needs can be met on an acute ward with additional advice and support from the critical care team.

Level 2

Patients requiring more detailed observation or intervention including support for a failing organ system or postoperative care and those 'stepping down' from higher levels of care.

Level 3

Patients requiring advanced respiratory support alone or basic respiratory support together with support of at least two organ systems. This level includes all complex patients requiring support for multi-organ failure.

Critical care resources within the hospital should provide increasing levels of care depending on the skills, staff and facilities available. Patients will move up or down the dependency levels according to their condition and may require inter-hospital transfer for clinical or non-clinical reasons if there is inadequate resource provision or a need for more advanced specialist care.

Identification of patients who require advanced respiratory support should be straightforward although it has been shown that a proportion of these patients have their treatment delayed. As dependency falls there is a greater overlap between the groups which may lead to difficulty in classifying patients particularly between levels 0-1 and 1-2. The vision for the future of Critical Care Services includes the provision of outreach to support care of level 1 patients on the general ward. The sudden collapse of a patient from an acute arrhythmia or a massive pulmonary embolism will not allow time for prior identification or intervention by an outreach team. The detection of deterioration in a patient's condition over hours or days, which is amenable to earlier intervention, is the challenge for outreach.

(a) A patient at risk of deterioration may be identified by:

1. Exhibition of abnormal physical signs.
2. Their condition or pre-morbid history (e.g. major emergency surgery).
3. Intuition: 'not quite right'.

When to call a critical care team? All cardiac and respiratory arrests and the conditions listed below.

Acute changes in: Vital signs: AIRWAY Threatened, All respiratory arrests, Respiratory rate <5 per minute, Respiratory rate >36 per minute, All cardiac arrests, Pulse rate <40 per minute, Pulse rate >140 per minute, Sudden fall in level of consciousness, Repeated or prolonged seizures.

The nurse should contact the responsible doctor and inform them of a patient with: Any 3 or more of the following:

Respiratory rate?25 breaths/min (or<10),
Systolic arterial pressure <90 mmHg,
Heart rate?110 beats/min (or <55),
Not FULLY alert and orientated,
Oxygen saturation <90%,

Urine output <100 ml over last 4h OR A patient not FULLY alert and orientated, and

Respiratory rate<35 breaths/min OR heart rate>140 beats/min.

(b) A doctor may call the team for any seriously ill patient causing concern. This will normally be done after discussion with the patient's consultant. The consultant responsible for the patient must be informed as soon as practical that the team has been called.

(c) Critical Care Liaison Service:

Heart rate <45 or >125 beats/min
Systolic arterial pressure <90mmHg
Respiratory Rate <8 or > 30 bpm

In certain instances blood tests or basic monitoring equipment such as a pulse oximeter are used. The patient developing critical illness on the ward will require focused and regular observations by staff, which appreciate and understand the significance of basic physiological parameters and derangement from normal values (including patients who may exhibit chronic or acute on chronic changes). The objective and dynamic measure of a patient's physiology will highlight deterioration to a greater extent than subjective assessments.

Specific Conditions

Patients Causing Concern

There are a proportion of patients who will mask critical illness by their physiological response and general demeanor. The development of any threshold criteria or simplified scoring systems to detect critical illness on the ward will never be totally inclusive. The ability to detect illness intuitively should never be underestimated. The clinical judgment of all staff will be of importance to the outreach team. Thus the patient who is 'not right', 'off colour' or 'agitated' must be considered at risk. The management and treatment of the patient developing critical illness should be initiated by ward based staff. Appropriate skills and resources for the management of patients with level 1 dependency should be available at ward level with an input from the Outreach Service. With additional assistance, it should be possible to achieve basic resuscitation and safe transfer of higher level dependency patients in a timely fashion to a critical care area.

The indications for asking for help from the Outreach Service should be determined and agreed locally, but aimed to ensure staff with the relevant competencies is involved in the management of patients at an early stage. This may require fairly simple and basic interventions. The importance of ward staff in the initial treatment of a patient with developing illness should be focused and enhanced by the process of outreach. Some patients will not benefit from the additional medical resources of the critical care team, either because their illness is beyond recovery or because co-morbidity would render treatment futile and inappropriate. Other patients, following discussion with staff experienced in intensive care medicine, may express a preference not to be admitted to a critical care area and these decisions require careful documentation.

Outreach is a multidisciplinary approach to critical illness and this should be reflected in the membership of that service. Inevitably the composition of the Outreach Service will vary depending on local critical care priorities, historical development and perceived needs by ward-based staff. The number of staff involved in the Outreach Service will be dependent on the size and geography of the hospital and whether it is planned to provide a team on a 24-hour, 7-day a week basis or only during 'daylight' hours. Aspects of outreach should be 'owned' by ward staff and hopefully skills learnt will then be passed on to the rest of the ward team. The support of senior ward staff at both consultant and nursing management level will be crucial to the successful introduction of outreach. It must be remembered that members of the outreach team will be visitors/ guests to the ward and it will only be in a way co-operative and supportive role that outreach will succeed. Any attempt to impose changes no matter how beneficial will be perceived to be a challenge to the 'autonomy' of the ward area and this could lead to confrontation.

Medical input should comprise consultants in critical care medicine with sessional commitment to the Outreach Service and trainee medical cover for critical care with no other responsibilities other than those directly related such as cardiac arrest, trauma calls or transfer calls. Nursing input should consist of critical care nursing staff, with a possible lead role for a nurse consultant or clinical nurse specialist, supported by other appropriately trained nurses. Physiotherapy support will add skills in the assessment and treatment of patients, and also help sustain the rehabilitation programme during recovery from critical illness. The physiotherapy team will be more aware of the respiratory status of patients and will often highlight deterioration at an earlier stage.

Other allied health professions will also have an important role in a hospital-wide delivery of services. These include dietetic, rehabilitation and pharmacy staff to provide advice and support. Critical care technicians should help with stabilisation of patients and have responsibility for standardisation of equipment throughout the hospital. The resuscitation officer should be involved in developing an integrated training programme. Support staff will be required to enable robust audit. The ability to audit service provision and clinical governance issues that may be highlighted by the introduction of outreach will require data collection for validation. One of the three stated aims of outreach in the 'Comprehensive Critical Care' document is the sharing of skills with ward-based staff. This aspect of outreach is of equal importance to the process of identification of the critically ill patient.

Education should be directed at the following levels

Ward

Involving all ward staff both nursing and medical. This should include details of out-reach and its purpose and will involve induction sessions on starting an appointment, as well as instruction on how the aims of outreach are achieved at the local level. Rotation of ward staff through critical care areas such as high dependency units should be encouraged to enable and consolidate re-skilling.

The importance of audit of services and joint morbidity and mortality meetings, not only between medical staff but also inclusive of nursing and allied health professions staff, are essential so that lessons from delayed or sub-optimal treatment can be shared, inadequacies highlighted and repetitive mistakes prevented. It will only be by developing a learning or safety culture that this will be achieved. Courses such as ALS (Advanced Life Support), CCrISP (Care of the Critically Ill Surgical Patient) and ALERT (Acute Life-threatening Events

Recognition and Treatment) should be actively promoted at the local level by Trusts for staff development and also by the responsible Royal Colleges.

The support of senior ward staff, and in particular the consultant body, is of great importance in the acceptance of these operational aspects. A considerable effort is required concentrating on why the service is being introduced. The aims of outreach should be presented to encourage ward staff to become involved in running aspects of the service. Standardisation of charts or incorporation of outreach objectives with existing documentation such as pain charts may be required. Outreach will need to be 'sold' to ward staff who are already short-staffed, inundated with forms to complete and who may feel threatened, under-valued or resentful that funding has been provided in such a manner. Experience has shown the benefit of selling the idea to nursing staff and stressing the advantage in the ability to focus attention on the right groups of patients at the right time with a mechanism to get an appropriate level of help. Initiation of the service in a defined area may be prudent as problems can be quickly identified and the number of staff that require training is limited. Loss of confidence in the system will happen readily if it is not continually monitored and any problems that arise are not addressed promptly. It will make a difficult task impossible if confidence is lost and disagreement ensues. The delivery and support of outreach medical specialist services has achieved considerable success over the last four years.

The Louisiana outreach Health Care model

The Louisiana Health Care describes the foundation of redesigned health care delivery as "accessible, integrated, community-based, ambulatory care, which is multi-disciplinary. This delivery system will be well suited to disease prevention, to the management of chronic illnesses and disability, and to episodic care. All primary care, specialty care, hospital services, after-care and community-based services will be effectively coordinated and patient-centered." In order to efficiently and effectively accomplish this coordinated delivery of comprehensive care, the various components must be formally organised into a true "system" of health care—across the entire continuum: preventive, primary, secondary, tertiary and long-term care; as well as, across providers and services: inpatient, outpatient, home-based, community-based, pharmaceutical, specialist, rehabilitation, diagnostic, and support services.

There is a need for health care system to one that is safe, effective, patient-centered, timely, efficient, and equitable regardless of gender, race, socioeconomic status, ethnicity, and geographic location. A strong preventive and primary care system will be the foundation on which the redesigned health care system will be built. This model will reduce the high costs associated with the current reliance on emergency departments for acute care.

The Medical Home Model

The medical home is not a "gatekeeper (who) restricts patient access to services," but rather facilitates and coordinates care. To be effective, medical homes must be accessible, comprehensive, continuous, coordinated, compassionate, and culturally effective. The medical home provides health promotion, disease prevention, health maintenance, behavioral health services, patient education, diagnosis and treatment of acute and chronic illnesses. The medical home is the base from which other needed services are managed and coordinated in order to provide the most effective and efficient care. This includes specialty care, inpatient care, community preventive services and medical home extension services for complex care needs. The medical home will use evidence-based practices, be quality driven, cost-effective, and promote strong medical management. Medical homes shall be closely linked to community preventive interventions. An evidence-based referral system will reduce the exclusive reliance on face-to-face specialist visits. Rather, the interoperability of the electronic medical record will allow the specialist to provide feedback to a medical home provider with recommendations that will make it more convenient for patients to benefit from expertise without attending additional appointments that may require unnecessary transportation.

The American Academy of Pediatrics describes the medical home to include family-centered care, through a trusting partnership with families, respecting their diversity. The medical home will address language and literacy barriers, including materials and teaching methods that address the language and developmental level of the patient. Medical homes will meet the following expectations:

- Prevention/primary care focused
- Patient centered, promoting patient responsibility

- Personal physician in collaboration w/other health professionals
- Formally tied to specialists and inpatient care
- Accessible 24/7
- Comprehensive
- Continuous
- Culturally effective
- HIT linked
- Evidence-based care

Preventive and primary care shall include:

- **Clinical preventive** services
- Acute ambulatory care
- **Diagnostic** services
- Behavioral health
- Disease management (see Appendix G)
- Care coordination/management
- Management of hospitalisation
- Home assessment/interventions for at-risk groups
- Alternative visits: telephone/email/group
- Patient education
- Nutrition counseling/education
- Oral health
- **Pharmacy** services
- **Access to specialised** extension **service systems**

Care Planning and Coordination:

- Assessment and monitoring of patient needs
- **Facilitate timely access to** services **and resources**
- Offer counseling, education, and listening
- Facilitate communication among the patient and the primary and specialty providers,
- **Have current knowledge of community support organisations, including health, education, and social** services **and connect the patient to these organisations**
- Develop, monitor, update, and follow-up with care planning and care plans
- Supply/provide access to referrals, information, and education across systems
- Maximize effective, efficient, and innovative use of existing resources
- Monitor outcomes for patient and practice
- Use evidence-based medicine and clinical decision support tools
- Organize the delivery of care according to the Chronic Care

Model (CCM), using the core functions of the CCM for patients with or without a chronic condition
- Provide convenient access not only through face-to-face visits but also via telephone, email, and other modes of communication
- Use health information technology to promote quality of care, to establish a safe environment in which to receive care, to protect the security of health information, and to promote the provision of health information exchange
- Measure key quality indicators to demonstrate continuous improvement in health status indicators for individuals and populations treated

Extension Service Systems for Complex and Special Populations

All individuals with complex, chronic illness, serious behavioral health care needs (mental illness and addictive disorders) or developmental disabilities will access primary care and specialised services through their medical home. For those individuals with severe, complex or multiple chronic conditions (typically 4 or more), services will be provided through a person-centered medical home extension service systems with an organizing structure consisting of 4 closely linked concepts (CHCS, 2005): the medical home, the care team, the care coordinator, and the care intervention.

- Within the medical home extension, the practice specialty of the coordinating physician, the skills and background of the care coordinator and the composition of the care team will vary depending on the needs and severity of the individual.
- The care team in most cases should include PCPs, specialists, behavioral health professionals and possibly pharmacists. It will also include the other care resources working with the individual. The individual patient/consumer will have a lead role in deciding who is on the care team, and may include family members or friends.
- The care coordinator will coordinate health care resources around the individual and help connect, navigate and interact with the delivery system. This person will have two primary responsibilities: (1) work with the individual to develop the care plan, and (2) organize and direct to care management process. The care coordinator will develop a shared care plan, coordinate providers and identify consumer needs spanning beyond the traditional medical model thereby ensuring fluidity in the care delivery process preventing anyone from "falling through the cracks."
- Care interventions and plans of care will focus on addressing medical, social and behavioral health issues. Interventions will

vary in intensity and length and will be dependent on the diagnosis, severity and complexity of the conditions. Pharmacy management and integration of physical and behavioral health will be included.

Adult-onset and Aging-related Disabilities

The delivery of long-term services and supports would be expected to be flexible enough to assure that all needed services are provided in the home and are varied as far as method of delivery. For example, a person choosing to receive supports and services at home should be offered the option to direct those services, by choosing, training and employing the workers who deliver the services and care in their home. Most persons who are elderly and/or have adult-onset disabilities will live in the community with primary care being delivered through their medical home. These persons may receive specialised supports and services in addition to medical care provided by the medical home.

Severe Behavioral Health Disorders

People with serious and complex behavioral health issues will have access to a full spectrum of needed consumer and family driven services though a medical home extension. Individuals will have timely and easy access through an integrated, person-centered system of care. Care will focus on increasing individual ability to cope successfully with life's challenges, on facilitating recovery, and on building resilience, not just on managing symptom" (From Study to Action: A Strategic Plan for Transformation of Mental Health Care.

Developmental Disabilities

Individuals with developmental disabilities will receive person-centered, integrated, comprehensive and portable care that conforms to the vision, values, and guiding principles of the Louisiana Long Term Care System Supports and Services for People with Developmental Disabilities (developed through the Long Term Care planning process.

Outreach and Engagement

Outreach and engagement of the community is essential. Non-traditional locations for outreach and enrolment will include grocery stores, beauty and nail salons, Vital Records locations, car license/Motor Vehicle offices, churches, libraries as well as nursing homes, hospital emergency departments and at discharge. Public information campaigns will be necessary.

How will medical homes be selected?—Patient Choice

Patients will choose their certified medical home from among those offered near their home, work or school. The neighborhood planning process led by the Louisiana Recovery Authority includes a health component. Citizens from each neighborhood have consultants working with them to plan for the rebuilding of their community. A summary of key elements of a healthy neighborhood has been incorporated into the planning materials. Information about the work of the Louisiana Health Care Redesign Collaborative is being distributed to each neighborhood planning group. LHCRC Guiding Principles emphasize the importance of easy access to a medical home as the key to improved health outcomes and cost containment. Citizens will acclimate to relying on their neighborhood medical home for health care instead of hospital emergency departments.

Transitioning to Certified Medical Homes

In order to move to the medical home model of health care delivery a phased process of implementation will be needed. Building on existing infrastructure and developing new structures such as HIT and negotiated linkages/system-building among primary, secondary and tertiary levels of care will enable the transition to the redesigned health care system. Reimbursement for the full set of required services must be at a level that enables the medical home model's success.

What is the relationship between specialists and hospitals with the Medical Home provider?

In order to efficiently and effectively coordinate the delivery of comprehensive care, the medical home, specialist providers and hospitals must be formally organised into a true "system" of health care—across the entire continuum: preventive, primary, secondary, tertiary and long-term care; as well as, across providers and services: inpatient, outpatient, home-based, community-based, pharmaceutical, specialist, rehabilitation, diagnostic, and support services.

Specialist and inpatient providers who participate are required to ensure there is two-way communication regarding the care of the person—between and among providers and ultimately linking back to the medical home. The exchange of information shall include but not be limited to:

- Referral from the medical home will include the reason for the referral, all related diagnostic procedures and results, as well as any treatments and prescriptions initiated.
- Specialist feedback to the medical home will include laboratory procedures, diagnosis, and recommendations of any following up care necessary.
- Inpatient provider feedback to the medical home at the time of discharge will include all treatment and laboratory procedures, specialist services and recommendations of any following up care necessary.

Quality-driven Preventive and Primary Care According to Life Cycle Groups

The purpose of this section is to describe the standards for the delivery of care, organised by life cycle groups including women's reproductive health, early childhood (birth—age 5), school age, adolescent, young adult, adult, and older adult. National guidelines were used for the life cycle groups including the American College of Obstetricians and Gynecologists, American Academy of Pediatrics, American Academy of Family Physicians, American College of Physicians, American College of Medical Genetics, and the Task Force on Community Preventive Services. Evidence-based interventions have been emphasized in order to address long-standing risk factors and health conditions prevalent in Louisiana and exacerbated in the New Orleans region by the devastation of Hurricane Katrina. The most prominent of these conditions is behavioral health problems.

Reproductive Health

(a) American College of Obstetricians and Gynecologists *Guidelines for Perinatal Care* (ACOG Guidelines)
(b) Family Planning Waiver services, along with community outreach to this population
(c) Sexually Transmitted Diseases (STD and HIV) screening, treatment, partner notification and treatment
(d) Depression and substance abuse screening and referral
(e) Folic acid education and supplements

Prenatal provider assures the following:

- 1st trimester prenatal care
- partner treatment for STDs
- screen for substance abuse and provide brief intervention; refer/follow up as indicated
- screen for tobacco use and provide brief cessation intervention; follow up as indicated
- screen for depression (pre and postpartum) and refer/follow up as indicated
- screen for periodontal problems and refer as indicated
- Nurse Family Partnership Program for low income, first time mothers: evidenced-based intensive home visitation programme
- Nutrition assessment and referral as indicated

Birth to Age 5

(a) American Academy of Pediatrics (AAP) *Recommendations for Preventive Pediatric Health Care*

(b) Use of *Bright Futures Guidelines for Health Supervision of Infants, Children, and Adolescents* (Sponsored by CMS and HRSA, DHHS)

(c) Screening to assure early intervention and referral to appropriate level of intervention, increasing in intensity according to the following:

Tier 1—Universal surveillance and screening for developmental and social-emotional problems using validated tools with referral/follow up as indicated to infant and early childhood mental health professionals.

(d) Adoption of the Research Diagnostic Criteria—Preschool Age as the basis for defining the need for mental health services

Tier 2—Targeted evaluations/interventions/supports for children whose rates of growth/performance are identified in Tier 1 surveillance/screening activities to be below those expected for similar-aged peers or targeted evaluations/interventions for children who are at known risk for primary or secondary disabilities.

Tier 3—Intensive, individualised interventions for children whose growth/performance trajectories do not appear to be changing, despite the delivery of Tier 1 and Tier 2 interventions (e.g., need for ongoing care by a tertiary care physician, specialised early intervention services, services through the Children's Special Health Services Program, Early Steps).

(e) American College of Medical Genetics' 2005 recommendation for new Newborn Screening testing and ensure follow-up care services including family education, treatment compliance monitoring, and genetic counseling

(f) Recommended immunisation schedule and participation in LINKS data system

(g) Depression screen of primary caretaker and referral as indicated

(h) Dental care

(i) Nutrition education and counseling with emphasis on obesity prevention using Institute of Medicine's Preventing Childhood Obesity-Health in the Balance School Age Children:

- (a) American Academy of Pediatrics (AAP) Recommendations for Preventive Pediatric Health Care
- (b) Use of Bright Futures Guidelines for Health Supervision of Infants, Children, and Adolescents (Sponsored by CMS and HRSA, DHHS)
  - • Obesity-related services
  - (a) Behavioral counseling
  - (b) Nutrition Education
  - (c) Physical activity education
  - (d) Physical activity environment changes
  - (e) Parental/family involvement
  - • Sedentary behaviors (decrease TV/video watching)

(c) Inclusion of mental health screening as part of preventive primary care and access to mental health treatment
(d) Access to oral health care with education about oral health
(e) Interventions with families aimed at decreasing abuse and increasing health promotion education to reduce injuries
  - Early identification of developmental delays/educational disabilities
  - Seat belt usage education

Adolescents

(a) Guidelines for Adolescent Preventive Services, American Medical Association, and Bright Futures
(b) Obesity related services including:
  - Behavioral counseling
  - Nutrition Education
  - Physical activity education
  - Physical activity environment changes
  - Parental/family involvement
  - Sedentary behaviors (decrease TV/video watching)

(c) Mental health screening and access to treatment
(d) Health education on reproductive health and risky behaviors which may lead to unintended pregnancy and sexually transmitted diseases
(e) Sexually Transmitted Diseases (STD and HIV) screening, treatment, partner notification and treatment, surveillance
  - Education on seat belt usage

Young Adults 18-24

(a) Obesity-related services including the following:
  - Behavioral counseling
  - Nutrition Education
  - Physical activity education
  - Physical activity environment changes
  - Parental/family involvement
  - Sedentary behaviors (decrease TV/video watching)

(b) Mental health screening and access to treatment
(c) Health education on reproductive health and risky behaviors which may lead to unintended pregnancy and sexually transmitted diseases
(d) Health education on tobacco use and other substance abuse
(e) Education on seat belt usage

Adults and Older Adults

Screening, counseling, and treatment for:

(a) Hypertension
(b) Cervical cancer
(c) Colorectal cancer
(d) Chlamydia
(e) Syphilis
(f) Breast cancer
(g) Osteoporosis
(h) Diabetes
(i) Aspirin for prevention of MI
(j) Lipid screening
(k) Obesity related services:
- Behavioral counseling
- Nutrition Education
- Physical activity education
- Physical activity environment changes
- Family involvement

(l) Sedentary behaviors (decrease TV/video watching)
(m) Tobacco use screening and brief intervention
(n) Alcohol use screening and counseling
(o) Education and counseling on reproductive health and risky behaviors which may lead to unintended pregnancy and sexually transmitted diseases
(p) Education on seat belt usage
- Mental health screening and access to treatment
- Influenza and pneumococcal immunisation

Assessment for At Risk Patients:

(a) Interdisciplinary geriatric assessment re: fall prevention, chronic confusion/disorientation
(b) In-home environmental barriers assessment
(c) Persons with developmental disabilities who are aging in place
(d) Persons with co-morbid psychiatric illness and chronic diseases

Chronic Disease Management:

(a) Type II Diabetes
(b) Congestive Heart Failure (CHF)
(c) Coronary Artery Disease (CAD)
(d) Hypertension
(e) Asthma
(f) Cancers

(g). HIV
(h) PCP Patient Population Profile, Utilisation, and Outcome Monitoring

Care Management:

(a) PCP/RN offers 24/7 advice; Care navigation services
(b) PCP/RN does post-ED visit follow-up with patient
(c) PCP/RN provides office visit within 5 days post-IP stay
(d) Telemonitoring w PCP/RN monitoring and contact
(e) Automatic patient reminders of appointments and preventive health cycle
(f) Coordination with church-based congregational wellness programme

Referral to Disability Extension Service System

The decision to refer a person to the aging and adult onset disability extension service system or an institutional setting is based on the clinical judgment of the primary care physician exercised in collaboration with the person and his or her family. Assessment tools that may be used to determine appropriateness of the referral include the Level of Care Eligibility Tool (LOCET), which on 11/20/06 will be required to determine if the level of care is met for entry into Louisiana's Long Term Care Programs (both home and community based services and nursing facility care) and Minimum Data Set (MDS) instruments (instruments have been devised for nursing facility and home care populations). When care offered through the medical home and home and community based supportive services no longer meet the needs of the person, a referral to an institutional setting may be appropriate. This institutional setting may become the new medical home for these persons

Aging and adult onset disabilities services that will be available through a medical home extension service system:

- Case Management
- Home health services
- Therapeutic services (physical therapy, occupational therapy)
- Housing services (e.g., assisted living, residential care, adult foster care)
- Personal emergency response system (an electronic device which enables participants to secure help in an emergency).
- Assisted Transportation (non-medical and medical)
- Family caregiver support (e.g., respite; training and education; peer support groups)
- Crisis Management
- Adult Day Health Care (including an array of nursing and social services to support greater independence and community involvement).

- Legal services (access to legal services to maintain independent living)
- Self-help or support groups
- Supported employment
- Education
- Assistive technology (e.g., motorized wheelchairs, listening devices)
- Adaptive services (e.g., home and vehicle modifications)
- Companion services (e.g., providing a personal attendant to enable the individual to attend community events such as worship services)
- Personal Care Assistance (for assistance with activities of daily living and instrumental activities of daily living)
- Transition Services (support for transition from institutional setting to home)
- Specialised health and nutrition counseling
- Nutrition services (home and congregate)
- Chore services (e.g., heavy housework, yard work)

Severe Behavioral Health Disorders

Care for individuals with serious and complex behavioral health care needs should be experiences as safe, effective, person-centered, timely, efficient and equitable (IOM Report). People with serious and complex behavioral health issues will have access to a full spectrum of needed consumer and family driven services though a medical home extension. Individuals will have timely and easy access through an integrated, person-centered system of care to the following:

- The appropriate level of care to treat their behavioral health care needs for as long as needed
- Primary physical health care
- Specialised care for those physical disorders which may be expected to occur as co-occurring conditions, including prevention, screening, early intervention, and treatment services
- Care that is reflective of best and/or evidence-based practices
- Care that improves and maintains quality of life in the community
- Care that eliminates disparities and is accessible in need regardless of ability to pay, race, gender, class, belief, geography.

"Services must be consumer and family driven geared to give consumers real and meaningful choices about treatment options and providers and not oriented to requirements of bureaucracies." The desired outcome is improvement in the person's quality of life. Care must focus on increasing individual ability to cope successfully with life's challenges, on facilitating recovery, and on building resilience, not just on managing symptom" (From Study to Action: A Strategic Plan for Transformation of Mental Health Care).

Behavioral health services that will be available through a medical home extension service system:

- case management (service coordination)
- counseling (individual, group, and youth; all modalities and ages)
- safe affordable housing/permanent housing programme (within the Road Homeplan)
- illness management and recovery
- medication management
- pharmaceutical services
- psychosocial rehabilitation
- family psychoeducation
- integrated treatment for co-occurring MH/SA disorders
- crisis line
- 24 hour face to face crisis screening and assessment services
- mobile crisis services
- crisis transportation
- crisis respite
- crisis intervention unit observation and stabilisation
- community-based acute inpatient beds
- crisis residential care
- medical detox
- medically supported detox
- social detox
- gambling treatment
- assertive community treatment
- intensive case management
- jail diversion
- day treatment
- health services (including tobacco cessation)
- independent living supports
- psychiatric consultation
- allied health services
- self-help or support groups
- small therapeutic group care
- transportation
- supported education
- vocational counseling
- peer support and mentoring
- residential treatment
- intermediate hospitalisation
- step-down placement following brief hospitalisation
- supported employment

Additional evidence-based and best practice services for children and youth:

- wrap-around services
- parent education and support
- education/special education services
- family support
- respite care
- therapeutic foster care
- tutoring
- life skills education/training
- intensive family-based counseling (in the home)
- school-based services
- transitional services from adolescence into adulthood

End-of-Life Care Requirements

The minimum requirements for a specialised medical home for end-of-life care shall include all basic medical home requirements as proposed in the Louisiana's.

Right-care programme as well as all the features listed below. Although advanced planning is a requirement of the specialised medical home for end-of-life care, it is strongly recommended the basic medical home provider provide as appropriate, end-of-life education and assistance with completion of an advance directive or (Physician Orders for Life Sustaining Treatment (POLST) either directly or indirectly through other parties.

Operations

- Interdisciplinary team delivering most services, including navigating any other parts of the service system; attending physicians shall have appropriate clinical skills especially in palliative care (including any nurse practitioners/physician assistants).
- 24-hour availability with response time within 5 minutes of a phone call; responder should generally be someone on the team and shall have at least the core elements of the plan of care. Emergency home visits—Responder shall be a member of the team and response time for shall be within 4 hours as medically necessary.
- Transportation services
- 24-hour medication availability
- Supply/Prosthetics processing/delivery
- Specialty referrals such as but not limited to pharmacist, cardiologist, pulmonologist, neurologist, oncologist, nephrology, psychiatrist, etc.
- "Occasional" back-up specialists
- On and Off-site HIT access

Core care plan must be available at all times—on call and during hours—

- Telemedicine services
- Telephone Management
- Home visits—routine and emergency
- Pathway to solicit and address shortcomings reported by any party

Clinical Services

- Advance Care Planning
- Disease Management
- Pain and symptom control
- Hospice and Palliative Services
- Family meetings, including counseling and education
- Respite
- Bereavement
- Wound Care Management
- Transitions of Care (multiple sites) management/collaboration
- Rehabilitative/Functional Maintenance
- Dental services
- IV treatments
- Mental health services, including counseling
- Ethics consultation

Adjunctive Services

- DME/Prosthetic processing and delivery, including (but not exclusive)
  Assistive walking devices
  Home O_2 with monitoring
  Hospital bed and specialty mattresses
  OT equipment (e.g. "reachers")
  Home safety devices (e.g. bathroom bars, bathtub bench, raised toilet seats)
  Home modifications (e.g. ramps for wheelchairs)
  Glucometers, home BP monitors
- Dietary Services/"Meals on Wheels"
- Lifeline Services
- Day care services (pediatric and adult), Community centers/services
- ADL/IADL assistance
- Respiratory services and maintenance
- Legal counseling/consultative services

Educational Services

- Provider
- Patient
- Caregiver
- Community agencies/services
- Students

HIV System of Services

Specialised Medical Home for Individuals Living with HIV/AIDS

The minimum requirements for a specialised medical home for individuals living with HIV/AIDS shall include all basic medical home requirements as proposed in Louisiana's Right-care programme, shall be consistent with the Public Health Service (PHS) guidelines for the clinical care of HIV infected individuals, and shall also include the features listed below:

Operations

- Availability of an interdisciplinary team to deliver services, with attending physicians who are experienced in treating patients with infectious diseases especially HIV care as well as palliative care (including any nurse practitioners/physician assistants)
- Team members must be able to navigate other parts of the service system
- 24-hour availability to address emergencies with a response time within 5 minutes of a phone call; responder should generally be someone on the team and shall have at least the core elements of the plan of care
- Mechanism to admit patients for inpatient care
- Availability of transportation services
- Access to medications to treat HIV and in particular, ability to coordinate with the Louisiana's AIDS Drug Assistance Program (ADAP)
- Specialty referrals such as but not limited to cardiology, obstetrics, gynecology, ophthalmology, pharmacy, pulmonology, neurology, oncology, nephrology, psychiatry, substance use treatment, etc.
- Telemedicine services
- Telephone Management
- Home visits—routine and emergency
- Mechanisms to solicit and address shortcomings reported by any party

Clinical Services

- HIV Antibody Counseling and Testing
- Primary Care
- Care of Chronic and Acute Diseases including:

Asthma, Diabetes, Hypertension, Cervical Displaxia, STDs, TB, Hepatitis B/C, Pediatric Care, OB-GYN/Prenatal Care, Dental Services, Radiology, Laboratory Services.

DISEASE MANAGEMENT

Disease management is a system of coordinated health care interventions and communications for populations with conditions in which patient self-care efforts are significant. It Supports the physician or practitioner/patient relationship and plan of care; Emphasizes prevention of exacerbations and complications utilizing evidence-based practice guidelines and patient empowerment strategies; and Evaluates clinical, humanistic, and economic outcomes on an on-going basis with the goal of improving overall health. Disease management components include:

Population identification processes; Evidence-based practice guidelines;

Collaborative practice models to include physician and support-service providers;

Patient self-management education (may include primary prevention, behavior modification programmes, and compliance/surveillance); Process and outcomes measurement, evaluation, and management; Routine reporting/feedback loop (may include communication with patient, physician, health plan and ancillary providers, and practice profiling).

Chronic Conditions Addressed by Disease Management

Asthma, Cardiac Arrhythmia, COPD, Coronary Artery Disease, Breast Cancer, Heart Failure, Diabetes, Lung Cancer, Cerebro-vascular accident (CVA), Anxiety/Depression, Colorectal Cancer, Dementia, Cervical Cancer, Ovarian Cancer, Injuries, Endometrial Cancer, Skin Cancer, Otitis Media, Neonatology, Peptic Ulcer Disease, Osteoporosis, Hypertension, Prostate Cancer, Pregnancy, Osteoarthritis, Urinary tract infections, Alcohol/ Substance Abuse, Pressure Ulcers, Weight Management, Irritable bowel syndrome, Musculoskeletal and chronic pain: Fibromyalgia/Somatoform, Migraine, Carpel Tunnel, Myalgia, Peripheral Nerve Damage (Neuropathy), Nerve Root Damage (Radiculopathy), Joint and Tendon Condition, Complex Regional Pain Syndrome.

Benefits of Disease Management

As more and more individuals face the symptoms, complications, and difficulties of chronic disease, disease management makes these challenges easier to manage, by helping individuals improve their health and avoid complications. A DM programme can utilize proactive educational programmes, proven clinical best practices and rigorously reviewed interventions to address the specific needs of each participant, promoting healthy changes that last and significantly reducing health care expenditures.

Ingredients of Disease Management Programs

Disease management programmes are designed to provide the right help at the right time in the right way. Participants in disease management programmes should have access to a range of resources and interventions. The intensity and frequency of interventions each participant receives is dependent on their needs and condition. The spectrum of services available to each participant may include:

- Welcome packets featuring a programme description and action plan, a comprehensive educational condition-specific clinical guide, a useful health information tracking calendar and programme reminder magnet.
- Welcome call to engage and enroll participants in the programme
- Mental and physical assessments that define both physical and mental risk on a real time basis to drive intervention frequency and intensity.
- A toll-free 24/7 line providing live response by registered nurses
- Online source for reliable and navigable health information and self-management tools.
- An array of targeted print educational media, including regular disease specific newsletters.
- For participants with the most acute needs, individualised outbound telephonic coaching and education by a registered nurse.
- Coordination of care with primary physicians.
- Medication monitoring through pharmacy claims with physician follow up as needed to promote compliance with guidelines.
- Screening for depression and physician alerts for patients identified as possible depression risk.
- Support for medication compliance.
- Support of physician's plan of care.
- Physician communications.
- Reporting systems.

Breast Cancer Foundation's Outreach Programs

This outreach programme is only illustrative. There could be several programmes on this pattern viz. related to other cancers, other chronic and acute ailments, ailments related to other organs/systems.

The Colorado Springs Affiliate of the Susan G. Komen Breast Cancer Foundation announced grants for 2005 totaling $422,494 for breast health education, screening, and treatment support programmes in El Paso, Pueblo and Teller counties. In addition, $107,000 has been contributed to the Susan G. Komen Breast Cancer Foundation Award and Research Grants Program.

The 2004 Komen Colorado Springs Race for the Cure and other year-round Komen fundraising events will provide funding for seventeen projects in 2005 including the Community Mammography Project (El Paso County Department of Health and Environment), Cancer Control for Women in their Forties (St. Mary-Corwin Medical Center, Pueblo), ANGELS: Enhancing Breast Health Education, Screening, and Prevention among African-American Women (Penrose Cancer Center, Colorado Springs) and The Breast Cancer Resource Center (Pikes Peak Library District, Colorado Springs).

Founded in 1982 in memory of Susan G. Komen, the Komen Foundation's mission is to eradicate breast cancer as a life-threatening disease through research, education, screening and treatment. In 2003, more than 100 Komen Affiliates nation-wide contributed over $30 million dollars to their local communities. Thanks to more than 75,000 volunteers dedicated to the fight against breast cancer, the Komen Foundation is the world's largest private funding source for community-based breast health education as well as breast cancer screening and treatment programmes. Together with its Affiliate Network, corporate partners and generous individual donors, the Komen Foundation has raised more than $600 million for the fight against breast cancer.

Swope Health Services

It is a member company of Swope Community Enterprises, which helps develop self-empowered, healthy people in healthy communities through health care, community development, and community and economic development planning.

Drug and Alcohol Rehab Choices

Find effective affordable rehab treatment, detox, dual-diagnosis centers or other behavioral treatment options nationwide. The services are free to the public and confidential.

Substance Abuse

There are locations throughout the united states that have options for specific drugs and detoxification needs that Outreach Services can explain in detail to each caller. If detox warrants a hospital stay then Outreach can refer to the most appropriate centers available. If detox is safe or inpatient treatment is the desired level of care, we have many resources that offer quality treatment options without hospital stays. The clients' needs are met on an individual basis and our in-depth screening helps to identify each case.

Co-Occurring Disorders

The network includes treatment centers that focus on dual-diagnosis. Most take insurance and are able to work with almost any case that we have come across. We also have resources for gender specific programmes that address these issues in a comfortable, safe and confidential environment.

Eating Disorders

Eating Disorders can be very complicated. Our staff is trained to understand the severity of each case. We provide direction for families that have loved ones afflicted with this disorder and are trained to understand whether hospitalisation is required or a free standing eating disorder programme would be appropriate.

Mental Health

Our network includes programmes that provide services in treatment centers and hospitals that focus on serious mental health issues regardless of drug dependence. We have learned that when the individual is compromised with a mental illness that it is imperative to recognize the illness and manage the affliction appropriately. With proper treatment, most mental illnesses can be managed so the individual can live a productive life. These cases are fragile and extremely important to handle appropriately. No one should be left behind. There are reputable organisations that can help and Outreach is proud to be of service to those in need.

Adolescents

Placing adolescents or teens into treatment can be one of the most difficult tasks for a placement agency. Outreach Services take great care in finding appropriate treatment for our young ones. The families are also so affected and need to know that they are sending their child to a safe place. Outreach researches in great detail the facilities we refer to. We will educate the family to the best of our ability and prepare them for the experience. Many adolescent treatment centers offer education components and that too is very important to maintain the clients self-esteem and progress when he or she is to return home. We are confident that the resources we have are accredited and appropriate for the individual. In addition to providing resources for the addict, we refer families to programmes to help them.

Conferences and Events

Outreach Services offers discounted rates to join us at national conferences by sharing our booth. Rates to advertise your organisation are very low. This helps treatment center keep their dollars where they belong; providing treatment services. Ask us about advertising for you or about how we can provide free website advertisements for special events you may want to share with the community. Networking at its best!

Resources are also available for Native American programmes, Pain Management, Older Adult programmes, Interventionists, and Gambling services. Outreach Services maintains a standard of excellence placing those suffering from Chemical Dependency, Dual Diagnosis, and other addictions into the appropriate treatment facility. We at Outreach Services have ongoing relationships with qualified treatment providers throughout the United States and Canada. Our goal is to be of service by informing callers of their available options based on the individuals needs.

Response time is usually 24 hours or less, and usually is performed by a telephone interview or a confidential online assessment. Outreach Services is designed to help addicts, alcoholics, chronic relapse victims, and their families find effective treatment and intervention for alcoholism and addictions of the highest quality. Information is gathered to help the placement specialist better determine an individual's needs and successfully match them with the best possible level of care available to them.

Outreach Services understands the complexity of successful treatment from addiction. Our staff reviews each individual case and provides information in order to place the person in need into the appropriate level of care. Services recommended may include Drug Rehab Centers, Medical Detox facilities, Residential Drug and Alcohol Treatment Programs, Extended Care programmes, Long-term and Short-term Rehab programmes, Outpatient Rehab Centers, and Sober Living environments.

Outreach Services strives to provide free resources to the public, reduce the stigma associated with addiction and support independent programmes that maintain a standard of excellence throughout all services provided. Founded in 2004 with compassion and love for people, serving those in need has been a rewarding experience. Understanding chemical dependency and other disorders and seeing that recovery works drives and inspires us to reach out across the world. Developing Outreach Services as a resource for networking, placement, education to reduce the stigma associated with addiction or mental health disorders is our passion because we believe that recovery is for everyone.

Service at doorsteps

The provisions relating to outreach services were inserted into the Act by the Australia Health Legislation Amendment Act (No. 1) 2001. These provisions were enacted to allow health funds to pay benefits for services that are provided to a patient as a direct substitute for hospital treatment, such as hospital in the home, under applicable benefits arrangements. Prior to these provisions being inserted, health funds could only pay benefits for such services if regulations modifying the Act were made under sub-section 140(2) of the Act. A facility that wishes a determination to be made in relation to an outreach service it provides makes an application to the Department of Health and Ageing. Each application is initially assessed by the Private Sector Outreach Services Working Party (the 'Working Party'). The Working Party members are drawn from: the Australian Health Insurance Association, the Australian Private Hospitals Association, the Committee of Presidents of Medical Colleges, the Royal College of Nursing Australia, Catholic Health Australia, Ambulatory Care Australia and the Consumers' Health Forum. The Working Party considers each application against guidelines that contain criteria about clinical standards and patient outcomes. The guidelines have been designed to assist the Working Party to assess whether the services to be provided are of a suitable quality. The Working Party makes a recommendation to the Minister as to whether the services meet the guidelines, and the Minister (or delegate) decides whether to make a determination under sub-section 5D(1) of the Act, taking into account the recommendation of the Working Party. This outreach service involves the provision of treatment (which may include nursing care, treatment by a medical practitioner or the provision of allied health services) to patients in their own homes.

Some hospitals that are in the outreach services are mentioned below.

Ballarat Health Services in Victoria

Hospital Health Services in the Home Service are outreach services for the purposes of sub-section 4(1) of the Act.

Knox Private Hospital

This item specifies that relevant health services provided to patients by, or on behalf of, Knox Private Hospital in Victoria as part of Knox Private Hospital in the Home Service are outreach services for the purposes of subsection 4(1) of the Act.

St Vincents and Mercy Private Hospital

This item specifies that relevant health services are provided to patients by, or on behalf of, St Vincents and Mercy Private Hospital in Victoria as part of St Vincents and Mercy Private Hospital. Other hospitals in such a service are:

The Wesley Hospital
Perth Clinic
The Northern Hospital
Ashford Hospital
Ortonville Area Health Services

Chemotherapy Ortonville Area Health Services offers chemotherapy services on a daily basis. Surgery Ortonville Area Health Services can provide surgery in your hometown for such procedures as laparoscopic gallbladder, hernias, colon surgeries, and many more. Varicose vein problems and consultations are also available for vascular problems such as aortic aneurysms and lower leg problems. They provide at least twice monthly outreach cardiology clinics at Ortonville Area Health Services providing care for "matters of the heart." They prescribe and set-up treatments for chest pain, heart murmurs, blood pressure, angiograms and stress tests. The urologist, Kevin Unger, M.D., specializes in urinary problems, bladder and prostate problems. Dr. Unger's home office is in Affiliated Medical Center in Willmar, MN. The podiatrist "de-feets" your foot problems. He provides treatment for those toenails, heel and ankle problems. The "bone doctors" diagnose and treat broken bones, arthroscopy procedures, total joint replacement (knee, shoulder and hips). Outreach orthopedic specialists are based at Northeast Orthopedic Center in Watertown, South Dakota and Slayton, Minnesota. They provide weekly outreach visits in Ortonville alternating between Dr. Michael Vener and Dr. Anthony Nwakama. Neurology specialist provides treatment and recommendation for neurological disorders such as seizures, strokes and Parkinson's. Lawrence Jedlicka, M.D., neurologist from a private clinic in Princeton, MN, also provides nerve conduction studies for arm and leg pain.

Two different outreach specialists provide Gastro-Intestinal services at Ortonville Area Health Services: Peter Meier, M.D.. and Rob Kruger, M.D. Dr. Meier is based at the VA Hospital in Minneapolis, MN and Dr. Kruger is based in Affiliated Medical Center, Willmar, MN.The specialists provide colonoscopies (exam of the colon) and UGI endoscopy (exam of esophagus and stomach). The "heads up doc" is Dr. Kenneth Rogotzke, M.D., from Lake Area ENT and Allergy, Watertown, SD. He diagnoses and treats ears, nose and throat problems such as recurrent ear infections, sinus problems, hearing problems, hoarse voice. Many of his surgeries can be performed at OAHS. An audiologist makes twice monthly visits to Ortonville Hospital to provide hearing services. Gina Kontz's scope of practice includes hearing exams and ordering/testing of hearing aid devices. Physician referrals are not needed and appointments can be made through the Madison Lutheran Home Audiology department.

The ophthalmology specialty offers consultation, exams and surgical procedures for eye ailments including glaucoma, cataracts and eye infections and injuries. The specialists are Curtis Wischmeier, M.D., based in Aberdeen, SD at the Ophthalmology Associate Clinic and Dr. Melvin Clark, based in Alexandria, MN. Visits are provided at least monthly by one or both of the specialists. An oncologist is a cancer specialist who diagnoses and prescribes treatment such as chemotherapy and/or radiation for patients with cancer. Many chemotherapy treatments can be given at OAHS. Preston Steen, M.D. from Meritcare, Fargo, ND, provides at least monthly oncology specialty clinics at OAHS. Obstetrics/Gynecology specialist provides care and treatment for women and those who are obstetrical patients. The specialist recommends treatment and/or surgery for gynecological (female) problems. Dr. Benson will also follow the obstetrical patient through the nine months of pregnancy. The OB/GYN specialist at OAHS is Kevin Benson, M.D. from Bartron Clinic, Watertown,

SD. Nephrology with the addition of the Dialysis Center at Ortonville Area Health Services, have two nephrologists that provide outreach services to patients. These nephrologists are Dr. Larry Burris from Sioux Valley Clinic in Sioux Falls, SD and Dr. Edward Zawada from the North Central Kidney Institute in Sioux Falls, SD.

A psychologist provides care for those seeking guidance in dealing with some of life's challenges and is on-site in the hospital facility one day per week. Dr. John Husted is based in Alexandria, Minnesota. Physician referrals are not needed and appointments can be made directly through Dr. Husted's Alexandria office. Unmet mental health treatment needs of children often "snowball," directly impacting multiple life domains. Researchers have found almost a threefold increase in children presenting to pediatric offices with psychosocial problems compared to 20 years ago, according to the Journal of Pediatrics (Vol. 105, No. 6, 6 June, 2000). Early identification helps children avoid many of the problems associated with early onset of mental health, substance abuse, and conduct related problems. The Report of the Surgeon General's Conference of Child Mental Health calls for a greater outreach and education effort to primary care physicians to help refer children for mental health services. Benefits of This Program: 1. Early identification of mental health issues that impact medical treatment compliance, 2. Patient's improved compliance with medications and doctor visits, 3. Reduced staff time, effort, and expense in handling mental health issues, 4. Full assessment of patient needs and measurable outcomes to track progress

Under section 1862(a)(1) of the Medicare law, claims submitted for service or supplies will only be paid if the service meets Medicare coverage criteria, and is "reasonable and necessary" for the beneficiary (patient), given his/her medical condition. If Medicare determines that a particular service, although it would otherwise be covered, is "not reasonable and necessary" under Medicare programme standards, Medicare will deny payment for that service.

MEDICARE will pay only for service or supplies that:

- are proper and needed for the diagnosis or treatment of the patient's medical condition according to coverage criteria,
- are used for the diagnosis, direct care, and treatment of the patient's medical condition according to coverage criteria,
- meet "frequency limitations",
- are not for experimental or research use, and
- are not mainly for the convenience of the patient and his/her doctor.

Physicians are required by Federal law to provide a diagnosis that medically justifies the laboratory test(s) at the time of the request. Prior to furnishing the service, the physician/provider must present to the patient an Advanced Beneficiary Notice (ABN) that Medicare will probably deny payment and that the patient will be personally and fully responsible for payment if Medicare denies payment.

Grief center/counseling

The Grief Center provides one-on-one counseling to persons of all ages who may be experiencing grief and loss. Brenda Wiese, Grief Center Coordinator, is the counselor for this service. Appointments can be made through the Rice Hospice Grief Center, Willmar, MN.

Free Medical Camps in India

AIMS provides free medical treatment in remote poor areas. In 2004, its departments ran 58 health camps. Eye camps screen for curable cataract conditions and send patients to AIMS for free operations. AIMS Mobile Medical Assistance takes free medical care out to remote tribal villages. The villagers are screened for major diseases and given free medicines. When necessary, cases are referred to AIMS for further free treatment.

Special Outreach Projects

Screening for cleft lip and lip-palate defects

Cleft palates and lip-palate defects are the fourth most common deformities in the world. 35,000 babies in India are born with such conditions every year. The Head and Neck Department provides reconstructive surgeries and runs regular free screening camps to locate and treat new cases.

Rheumatic heart disease

The Indian Council of Medical Research has identified AIMS as one of the three national centers for the monitoring of rheumatic fever and rheumaticheart disease. Under the guidance of the Pediatric Cardiac Services, the project determines the trends of the diseases in school children and educates the public about preventative measures.

Diabetes prevention

Diabetes is one of the major life-threatening diseases in Kerala. AIMS Department of Endocrinology set-up the Amrita Diabetes Welfare Society to increase awareness of the disease and to provide free insulin for poor patients. The Association holds exhibitions, and medical camps are regularly held to promote preventive measures.

The Community Medicine Department of AIMS School of Medicine is training dedicated doctors through its innovative education policy "SOPAL," which promotes "Sharing, Observation, Participation and Action by students in Local communities." The department has trained hundreds of tribal villagers as health care workers, bringing them to the school to learn basics in medical care. In turn, the community-medicine students and their teachers go to the trainees' tribal villages to provide them appropriate medical care.

Pain and Palliative Home Care

The department gives loving care to patients with terminal diseases, especially those who are unable to travel to the hospital and who need pain relief. The home-care unit offers its services free, providing home-based psychological support for the whole family, as well as medical care for the patient.The department started in 1999. It treats 75,000 patients annually, all of whom receive free treatment. Most hospitals are not interested in providing such a service since it is not financially remunerative.

Telemedicine

In 2002, AIMS established the first Telemedicine Centre in Kerala in partnership with the Indian Space Research Organisation (ISRO). The centre allows medical information to be processed from remote centers throughout India via satellite, including Sabarimala, Amritapuri and the Andaman Islands. Telemedicine was used extensively to facilitate MAM's relief work following the 2004 Indian Ocean Tsunami. AIMS also operates

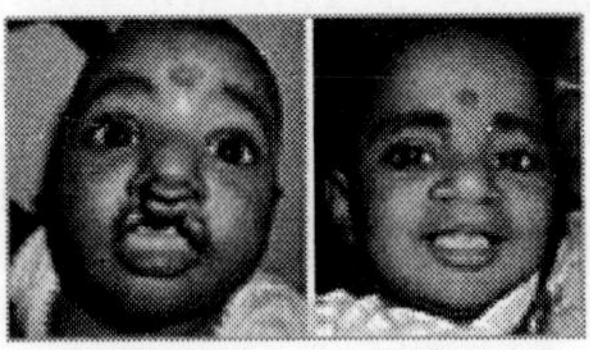

Before After

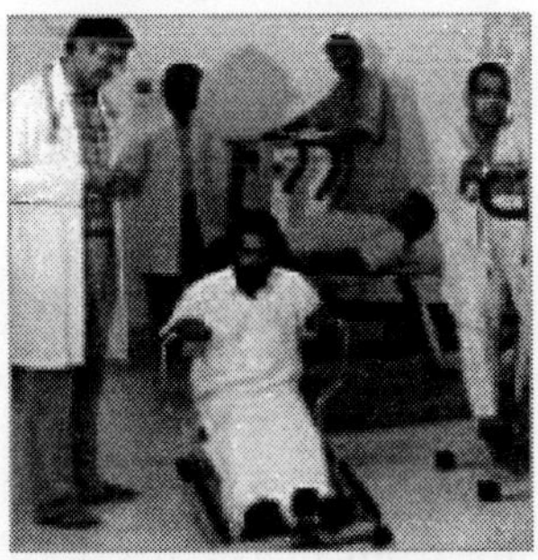

a Mobile Telemedicine Unit, the size of a city bus, which brings sophisticated medical care to remote areas. The Telemedicine Unit was sent to Bihar by train to assist MAM's flood-relief operations in 2008.

Harm Reduction Outreach Services for People Living with HIV/AIDS California

This study examines service utilisation patterns among a socially vulnerable population of homeless people living with HIV/AIDS and who have a history of chemical dependence, as they are engaged through outreach services. Citi-Wide Harm Reduction collaborates with Montefiore Medical Center to connect homeless people with health care through harm reduction outreach and low threshold medical services. Analysis of two cohorts—individuals engaged through harm reduction outreach and individuals who "walk-in" to engage in services at CitiWide Harm Reduction's drop-in center assesses the program's theory that outreach engagement is a mediating variable increasing service utilisation. These results demonstrate that low-threshold harm reduction outreach, a brand of outreach designed to reduce barriers to services, does increase access to health care and related services for a socially vulnerable, traditionally "hard-to-reach," population. Harm reduction outreach is a valuable intervention for increasing service utilisation among this highly marginalised group.

What is harm reduction approach?

It can be defined as a set of interventions which seek to "reduce the negative consequences of drug use, incorporating a spectrum of strategies from safer use, to managed use to abstinence" (HRC, 2004). Rooted in pragmatism, harm reduction acknowledges the risks which accompany drug use, but recognizes the reality that drug use is a part of life. "Harm reduction is not making drug use solely acceptable, but its accepting that people use," notes Allan Clear, the executive director the NY based Harm Reduction Coalition (Richardson, 2004). Thus, rather than condemn or condone, harm reduction practitioners seek to work collaboratively with the client. Harm reduction aims to build on the ability of individuals to make decisions about their own lives. Unfortunately, countless social and economic barriers reduce the possibilities for client self-determination and diminish the individual capacity to limit drug-related harm. Social and economic inequalities present countless barriers to care for low-income people, including those with HIV/AIDS (Adler *et al.*, 1993; Cunningham *et al.*, 2005, Moore *et al.*, 1994; Smedley *et al.*, 2002; Williams, 2000).

Harm reduction recognizes that admonishments about failure to "adhere" or "comply" often function as thinly veiled narratives of social control (Keefe, 1978). Harm reduction-based interventions focus on minimizing harmful effects of drug use, rather than insisting on abstinence as the only viable treatment goal. Drug use is thus viewed along a spectrum, ranging from heavy use to abstinence.

By emphasizing choice rather than coercion, harm reduction functions as a deeply humanistic, democratic mode of practice. Rather than advance approaches which serve the interests of the dominant culture over client needs, harm reduction practitioners promote an egalitarian spirit of partnership between provider and client (Keefe, 1978). Rather than call for clients to passively adhere to provider treatment plans, harm reduction practitioners work to avoid being viewed as authority figures (Marlatt, 1998). Four basic steps are involved in this approach: (1) engaging participants 'where they are at' by discussing and learning about their life, their drug use, and asking questions like 'tell me about your dreams and goals', (2) reducing barriers to health care for participants; (3) emphasizing participant rather than provider goals; and (4) helping clients reach these goals.

Levy (2000) delineates five principles of outreach to homeless people: (1) promote safety; (2) relationship formation; (3) develop common language; (4) promote and support change; (5) cultural and ecological effects. Based on the literature, outcomes for these interventions can be broken down into three major categories: (1) behavior change with an emphasis on risk reduction, (2) entry into testing and counseling, and (3) engagement into health and social services (Tobias, 2003). The model's key features include: integrated staffing (medical providers and peer workers), evening outreach hours, useful tools (e.g. syringe exchange, self care kits), tailored service options, consistent services, and a supported transportation provision. Program theory is grounded in the belief that this model increases access to and engagement in, care for this marginalised population. Once trust is established, participants are provided access to health care services in their rooms or at Montefiore Hospital and/or social services at CitiWide's drop-in center. The aim is to create a comfort level with participants who may be wary, distrusting, or uncomfortable with service providers after negative experiences or interactions in the past. Given the social isolation, stigma, and shame experienced by individuals residing in the SRO hotels targeted by outreach, and the frequently chaotic and unsafe environment of the SRO hotel setting, it is essential that the team set out to build trust with this

Community. Thus, participants are engaged for their health care needs and connected to services on their own terms. As a result of connection to syringe exchange services the transmission of HIV infection in communities is reduced (Des Jarlais *at al*, 1996)

The Ethiopian Health Extension Program

In 2003, the Ethiopian Federal Ministry of Health (FMOH) launched a new health care plan, the "Accelerated Expansion of Primary Health Care Coverage," through a comprehensive Health Extension Program (HEP). Recognizing the huge gap between need and health care services available, the FMOH has focused on "providing quality promotive, preventive, and selected curative health care services in an accessible and equitable manner to reach all segments of the population, with special attention to mothers and children. The policy places particular emphasis on establishing an effective and responsive health delivery system for those who live in rural areas." More than 84 percent of Ethiopians live in rural areas, many remote and difficult to access. The government recognized the need to develop health care delivery capacity, "designed to improve the health status of families, with their full participation, using local technologies and the community's skill and wisdom."

At the core of Health Extension Program implementation is a sizeable cadre of new Health Extension Workers (HEWs), who are trained to implement a Health Extension Package of 16 health care activities at the village level. The Government of Ethiopia (GOE) plans to train 30,000 HEWs by 2010. All HEWs are women, at least 18 years of age, with a minimum of 10th grade education and recruited from the communities in which they will work. As a preventive health programme, the HEP promotes four areas of care: Disease Prevention and Control, Family Health, Hygiene and Environmental Sanitation, and Health Education and

Communication. To address strong community demands for basic curative care, HEWs are trained to provide first aid; treat malaria, dysentery, intestinal parasites, and other ailments; and to refer cases to the nearest health center when more complicated care is needed.

References

'Interim report on encroachments on the sphere of private practice by the activities of local authorities', Br. med. J., Supplement, Nov. 1928, pp. 185–95, esp. paras 16, 17.

Adler NE, Boyce WT, Chesney MA, Folkman S, Syme SL. (1993) Socioeconomic Inequalities in Health: No Easy Solution. *JAMA* 269(24):3140-5.

Aidala A. and Lee G. (2000) Housing Services and Housing Stability among Persons Living with HIV/AIDS. Community Health Advisory and Information Network Update Report # 32. New York.

AIDS. Who's Paying the Price? A Report of the New York City AIDS Housing Network.

Al-Sabir A *et al.* Evaluation of FWVs skills as MCH-FP services providers in Bangladesh. Dhaka, National Institute of Population Research and Training, 1995.

Andersen RM: Revisiting the behavioral model and access to medical care: does it matter? *Journal of Health and Social Behavior* 36:1-10, 1995.

B Harris, The origins of the British welfare state: society, state and social welfare in England and Wales, 1800–1945, Basingstoke, Palgrave Macmillan, 2004, pp. 180–1.

B Webb and S Webb (eds), The break-up of the Poor Law: being part one of the minority report of the Poor Law Commission, London, Longmans, Green, 1909, p. 584, paras 29, 30.

Barnett B. Womens views influence choice. Network, 1995, 16(1): 14–18.

Barrow SM, Hellman F, Lovell AM, et al: Evaluating outreach services: lessons from a study of five programmes. *New Directions for Mental Health Services* 52:29-45, 1991.

Bien TH, Miller WR, Boroughs JM: Motivational interviewing with alcohol outpatients. *Behavioral and Cognitive Psychotherapy* 21:347-356, 1993.

Blumenfeld SN. Quality assurance in transition. *Papua New Guinea Medical Journal,* 1993, 36(2): 81–89.

Brian W. Patient satisfaction: a valid concept? *Social Science and Medicine,* 1994, 38: 509–516.

British Hospitals Association, Report of the Voluntary Hospitals Commission, London, British Hospitals Association, 1937, pp. 9, 63–5.

Brown JM, Miller WR: Impact of motivational interviewing on participation in residential alcoholism treatment. *Psychology of Addictive Behaviors* 7:211-218, 2001.

C Webster, 'Conflict and consensus: explaining the British Health Service', Twentieth Century Br. Hist., 1990, 1(2): 115–51.

C Webster, The health services since the war. Volume I: Problems of health care, the National Health Service before 1957, London, HMSO, 1988, ch. 1.

Calnan M *et al.* Major determinants of consumer satisfaction with primary care in different health systems. *Family Practice,* 1994, 11(4): 468–478.

Calnan M. Towards a conceptual framework for lay evaluation of health care. *Social Science and Medicine,* 1988, 27: 927–933.

Cioffi J. Recognition of patients who require emergency assistance: a descriptive study. *Heart Lung* 2000; 29: 262-68

CitiWide Harm Reduction (2002) http://www.citiwidehr.org. Accessed December 11 Cohler, B. (1993) Intent and meaning in psychoanalysis and cultural study. In New Directions in Psychological Anthropology Ed. by Theodore Schwartz T. White. G.M., Lutz CA., (eds.), Cambridge University Press, New York pp. 269-93.

Consultative Council on Medical and Allied Services, Interim report on the future provision of medical and allied services (hereafter Dawson Report), Cmd. 693, London, HMSO, 1920, pp. 5–6.

Cowan went on to be MOH for Essex County Council, 1949–54, then Chief Medical Officer to the Scottish Department of Health, 1954–64, Who was who, 1971–1980, London, Adam and Charles Black, 1981, p. 177.

Cunningham, C. *et al.* (2005) An Evaluation of a Medical Outreach Program Targeting Unstably Housed HIV-Individuals. *J Health Care Poor Underserved,* 16: 127- 138.

D Ritschel, The politics of planning: the debate on economic planning in Britain in the 1930s, Oxford, Clarendon Press, 1997.

De Geydnt W. Managing the quality of health care in developing countries. Washington, DC, The World Bank, 1995.

DeCarlo, P.; Susser, E.; Tulsky, P. (1996) What Are Homeless People's HIV Prevention Needs? Retrieved 1 January, 2005 http://www.caps.ucsf.edu/home-lesstext.html

Denning, P. (2000). Practicing Harm Reduction Psychotherapy: An Alternative Approach to Addictions. The Guilford Press, New York.

Dennis DL, Buckner JC, Lipton FR, et al: A decade of research and services for homeless mentally ill persons: where do we stand? *American Psychologist* 46:1129-1138, 1991

Des Jarlais, D. (1998) Systems Issues. In Management of Drug Users in the Community: A Practical Handbook. Robertson, R. (ed.), Co published by Arnold/

Des Jarlais, DC, Marmor, M., Paone, D., Titus, S., Qiuhu, S., Perlis, T., Jose, B., and. Friedman, S. (1996) HIV incidence among injection users in New York City syringe exchange programmes. *Lancet* 348: 987-991.

Donabedian A. The quality of care: how can it be assessed? *Journal of the American Medical Association,* 1988, 260: 12.

Epstein A. Sounding board: the outcomes movement, will it get us where we want to go? *New England Journal of Medicine,* 1990, 323 (4): 266–269.

Epstein, I. (2001) Using Available Clinical Information in Practice Based Research: Mining for Silver While Dreaming of Gold. In Clinical Data-Mining in Practice Based Research: Social Work in Hospital Settings.

Epstein, L. (1992) Brief treatment and a new look at the task-centered approach (3rd ed.). New York: MacMillan.

Fisher AW. Patients evaluation of outpatient medical care. *Journal of Medical Education,* 1971, 46(3): 238–244.

Fitzpatrick R. Surveys of patient satisfaction: I. Important general considerations. *British Medical Journal,* 1991, 302: 1129–1132.

Franklin C, Mathew J. Developing strategies to prevent inhos-pital cardiac arrest: analyzing responses of physicians and nurses in the hours before the event. *Crit Care Med* 1994; 22:244-47.

GA, CM/M/16/1 GEMSS MB, 20 Dec. 1919, 27 March 1920, 24 April 1920.

Gamache G, Rosenheck RA, Tessler R: Factors predicting choice of provider among homeless veterans with mental illness. *Psychiatric Services* 51:1024-1028, 2000.

Germain, C. and Gitterman, A) (1980) The Life Model of Social Work Practice. New York: Columbia University Press.

Gloucestershire County Council, Annual report of the Medical Officer of Health, 1936 (hereafter GCC MOH), Gloucester, 1937, p. 40.

Goldhill DR, White SA, Sumner A. Physiological values and procedures in the 24 h before ICU admission from the ward. *Anaesthesia* 1999; 54: 529-34.

Goldhill DR, Worthington L, Mulcahy A, Tarling M, Sumner A. The patient-at risk team: identifying and managing seriously ill ward patients. *Anaesthesia* 1999; 54: 853-60.

Harrison GA, Hillman KM, Fulde GWO, Jacques TC. The need for undergraduate education in critical care. *Anaesth Intensive Care* 1999; 27: 53-58.

Hasan M *et al.* Accessibility and services in satellite clinics: findings from exit interview. Dhaka, Bangladesh, ICDDR/B, 1994 (Working Paper No. 98, MCH-FP Extension Project).

Hashemi S, Hossain Z. Evaluation of knowledge and skills of field level workers of health and FP programmes, Dhaka, Bangladesh. Dhaka, PDEU, Implementation Monitoring and Evaluation Division, Ministry of Planning, 1995.

Heller, D, McCoy K, Cunningham C. (2004) An Invisible Barrier to Integrating HIV Primary Care with Harm Reduction Services: Philosophical Clashes Between the Harm Reduction and Medical Models. *Public Health Rep.* 119(1):32

Heller, D. and Shepard, B. (2001) The CitiWide Harm Reduction HOME Model of Services. Position Paper.

Helping mentally ill people break the cycle of jail and homelessness: the Thresholds, State, County Collaborative Jail Linkage Project, Chicago. *Psychiatric Services* 52:1380-1382, 2001.

Hickey C, Allen MJ. A critical care liaison service. Br J Anaesth 1998; 81: 650P.

Hodder Headline Group and Oxford University Press Inc, New York. pp. 39-53.

Hossain MB, Mita R, Haaga JG. Quality of care and contraceptive adoption in rural Bangladesh: MCH-FP extension project areas. Dhaka, Bangladesh, ICDDR/B, 1991 (Working Paper No. 61, MCH-FP Extension Project).

Housing Works Inc., Advocacy Department. (1999) September 29. Survey of the Conditions in the Singe Room Occupancy Hotels Utilised by the New York City Division of AIDS Services Income Support to House Its Clients

HRC (Harm Reduction Coalition) (2004) The Principles of Harm Reduction. Retrieved February 2004 from www.harmreduction.org/prince.html.

Humphreys K, Huebsch BA, Moos RH, et al: Alcohol and drug abuse: the transformation of the Veterans Affairs substance abuse treatment system. *Psychiatric Services* 50:1399-1401, 1999.

J Middleton Martin, 'An analysis of Gloucestershire statistics, 1901–10', Proceedings of the Royal Society of Medicine, Section of Epidemiology and State Medicine, 1915–16, 9: 1–32; idem, 'Scarlet fever outbreak at Stroud due to milk', Public Health, Dec. 1901, 14: 138–42; idem, 'Schools and infectious disease', Public Health, July 1902, 14: 608–11; idem, 'An inquiry into the distribution of certain diseases (cancer, phthisis, and pneumonia) on the western slopes of the Cotteswold Hills', Public Health, Oct. 1904, 17: 4–31; Eyler, *op. cit.*, note 23 above, pp. 27–41.

J Middleton Martin, 'Poor law reform and public health', Br. med. J., 28 Aug. 1926, ii: 376–80, on pp. 378–9; Report of the Royal Commission on the Poor Laws and Relief of Distress (hereafter Majority Report), 5 Vols, Cd. 4499, 1909, Vol. 1, pp. 371–2, 380–1.

J Middleton Martin, 'The medical profession and rate-provided hospitals', Br. med. J., 6 Aug. 1921, ii: 191–2, on p. 191.

J Mohan, Planning, markets and hospitals, London, 2002, ch. 3.

J Welshman, Municipal medicine: public health in twentieth-century Britain, Oxford, Peter Lang, 2000; M Powell, 'An expanding service: municipal acute medicine in the 1930s', Twentieth Century Br. Hist., 1997, 8 (3): 334–57; A Digby and N Bosanquet, 'Doctors and patients in an era of national health insurance and private practice, 1913–1938', Econ. Hist. Rev., n.s., 1998, 41 (1): 74–94, pp. 81–2, 90–1.

Kamal GM *et al.* The quality of NORPLANT services in Bangladesh. Dhaka, Associates for Community and Population Research (ACPR), 1991.

Keefe, T. (1978) The Economic Context of Empathy. Social Work. 11: 460-65

Khanun P *et al.* Service delivery at the union health and family welfare centers: the clients perspective. Dhaka, Bangladesh, ICDDR/B, 1994 (Working Paper No. 110, MCH-FP Extension Project).

Kippler, S.; Flynn, J.; Schafran, A.; Branch, L. (2003) Too Little for Too Much for Too Long: Emergency Housing for Homeless New Yorkers Living with

Koegel P, Burnam MA, Farr RK: The prevalence of specific psychiatric disorders among homeless individuals in the inner city of Los Angeles. *Archives of General Psychiatry* 45:1085-1092, 1988.

Kuhlman, T.J. (1994) Psychology on the streets: Mental health practice with homeless persons. John Wiley and Sons, Inc, New York.

Kwan M. When the client is the king. Planned Parenthood Challenges, 1994, 2:37–39.

Lam JA, Rosenheck R: Street outreach for homeless persons with serious mental illness: is it effective? *Medical Care* 37:894-907, 1999

Lamb HR, Weinberger LE: Persons with severe mental illness in jails and prisons: a review. *Psychiatric Services* 49:483-492, 1998

Levy, J.S. (2000). Homeless outreach: On the road to pre-treatment alternatives. *Families in Society*, 81(4), 360-368.

Lupton D, Donaldson C, Lloyd P. Caveat emptor or blissful ignorance? *Social Science and Medicine*, 1991, 33: 559–568.

M Gorsky, '"Threshold of a new era": the development of an integrated hospital system in northeast Scotland, 1900–39', *Soc. Hist. Med.*, 2004, 17(2): 247–67.

Mabub F, Huq Md N, Rashid MA. An assessment of counselling for clinical FP methods in GOB clinics. Dhaka, National Institute of Population Research and Training, 1991.

Majority Report, pp. 384–8; S Sturdy, 'Alternative publics: the development of government policy on personal health care, 1905–11', in S Sturdy (ed.), Medicine, health and the public sphere in Britain, 1600–2000, London, Routledge, 2002, pp. 241–59.

Marlatt, A. (1998) Highlights of Harm Reduction: A Personal Report from the First National Harm Reduction Conference in the United States. Harm

Marlotte, C.K. *et al.* (2002) Stage of change vs. an integrated psychosocial theory as a basis for developing effective behavior change interventions. *AIDS Care* 12(3):357-364.

McLellan AT, Luborsky L, Woody GE, et al: An improved diagnostic evaluation instrument for substance abuse patients. *Journal of Nervous and Mental Disease* 168:26-33, 1980.

McQuillan P, Pilkington S, Allan A *et al.* Confidential inquiry into quality of care before admission to intensive care. *BMJ* 1998; 316:1853-58.

Middleton Martin, 'Poor Law reform', *op. cit.*, note 56 above, p. 380.

Middleton Martin, 'The problem of medical services', *op. cit.*, note 32 above, pp. 364–7; idem, 'Poor Law reform', *op. cit.*, note 56 above, pp. 376–8.

Middleton Martin, Gloucestershire scheme, op. cit, note 28 above, p. 6; Br. med. J., 1918, ii: 23–6, 56–9; intriguingly Dawson and Middleton Martin both trained at University College London, though Dawson was six years the elder: C Webster, 'The metamorphosis of Dawson of Penn', in Dorothy Porter and Roy Porter (eds), Doctors, politics and society: historical essays, Amsterdam, Rodopi, 1993, pp. 212–28.

Miller, W. and Rollick, S. (1991) Motivational Interviewing: Preparing People to Change Addictive Behavior. Guilford Press, New York.

Ministry of Health, Department of Health for Scotland, A national health service, Cmd. 6502, London, HMSO, 1944, pp. 7–8.

Ministry of Health, Voluntary Hospitals Committee, final report, London, HMSO, 1921, Cmd. 1335, pp. 12–16.

Moore, R.D., David Stanton D., Gopalan R., and Chaisson R. E.(1994) Racial Differences in the Use of Drug Therapy for HIV Disease in an Urban Community. *N. Engl. J. Med.* 330(11): 333-334.

Morse, G.A., Calsyn, R.J., Miller, J., Rosenberg, P., West, L., and Gilliland, J. (1996) Outreach to homeless mentally ill people: Conceptual and Clinical Considerations. Community Ment. Health 32(3):261-74.

Mullaly, R. (1993) Structural Social Work. McClelland and Stewart, Toronto.

Murray, Stephen O. and Paine, Kenneth W. 1988. Medical Policy without Scientific Evidence: The Promiscuity Paradigm of AIDS. *California Sociologist* 11:13-54.

Nuffield Provincial Hospitals Trust, The hospital surveys: the Domesday Book of the hospital services, Oxford, Nuffield Provincial Hospitals Trust, 1946, p. 4.

O'Flaherty B: Making Room: The Economics of Homelessness. Cambridge, Massachusetts, Harvard University Press, 1996

Palmer RH, Adams MME. Quality improvement/quality assurance: a framework. In putting research to work in quality improvement and quality assurance. Washington, DC, Agency for Health Care, Policy and Research, 1993, 90-0034.

Parsons, T. (1951) The Social System. The Free Press, New York.

Peele, S. (1998) The Meaning of Addiction: An Unconventional View. Jossey-Bass, New York.

Reduction: Pragmatic Strategies for Managing High Risk Behaviors. Marlatt A (ed.), Guilford Press, New York. pp. 3-29.

Richardson, L. (2004) From Punk Rock and Drugs to the War on Drugs. *New York Times*. (3 March): B2.

Rock M: Emerging issues with mentally ill offenders: causes and social consequences. *Administration and Policy in Mental Health* 28:165-180, 2001.

Rosenheck R, Gallup P: Involvement in an outreach and residential treatment programme for homeless mentally ill persons. *Journal of Nervous and Mental Disease* 179:750-754, 1991.

Rosenheck R, Seibyl CL: Homelessness: health service use and related costs. *Medical Care* 36:1256-1264, 1998.

Rosenheck RA, Koegel P: Characteristics of veterans and nonveterans in three samples of homeless men. *Hospital and Community Psychiatry* 44:858-863, 1993.

Roth D: Homeless veterans: comparison with other homeless men, in Homelessness: A National Perspective. Edited by Robertson MJ, Greenblatt M. New York, Plenum, 1992.

Seeley, K. (2004) Short Term Intercultural Psychotherapy: Ethnographic Inquiry. Social Work. January. 49(1):121-130.

Sender, K.; Sherman, J.; and Newman, R. (2004) June. Transitional and Emergency.

Shepard, B. (1997) White Nights and Ascending Shadows: An Oral History of the San Francisco AIDS Epidemic. Cassell Press, London.

Shernoff M. (ed.), Harrington Park Press: Binghamton, NY pp. 141-58.

Sir A Newsholme, Medicine and the state: the relation between the private and official practice of medicine with special reference to public health, London, 1932, p. 29; for Newsholme, see notes 23 and 57 above.

Smith WA. Consumer demand and satisfaction. The hidden key to successful privatisation. Washington, DC, Academy for Educational Development, HealthCom, Communication for Child Survival, 1989.

Solomon P, Draine J: Issues in serving the forensic client. Social Work 40(1):25-33, 1995

Springer, E. (Undated Interview). HIV Counseling: Practicing Harm Reduction with Substance Abuse Clients, an Interview with Edith Springer.

Springer, E. (Undated) The Psychological and Cultural Factors in Drug Use, "Drug, Set, and Setting" (The Basis for Controlled Intoxicant Use) Dr. Norman Zinberg's Work. Workshop Handout.

Stewart, *op. cit.*, note 20 above; J Harris, Private lives, public spirit: Britain 1870–1914, Oxford University Press, 1993; Harmondsworth, Penguin, 1994, pp. 237–41.

Stovall JG, Cloninger L, Appleby L: Identifying homeless mentally ill veterans in jail: a preliminary report. *Journal of the American Academy of Psychiatry and the Law* 25:311-315, 1997

Susser, E., Goldfinger, S., and White, A. (1990). Some clinical approaches to the homeless ill. *Community Ment. Health J.* (26):463-480.

T Willis, 'The Bradford Municipal Hospital experiment of 1920: the emergence of the mixed economy in hospital provision in inter-war Britain', in M Gorsky and S Sheard (eds), Financing medicine: the British experience since 1750, London, Routledge, 2006; Gorsky, *op. cit.*, note 13 above; Pickstone, *op. cit.*, note 13 above, pp. 276–83.

Tartarsky, A. (2002) Harm Reduction Psychotherapy In Harm Reduction Psychotherapy: A New Treatment for Drugs and Alcohol Problems. Tartarsky, A, (ed.), Jason Aronson: New Jersey. pp. 15-49.

Tobias, C.; Rajabium, S.; Shiu, I; Abuchar, V. (2003) Outreach Strategies to Engage Individuals with HIV in Health Care: a Review of the Literature. Prepared by the Center for Outreach and Evaluation, Health and Disability Working Group, Boston University School of Public Health.

Ware JE *et al.* Defining and measuring patient satisfaction with medical care. *Evaluation and Program Planning,* 1983, 6: 247–263.

Whittacker and MacLeod. (1998) Care in the Community. In Management of Drug Users in the Community: A Practical Handbook. Edited by Roy Robertson. Co published by Arnold/Hodder Headline Group and Oxford University Press Inc., New York. pp. 353-95.

Whittaker M *et al.* Rural womens perspectives on quality of family planning services. Dhaka, Bangladesh, ICDDR/B, 1993 (Working Paper No. 85 MCH-FP Extension Project).

Williams T, Schutt-Aine J. Meeting the needs, client satisfaction studies: a simple, inexpensive way to measure quality. *Forum,* 1995, 11(1): 22–24.

Williams, David R. 2000. Race, SES, and Health: The Added Effects of Racism and Discrimination. In Perspectives in Medical Sociology, Third Edition. Edited by Phil Brown. Waveland Press, Long Grove, Illinois. pp. 21-39.

Woods, M. and Hollis, F. (1999) Casework: A Psychosocial Therapy McGraw-Hill Humanities, New York.

Zinberg, N. (1984) Drug, Set, and Setting: the Basis for Controlled Intoxicant Use. Yale University Press, New Haven.

Zweben, J. with Denning, P. (1998) The Alcohol and Drug Wildcard: Substance Use and Psychiatric Problems in People with HIV. UCSF AIDS Health Project Monograph Series Number Two, Caregiver and rehabilitation services.

2

Non-communicable, Lifestyle and Lifetime Diseases: Role of Hospitals

Non-communicable diseases are usually thought of as chronic conditions that do not result from an acute infectious process. These conditions cause death, dysfunction, or impairment in the quality of life, and they usually develop over relatively long periods—at first without causing symptoms; but after disease manifestations develop, there may be a protracted period of impaired health. Generally, these conditions or diseases result from prolonged exposure to causative agents, many associated with personal behaviors and environmental factors. The major non-communicable diseases are listed below. Non-communicable diseases also include injuries, which have an acute onset, but may be followed by prolonged convalescence and impaired function, as well as chronic mental diseases.

Non-communicable diseases group is the leading cause of functionary impairment and death worldwide. These conditions have been the leading causes of death in the United States and other high-income countries over the last fifty years, and they are emerging as leading causes of deaths in low- to middle-income countries.

In addition, these diseases cause pain, disability, loss of income, disruption of family stability, and an impaired quality of life.

Disability-adjusted life years (DALYs) constitutes one means of assessing the effect of disease as shown in Table 1. (DALYs are a measure accounting for years of life spent with diminished function resulting from health conditions of varying severity.) Over the past century, dynamic changes have occurred in the worldwide prevalence of non-communicable diseases, and even more rapid transitions are expected in the twenty-first century. These changes have been driven by social, economic, and public health progress, and the strategies for change have been illuminated by research.

TABLE I

Causes of Death Worldwide: Estimates for 1999 (in thousands)

Total Deaths	**55,965**
Communicable Diseases	17,380 (31%)
Non-Communicable Diseases	33,484 (59.8%)
Injuries	5,101 (9.1%)
Cardiovascular Diseases	16,970 (30.3%)
Cancers	7,065 (12.6%)
Respiratory Diseases	3,575 (6.4%)
Digestive Diseases	2,409 (3.7%)
Neuropsychiatric Disorders	911 (1.6%)
Genitourinary Diseases	900 (1.6%)

Source: Adapted from The World Health Report, 2000: Health Systems: improving performance. Geneva: World Health Organisation, 2000.

South Asia (SA) region and NCDs

The rising epidemic of NCDs in the South Asia (SA) region is fuelled by demographic ageing and globalisation resulting in changing lifestyle, eating habits, and working patterns with less physical activity. In 2000, 44 of the burden of disease in this region measured in disability-adjusted life years (DALYs) lost was attributed to NCDs, and these figures are expected to rise. Yet this growing epidemic is a neglected health issue in these countries to a greater extent. Cardiovascular diseases are the major contributors to premature mortality and morbidity in the SA region. The prevalence of diabetes has risen more rapidly in South Asia than in any region of the world. By the year 2030, India will have the highest number of persons with diabetes (79.4 million); similar trends are also projected for other SA countries. Overall, prevalence of hypertension among Pakistani adults (greater than or equal to 15 years) is about 19, and this is likely to be the pattern in other SA countries. In South Asia, one third of the adult population is classified as obese and the trend is also increasing in SA children. Large number of South Asians use tobacco in various forms: it is estimated that up to 65 of all men use tobacco in some form. Tobacco use is responsible for approximately half of the tumors in males. South Asians have one of the highest rates of oral cancers reported worldwide, and the rates are still increasing. Due to the lack of reliable data and under-reporting of injuries, it is difficult to estimate their prevalence and future projections; nevertheless, the burden is substantially high enough to be one of the major health concerns in South Asia. In Sri Lanka alone, a smaller SA country, road traffic injuries result in 2,000 deaths and 14,000 injuries each year.

NCDs are expensive diseases to manage, and SA countries, which already have poor health and economic indicators, cannot afford this emerging costly epidemic. South Asians have a tendency to develop cardiovascular diseases at relatively earlier ages compared to other parts of the world, resulting in the highest potential of loss of productive life years. For a low-income Indian family with an adult with diabetes, as much as 25 of family income may be devoted to diabetes care.

Like the LAC region, SA countries have social and cultural disparities and inequalities. People of higher socioeconomic status and men who are the major economic contributors of their families are usually able to access the best available health-care facilities. As in LAC countries, South Asians of lower socio-economic levels have the highest prevalence of mental health problems. The SA countries are well-equipped with highly qualified human resources and have common culture and languages, which can enhance more meaningful research, but are often unable to produce significant levels of quality research due to lack of funding and financial resources. With some exceptions, much of the research on NCDs has been descriptive or observation and on a small scale. Hence, the generalizability of existing research for the whole region is questionable and translating this research into practice is also difficult.

Lifestyle-related diseases

These diseases are on the rise and the victims are executives with high pressure jobs, the professionals with ambition and even the common man struggling to make his both ends meet. According to a study, now 65 percent of the diseases are accounted by non-communicable diseases (NCDs), which proportion earlier used to be of communicable diseases. Seeing this epidemic of NCDs it appears that our hospitals and health care system will fall inadequate to meet the requirements and the cost of hospital treatment will become un-affordable for the community. In fact this trend is already visible in the corporate hospitals, where the 'house full' scene prevails and the hapless patients are incurring huge debts even after single hospital admission.

Today, there are a host of diseases and health related problems that are being increasingly detected amongst executives and others: Colon cancer, high cholesterol, gum diseases, hair loss, hearing loss, overweight, early ageing, prostate cancer, fading libido, joint and muscles weaknesses and early menopause and breast cancer among women are but a few examples. The role of food and exercise in health development and prevention of diseases is paramount. Lack of food will give rise to malnutrition related diseases, which a segment of Indian population is suffering from. More worrying aspect is overeating of junk foods and those foods, which contain a lot of saturated fats and salt. On the top of it they lead a life of comforts and avoid inconvenience of exercise or doing any household work.

It is now well known that style of living of the people of a nation determines the level of health of that nation. The lifestyle our people adopt for their living is important for the quality of health they enjoy. Thus India's future health needs would be driven by three factors: population growth, economic growth aspirations and a transition from communicable to lifestyle diseases for a large segment of the population. By the year 2015, India's population will increase to 1.24 billion and its ageing population will increase by 60% to 112 million. We have to see that our senior citizens do not become a burden on health infrastructure, by promoting a healthy lifestyle among them. The worst possible scenario is already beginning to unfold in India. One segment of society is making the transition and has begun to require costly hospital treatment for chronic illnesses. On the other hand, a very significant population remains mired in communicable diseases profile. It is imperative that India avoids merely investing in health care that addresses diseases of development. India has to battle with life threatening diseases for a large component of its underprivileged, while simultaneously caring for lifestyle diseases for a large segment of relatively well-off people. It is this so-called 'well off' segment, which is more scaring. In the battle for better health, India can face loneliness. This west is concerned primarily with lifestyle diseases. The world Health Organisation estimates that more than 56 billion US dollars are spent on health research but less than 10% of it is spent on diseases that afflict 90% of the world's population. Between 1975 and 1997, 1,223 drug compounds were launched but only eleven of them were designed for tropical diseases. India, a poor country is caught in a special paradoxical situation. No doubt, we have well developed and advanced state of the art hospitals to take care of serious ailments, but only for a few. Here good facilities are available, but at a price which only a small percentage of people can afford. More so the capacity of hospitals and the number of beds available is limited, as compared to ever growing demand, due to our newfound prosperity. Unfortunately the prosperity is manifesting in overeating of a large quantity of food with high content of saturated fat and salt, alcohol and other intoxicants and total neglect of any physical activity. Thus an epidemic of serious diseases like heart attacks is lurking. We are ill prepared for that situation.

Dismal state of India's health care

Most of the Indian population is devoid of even basic hospital services. With the spurt in non-communicable ailments on the one hand and communicable ailments still being one of the frequent causes of death, India is suffering from a double whammy. To realize the vision of a healthy society, India has to focus on health development with the mission of 'creating an affordable and efficient health care system, balancing preventive and curative measures and establishing an enduring public private partnership. Besides that we have to use the weapon of public education on health matters in a big way to alter the lifestyle of our people. This single intervention can go a long way to lay the foundation of healthy life for its citizens.

India has the potential to be at the forefront of modern health care, given its strong base in quality health care professionals and cost effective world-class drug research. India has the opportunity to harness these strengths to deliver quality health care not only for its people but to larger geographical regions as well. What strategy needs to be adopted?

1. Strategic Objectives

(i) Increase Government expenditure on health care to improve equitable distribution among all segments of the population.
(ii) Ensure a health care safety net for the poor and indigent to ensure that every citizen of India has access to affordable and appropriate health care.
(iii) Reduce the health and health care disparities between urban and rural areas.
(iv) Encourage evolving new range of health financing mechanisms that ensure financial viability of India's health care system.
(v) Ensure saving on wastage of scarce funds in health sector and proper spending of funds for health care, based on outputs and outcomes and to promote and reward efficiency and quality.
(vi) Increase the role of the private sector.
(vii) Support the establishment of world class, tertiary, multi-disciplinary health care facilities at every district headquarters. Also to encourage the creation of state of the art medical institutions for education, research and care in all disciplines of medicine.
(viii) Legislate and enforce adequate regulations to ensure minimum levels of quality standards and accreditation for both public and private health care services.
(ix) Create institutional linkages with other sectors of social development such as education, sanitation and civic amenities.

2. Guiding Principles

India's journey to achieve a world-class health care system needs to be guided by the following principles:

(a) India's emphasis should shift to improving lifestyle of its people for better health.
(b) Health care services should be affordable—by subsidy or other means to all sections of Indian society.

(c) Health care services and delivery should comprise a healthy mix of state supported health care systems and private sector initiatives.
(d) Health care services should be equitably distributed between urban and rural India.
(e) Health care services should be aimed at maximizing health gain.

To achieve the above mission, a radical reform of the existing health system and infrastructure is called for. The major challenges in this mission lie in rallying the existing system to fully meet the health care needs of the indigent, funding the vast resources required for public health expenditure and encouraging the private sector to substantially invest in the health sector.

3. Healthy lifestyle

In many ways health trends have never looked brighter. A 1998 report by the World Health Organisation (WHO) says: "More people than every before now have access to at least minimum health care, to safe water supplies and sanitation facilities." British Broadcasting Corporation reported, "poverty around the world has been reduced more in the last 50 years than in the previous 500 years Improvements in the world's health care systems have added years to the worldwide average life expectancy at birth. In 1955 the average was 48 years, by 1995 it had jumped to 65 years". One reason for this increase is the advances made against childhood diseases. Just over 40 years ago, children under five years of age accounted for 40 percent of all deaths. By 1998, however, thanks to vaccines, many of the world's children had immunized against the major childhood diseases. Thus, the number of deaths for children under the age of five fallen to 21 percent of all deaths. According to WHO, there has been "an unmistakable trend towards healthier, longer life."

However, a longer life with little improvement in its quality would be a hollow victory. In a search for better living conditions, many people place great emphasis on material pleasures. Such a life-lifestyle, however, can carry its own set of health risks, which means high morbidity and untimely deaths. Advent of automobiles and their increasing use is being touted as a better lifestyle, while it may offer temporary comfort, long-term effects will be devastating to health. Thus a large number of our people are spending a good percentage of their increased buying power to purchase such things as addictive drugs, alcohol, and tobacco. Sadly, the results have been all too predictable. Within 25 years, tobacco-induced illnesses are expected to overtake infectious diseases as the leading threat to human health worldwide. So are the devastating effects of alcohol and other intoxicants. Moreover, scientific American says: "An astonishing 30 percent of fatal cancers can be blamed primarily on smoking, and an equal number on lifestyle, especially dietary practices and lack of exercise. Without a doubt, the choices we make about the way we live have a major impact on our health. How, then, can we maintain or improve our health? No doubt, diet and exercise have a big role. Additionally, what part do mental and spiritual factors play in a healthy lifestyle?

4. Need for broader perspective: WHO

People in the developing world would carry over 90 percent of the disease burden—with access to only 10 percent of the resources used for health. Changing this equation is the core of our challenge. Health is not only a vital asset for each individual; it is the very core of human development. We cannot point to more doctors and more affordable drugs along and say that this is what we need to change the course in our world. The deep root of global health challenges are still linked to poverty, ignorance and underdevelopment. Poor health leads to poverty and poverty breeds ill health. Unless we can help break that vicious circle, our effort will matter only marginally. Similarly, lack of public education is a great impediment to better health for different communities of the world. Most determinants of better health lie outside the health system. They include better education, a cleaner and safer environment, sustained reductions in poverty, a stop to armed conflict and excessive military expenditures.

Dr. G.H. Brundtland, Director General WHO says, we have grouped the ailments into communicable diseases, and non-communicable disease. Our fight against the communicable diseases, such as HIV/AIDS, polio, malaria, TB and leprosy—must go on with renewed dedication. At the same time we need to prepare for the epidemic of non-communicable diseases—now hitting the poor countries and putting their health systems under great strain.

Dr. Brundtland singled out tobacco use as a great danger to health. Speaking in context of China, he observed Annual Chinese Cigarette consumption has been about 1800 billion in recent years. Tobacco may kill about 100 million of the 300 million Chinese men now under twenty-nine years of age, with half these deaths in middle age and half in old age. WHO cannot remain indifferent? We need to free our population—in particular the young—of the tobacco pandemic. Tobacco should not be advertised, subsidized or glamorized. Substance use, particularly alcohol and tobacco, is a major health risk for many of the estimated 200-300 million indigenous and tribal people from around the world.

5. Non-infectious diseases

Non-infectious diseases take an enormous toll in lives and health worldwide. Nearly 60% of deaths globally are now due to heart disease, diabetes, stroke, cancer and lung disease. It is this area, where the emphasis has to be the most. The emphasis will not be so much on treatment, as on prevention. The role of public health education in prevention is paramount.

Epidemic of top killers

WHO experts have identified close links between certain nutritional factors and risk of major cardiovascular diseases (CVD) and brain strokes. Important nutritional risk factors are high blood LDL cholesterol, elevated blood pressure, elevated blood glucose tolerance and obesity. It has also been shown that the links between nutritional factors and many forms of cancer, musculo-skeletal problems, diabetes, etc. exist. Worldwide, the unfortunate trends are towards a reduced intake of fruit and vegetables and increased intake of meat, animal fats (especially saturated fats) and sugar. When associated with reduced physical activity, this leads to increasing weight and growing problems of obesity. Salt consumption is also high in our population, greatly contributing to elevated blood pressure level and risk of cerebro-vascular strokes. Also intake of fibre is decreasing. Basically, it is a question of communicating health information and skills to people, persuading them of the benefit of healthy lifestyle changes and providing them with social and environmental support for such changes. Major changes in national NCD rates can only be based on a population approach—that is on influencing general dietary habits in the population—because risks usually concern a great proportion of the population and lifestyle changes cannot be isolated for only a fraction of the population. Instead, they have to concern general dietary habits of the nation in general. In India, if Punjab is showing signs of obesity-related epidemic of heart disease due to excessive intake of saturated animal fat and salt, Tamil Nadu is suffering from high incidence of heart attacks due to excessive edible oils intake—the oils being derived from (Coconut) Narial and Palm.

Regular health check ups in Hospitals

The executives not having a family history of heart diseases, diabetes, and blood pressure should get a preventive health check up once in two years till the age of 30 if everything is normal. However, in case of abnormality, checkup should be done every year. If the person is not in the high risk category an executive check-up can be done once in every five years till the age of 45. Thereafter, it can be done once every year in case the executive has problems of hypertension, blood sugar, cholesterol, etc. and once every two years in normal cases. It was generally believed that non smokers are not very prone to lung tumors and those who avoid non-vegetarian food and exercise daily have significantly lower risk of cancer, particularly that of colon.

Women executives, however, have some cause for comfort; since they are protected by a special hormone (before menopause preventing them from falling prey to heart attacks as much as men. But doctors suggests that women executives however need to go in for mammography for detecting and preventing breast cancer, ultrasound for uterine abnormality and PAP smear for cervical cancer. They recommend women with no case history and abnormalities in breasts and the uterus to go in for a PAP smear, mammography and ultra-sonography once every 5 years between age category 35-40 and once every 2 years after the age of 40. Awareness of preventive medicine is still very low and that people tend to postpone their health check-ups till serious complications arise. Private companies, as well as Government should mandate periodic health checkups for its employees. This, it believes will help the companies keep a track of the health condition of their employees, reduce the cost of health care requirement and increase productivity of employees. The muscle strength of a 40 year old can be toned up-to be as agile as that of a 20 year old. Not surprisingly, those who don't exercise pay the price of laziness.

Secret of staying healthy

With early detection it is easier to manage any condition. At what age and how frequently must you start taking routine clinical exams? Use the chart below as a guide. People with a chronic condition such as diabetes or those at high risk for any other ailment should discuss their screening needs with a doctor

Age in years 18 20 25 30 35 40 45 50 55	60 65 and up
Blood pressure	every two years
Cholesterol	every 5 years
Blood sugar	yearly
Gynae check up	yearly
Pap smear	1-3 years
Glaucoma/Eye check up	every 1-2 years
Cardiac checkup/treadmill test	yearly
Colonoscopy	every 5-10 years
Stool occult blood	yearly
Body weight	3 monthly
Mood	daily.

Healthful foods

Healthful foods are available in abundance in nature and they are not expensive either. It is recommended that we eat a variety of vegetarian food, with the largest portion of our calories coming from complex carbohydrates, especially those found in whole grains, beans, vegetables and fruits. It is important to eat in moderation. Taking in more calories than our body can burn, lead to obesity. This in turn, can cause strain on the heart, weaken the body, and make a person more susceptible to heart disease, diabetes, rheumatoid arthritis, and several other disorders. A diet high in saturated fats raises the risk of heart disease and certain types of cancers. A good approach is to reduce both fats and carbohydrates in your diet. Meat diet has to be minimal. Overall intake of food is for living a healthful life and not to satisfy palate or cravings for gluttony. Exercise restraint, as you eat.

Establishing healthy eating habits at a young age is critical because changing eating patterns in adulthood can be difficult. Schools community and health facility can help young people improve their eating habits. Elevated blood pressure and insulin resistance appear in these children. Sleep disorders and orthopedic problems can also occur. In addition, as long-term consequences, obese children are more predisposed to obesity later in life. Obesity in adults is known to be a risk factor in several top killers, e.g. hypertension, cancer and premature death due to heart disease and diabetes. Obesity is unwelcome for son as well as father.

1. Benefit of Adequate but Proper Eating

(i) Helps young people grow, develop, and do well in school
(ii) Prevents childhood and adolescent health problems such as obesity, eating disorders, dental caries, and iron deficiency anemia.
(iii) May help prevent health problems later in life, including heart disease, cancer, and stroke—the three leading causes of death.
(iv) Hungry children are more likely to have behavioral, emotional, and academic problems at school
(v) Research suggests that not having breakfast can affect children's intellectual performance.
(vi) Poor eating habits and inactivity are the root causes of overweight and obesity. The percentage of young people who are overweight has almost doubled in the past 20 years. We are heading for a health disaster, if the epidemic of obesity is not controlled
(vii) Eating disorders such as anorexia (not eating, willfully) can cause severe health problems.
(viii) Poor diet and inactivity can cause several deaths among young people.

2. Eating habits of the Nation's Children

- Children, youths and even adults belonging to upper strata eat too much fat, and more than 91% eat too much saturated fat. Many of them take meals in excess of need and even drink alcohol regularly.
- Only one in five young children eats the recommended daily servings of fruits and vegetables.
- The average calcium intake of adolescent girls is considerably less than the recommended dietary allowance for adolescents of 1,200 mg of calcium a day.
- Most students aged 15-18 regularly skip breakfast.
- A percentage of high school girls vomit, takes laxatives, or take diet pills to lose or keep away from gaining weight. Harmful weight-loss practices have been reported among girls as young as 9 years old. This also leads to loss of health.

3. The Opportunity

Schools are ideally suited to give children and adolescents the skills and support they need to adopt healthy eating behavior for life. Most of children and adolescents aged 5-17 are expected to be enrolled in school, so they should be given an opportunity to learn the following:

(a) Eat a variety of foods.
(b) Balance the food they eat with physical activity.
(c) Eat plenty of grain products, vegetables, and fruits and less of meat and eggs.
(d) Choose a diet that is—Low in fat, low in saturated fat, and cholesterol and rich in unsaturated vegetable oils.
(e) Moderate in sugars, salt and sodium.

4. Guidelines

School-based nutrition education programmes are most likely to be effective to;

(i) Help young people learn skills (not just facts).
(ii) Give students repeated chances to practice healthy eating.
(iii) Make nutrition education activities fun.
(iv) Involve teachers, administrators, families, community leaders, and students in delivering strong, consistent messages about healthy eating as part of school health programme viz.: (a) *Policy:* seek input from all members of the school community to develop school nutrition policy, it should provide adequate time for nutrition education, offer healthy, appealing foods (such as fruits, vegetables, and low-fat grain products) wherever available and discourage the availability of foods high in fat, sodium, and sugars (such as soda, candy, and fried chips) on school grounds and as part of fund raising activities, discourage teachers from using food to discipline or reward students, provide adequate time and space for students to eat meals in a pleasant and environment. (b) *Links*: Establish links with professionals who can provide counseling for nutritional problems, refer families to nutrition services, and plan health promotion activities for staff. (c) *Curriculum*: As part of health education, curriculum that begins in preschool and continues through secondary school, should help students learn specific nutrition-related skills, such as how to plan a healthy meal. Ensure that students learn general health skills, such as how to assess their health habits, set goals for improvement, and resist for pressures to make unhealthy eating choices. (d) *Instruction*: Provide nutrition education through activities that are fun, participatory, developmentally appropriate, and culturally relevant, e.g. emphasize the positive, appealing aspects of

healthy eating. Present the benefits of healthy eating in the context of what is already important to students. Give students many chances to taste foods low in fat, sodium, and sugars and high in vitamins, mineral and fiber. (e) *Program Coordination*: with the available food and also the service of experts for staff training and student education. (f) *Family and Community Involvement*: Involve family members and the community in supporting and reinforcing nutrition education.

5. Overweight kids

As said earlier, excess weight in childhood is likely to be carried over into adulthood, and it will predispose children to high blood pressure, heart disease, diabetes and several other obesity related chronic illnesses. Major environmental factors, such as a sedentary lifestyle and a high fat diet, must be in effect for obesity to take hold. There are plenty of fat prone kids out there who never get fat because they practice good health habits. For most overweight children, the problem can be attributed directly to the environmental causes. That's good news, because it means there is a lot you and your child can do to get that excess weight, the deadly cargo off.

However, if the child is overweight, restricting calories until the child loses weight is, at best, impractical, and at worst, potentially dangerous. What overweight children need is a flexible, low fat eating plan (low calorie foods) to follow, in which portion size and between meal snacking are kept to moderate levels. Losing weight shouldn't be a goal at all for most plump children. The goal should simply be to get the child to stop gaining weight. If a child's weight stabilizes while he is still growing and his problem isn't too severe, he will grow out of his obesity. (Most girls grow until they are about 16, boys until they are 19). Make sure that you are buying and preparing only low fat, high fibre foods and that the cabinets are clear of fatty chips and sweets and the freezer has been declared an ice-cream free zone. Make a new rule, no eating anywhere in the house except at the dinning table and that too at stipulated time. Everyone has to abide by this rule, including the grown ups.

If a child's weight problem continues, both the parents and child may need counseling separately. The children need to learn new eating habits and to enjoy physical activity. But remember, any formal programme for overweight children and their families should focus on appropriate behaviour and healthy foods, not on dieting and calorie counting. Only if a child's obesity is severe, should weight loss be on agenda. Weight loss diets for children must be constructed carefully by pediatricians and should always include a 10 percent increase in physical activity. Starving a growing child, to shed the weight may be unwise.

6. You hate being couch potato

You have struggled with one miracle diet after another and watched helplessly as the weight inevitably crept back on. You hate being fat and you hate yourself for being fat. And now you are beginning to feel totally out of control. Are you a couch potato? If you are careful about yourself, you will be inclined to embrace healthful eating and regular exercise regimen because it will make you look, and feel better. The sensible route to losing and keeping the kilos off is through: (i) low fat, low carbohydrate diet; ii) moderate exercise, and (iii) behaviour modification. While cutting down on fats, keep your diet adequate in carbohydrates, it's your body's primary fuel and the one that is most easily burned up in activity. Recent studies have shown that you can lose weight even if take calories from complex carbohydrates—like whole grain cereals, beans and vegetables, as long as you cut down on fat calories. By eating small amounts of low fat dairy produce (such as skimmed milk) and lean meat along-with generous amounts of carbohydrate rich foods, you will easily satisfy your daily protein requirement too. This is important because a moderate amount of protein is needed to maintain muscle mass while losing weight.

Once you accept that you will also stop looking for quick, easy results, you will be ready to lose weight slowly, taking years rather than weeks to reach your weight goal. You will be looking for permanent solution, not a quick fix. What is important is the kind of exercise you do, and how regularly you do it. Aerobic exercises—like brisk walking, jogging, swimming, cycling or running or weight training exercises are best at reducing overall body fat and improving muscle tone.

Myths in food

Several foods have been named from time to time as health promoters and providers for prevention of diseases. While we can't take up a comprehensive list, we will dwell up a few of them. Let us see if they have any role in preventing obesity?

(a) Neem (Margosa)

Neem tree is generally considered to be an air purifier and a preventive against malarial fever and cholera. The leaves are useful in relieving flatulence, in promoting the removal of catarrhal matter from the bronchial tubes, and in increasing secretion and discharge of urine. To check profuse bleeding from piles, three or four neem fruits should be administered with water. Neem is very valuable at the time of childbirth. It facilitates easy and normal delivery. The leaves applied externally are useful for skin diseases, e.g. boils, chronic ulcers, eruptions, syphilitic sores, glandular swelling and wounds.

The juice of Margosa leaves is helpful in controlling diabetes. One tablespoon of this juice should be taken early in the morning on an empty stomach for this purpose. This treatment should be continued for three months. In the alternative, 10 leaves should be chewed daily in the morning. Neem twig is used as a tooth brush, and its juice as toothpastes. While neem is useful for a few things, as given above, its role in prevention of obesity is yet to established.

(b) Tea

Tea is used as a beverage all over the world for refreshing oneself. What is its role in obesity prevention? is it useful as a food? It has been linked with a lowered risk of everything from tooth decay to heart disease or stroke. The tree plant is a rich source of flavonoids, the same substance which make oranges and tomatoes potential disease fighters. Studies show these antioxidants may protect the heart by lowering cholesterol. In a study of more than 1000 Japanese men, the more green tea they drank, their concentration of blood cholesterol dropped. Tea may even help fight cancer. Recently, researchers found a link between tea consumption and a decreased risk for cancers of digestive and urinary tract organs in women. How tea can prevent obesity is not clear. If green tea is taken without sugar and without milk and the leaves are not boiled (but put in boiled water) it becomes a calorie free drink. It may act as filler, thus reducing the urge to eat. Antioxidants in the tea can also help. However several cups of tea taken daily containing plenty of sugar, can add to obesity.

Beware of excessive intake of caffiene, lest you get addicted to it.

(c) Papaya

Besides being effective in settling upset stomach, papaya has so many other curative properties. Pure papaya contains—Sucrose 0.5-1.49%; Glucose 2.91-5.23%; Fructose 2.34-3 18%, Crude fibre 0.3 – 0.5%, Phosphorus 4-7%; Potassium 0.36-0.6%; Calcium 8-21%; Vitamin C 46-125 mg/100 g and Vitamin A (IU), 599-6,347. Papaya is a good fruit, like others. If you take a meal of the fruit, you may not ask for paranthas or burgers. So it may prevent obesity.

(d) Hot spices aid weight loss

Hot spices such as cayenne pepper, paprika and chillies can help you lose weight according to the German Institute for Nutritional Medicine and Dietetics (DIET). Hot spices make the body sweat, thereby increasing the need for energy, say the experts. People wanting to lose weight after summer holiday excesses should not resort to crash diets, says DIET. They advise starting the day with a fruit or vegetable juice and eating plenty of fruits and vegetables and chillies.

(e) Garlic

A Clove a day may fight Cancer, Heart Disease and Infection. It is widely known that garlic lowers the level of blood cholesterol and other fats and saves from ill effects of obesity. If it sounds that garlic is a wonder drug, well, it has been the wonder drug of traditional medicine for over 2000 years. A safe bet, then, is to get more garlic into your diet both ways—cooked and raw. Today several medical researchers themselves say, they eat it frequently and the social consequences be damned. We eat garlic several times a week in my family, says Penn State's Dr. Yeh. Of course, it is a staple of Chinese cooking, but we work it into other meals, too. It certainly won't hurt to get a bit more garlic into your meals regularly (A tip: Minimize the potential damage to your social life by brushing your teeth and tongue after indulging). It is hard to imagine overeating garlic, but don't go overboard. How can it reduce obesity itself?

(f) A fruit bowl

A fruit bowl contains apples, oranges, bananas and also papaya, pomergranate, custard apples and vast array of other exotic fruits that will add more than just a splash of colour to your fruit salad. The exotic fruits that we can buy today are also low in fat, sodium and cholesterol and full of minerals and trace elements. A single amla provides more immune-boosting Vitamin C than the average adult needs a day and plenty of other antioxidant vitamins. Some fruits offer more unusual therapeutic benefits. Pineapple is rich in bromelain, a powerful digestive enzyme thought to have healing properties. It may help to reduce the risk of blood clots, ward off urinary tract infections and sinus problems. Pineapple and papaya contain enzymes that can ease stomach ulcers and can help people digest protein more easily. 5 servings of fruits can reduce your fat and bring energy. Fruits are a rich source of fibre. They ensure that you don't feel hungry after a meal. They act in three ways. Since they absorb water, they give you that feeling of being full. They also act as internal security gaurds against fat. Due to their absorption powers, they soak in stuff that could turn into fat-thus preventing it from being digested and turning into flab. And finally, they are your internal cleaners, they help the movements of unwanted food through your intestinal track so that it can be eliminated. In short, they satisfy your appetite, soak in potential fat troublemakers and clean up your system.

(g) Dieter's delight: Dishes low in fat and calories

Steamed Salmon

Ingredients
250 gms. salmon steak (ravas or pomfret fillet)
5-6 vine leaves
20 gms. ginger juliennes
20 gms. garlic flakes
15 gm. celery (ajwain-ka-patta)
20 gms. leeks
2 tbsp. white wine
20 gms. carrot
15 gms. fresh dill (suva)
Salt and lime juice
2 tbsp white wine

Method:

- Cut the vegetables into juliennes and keep aside

- Marinate fish with salt and lime juice
- Wrap each fish slice in a vine leaf
- Place in a baking dish, surround with the vegetables, ginger, garlic and dill. Pour the wine over the lot.
- Cover with a foil and steam.
- To serve, using a slotted spoon, place the fish in the centre of a plate and surround with drained steamed vegetables.
- Keep aside the residual stock for the sauce.

Recipe for sauce

Ingredients:

- Fish and vegetable stock from above
- 2 tbsp lemon juice
- A few garlic flakes
- ½ tsp arrow root powder

Method:

Mix the vegetable stock, lemon juice and garlic flankes. Bring to a boil and add arrowroot to thicken the sauce.

Pour the sauce over the fish and vegetables or serve on the side.

No. of servings: 2 portion

Calories per serving: 145

Kcals, carbohydrates 10 gms

Protein 22.3 gms

Fat—1.8 gms.

(ii) Gourmandine

Ingredients:

200 gms.iceberg/ramaine lettuce

75 gms. Paneerflow fat cottage cheese.

50 gms. cherry tomatoes (fresh)

50 gms. asparagus/baby corn

30 gms. bell peppers (red, green, yellow capsicum)

75 gms. grap fruit

10 gms. crushed pepper

100 ml orange juice

50 gms. Pmergranate seeds

Lime juice and salt as required

Method:

- Wash the lettuce, cut into big squares
- Blanch asparagus tip if using. Steam baby corn; keep aside. Cut cheese/paneer and peppers into cubes
- Skin and deseed grape fruit.
- Make a sauce by simmering orange juice with pepper and strain.

- Mix all the vegetables, grapefruit, pomergrenate seeds and paneer together, add the reduced orange sauce, salt, and lime juice and toss. Serve chilled.

No. of servings: 3

Calories per serving: 75 kcals; carbohydrates—7 gm; protein 9.3 gms; fat: 1 gm.

(iii) Guava nector

Ingredients: 5-6 ripe guavas, 50 ml. rasphery/strawberry syrup, 20 ml. fresh lime juice, crushed ice as required.

Method:

- Wash guava, remove skin, dice and run in a blender to liquefy. Strain and remove the seeds. Combine with the rest of the ingredients in a shaker and shake well. Pour into chilled Collins glasses. Serve:
  No. of servings A:3
  Calories per serving: 215 kcals;
  Carbohydrates: 48.7 gms;
  Protein: 3 gm; fat: 1 gm.

(iv) Oatmeal dish

If you have got high blood pressure (BP), a daily dish of oatmeal may help you decrease or even eliminate—your need for BP lowering drugs. Soluble fibre is also present in barley, ragi and other millets like sanwa, varagu etc, so take advantage of these cheap options. Don't stop your BP medication without consulting your doctor.

(v) A low fat spread that's better than butter

Roasted garlic, an Italian restaurant staple, can easily be transformed into a savory spread at home. Here's simple technique that yields a rich, buttery taste: Break a head into unpeeled cloves. Mix the cloves with a pinch of salt and sugar and one tablespoon olive oil (coriander and fennel seed are optional). Place on a sheet of aluminium foil, roughly three times the size of the head. Cover with another sheet and fold sides in three times, leaving enough room for steam. Bake at 200°C for 45 minutes to an hour. When cool enough to handle, squeeze the surprisingly mid-tasting garlic "meat" out of the skins for easy spreading on toast or bread.

(vi) Dear Honey

According to research from the US National Headache Foundation, a couple of spoonfuls of honey immediately before or after drinking may help prevent a hangover. Honey contains fructose, a type of sugar that helps your body process alcohol more quickly, according to headache experts. Tomato juice is another good source of fructose—partially explaining why a Bloody Mary in the morning is sometimes considered a hangover remedy.

(vii) Humble potatoes

Researchers in Washington are developing red and purple tomatoes that taste just like regular potatoes but pack up to four times the level of disease fighting antioxidants. These potatoes contain such high levels of nutrients that eating them is comparable to eating leafy greens like Brussels sprouts and spinach. Potatoes are useful ingredients of our diet even now, when taken in moderation.

(viii) Instant Energy

Oats is one of the best energy foods around. Certain chemicals in oats are actually very similar to the active ingredient in natural stimulants such as ginseng. Try to eat a cup of oats daily to keep energy levels high, make sure that you re eating plenty of C-rich foods. Amla, guava, oranges and orange juice are excellent choices, but green peppers (capsicum), moong sprouts, and cabbage are also naturally high in vitamin C. You wouldn't have much energy without water. If your body is even ½ cup shy of the amount it normally needs, your physical and mental energy will dip sharply. Drink at least eight glasses of water per day. The risk of heart attack jumps tenfold during the first hour following a heavy meal—never take a large meal.

WATER AS A FOOD

Remember, water is not a food, since it contains no calories, but as a vehicle of food, it is the most vital source. No life is possible without water, so never neglect intake of water. Do not allow its deficiency, what is called dehydration. No amounts of vitamins, proteins, fats, etc. restore your health, e.g. after a febrile illness, if there is deficiency of water. It is the very essence of life. It is important that water you take is adequate in quantity and is of good quality, i.e. free from impurities and germs. The Tribune dated July 14th, 2002 wrote the perils of usage of infected water and inadequate water supply.

The combination of unsafe water and poor sanitation is responsible for 4 billion cases of diarrhea with 2.2 billion deaths every year. Intestinal parasitic infections, trachoma and schistsoma infection devastate a large population in developing countries. In India, we have the dubious distinction of having the highest percentage of population, nearly 80 percent without adequate sanitation and about 25 percent without safe drinking water. The report paints a very discouraging picture of the situation in Punjab. The amount of industrial discharge and urban sewerage which enters the Sutlej after the Gobind Sagar at Nangal makes this river seem like a sewerage drain. The river supports over 50 aquatic species in the Nangal Dam, but soon after the effluent from various industrial units and Budha Nala of Ludhiana enters the river, it is unable to support any life at all. Unlcean water is known to carry water borne diseases. Water borne infections manifest themselves in the summer and rainy seasons as diarrhea and dysentery. These include various virus infections like hepatitis, bacterial infection like typhoid, dysentery, cholera and the common bacteria E.coli, protozoal infection like ameobiasis and giardia and worms like round worms.

Hazards from the toxic effluent from industries become evident over a longer period of time and might even be responsible for the spurt in cardiovascular diseases like coronary artery diseases and hypertension. Their role in causing cancer has always been a cause for concern. An epidemic of cholera has broken out in Chandigarh today, the August 26, 2002, as I am writing this piece, due to water brone infection.

WHAT TO WATCH WHEN DINING OUT?

Don't make it an opportunity to overeat or compromise on your dieting programme. While eating out, don't use this opportunity to overeat. If you are on a special diet and planning to visit restaurant, call ahead to see what choices or substitutions can readily be made. Most restaurants agree to modify their dishes by changing the cooking method, as per your need or direction. If you have a food allergy or sensitivity, you should be extremely careful about eating out. Common allergens and irritants include milk, eggs, shellfish (crab, lobster, shrimp), some fruits, legumes (soyabeans, lima beans), peanuts, spices, artificial food dyes, molds wheat, etc. Ask specific questions, and be sure your waiter understands you. Also keep these eating out tips in mind:

(i) Translate menu language. Look for broiled, grilled, steamed, roasted or baked, and avoid foods such as fried, crisp, creamy or breaded.

(ii) Share with a friend. You won't tend to overeat if you split your appetizer and main servings and share them with your friend.

(iii) Watch portion size. If you know you will be tempted to eat more than you should, get a half order at the table.

(iv) Eat low-calorie food first. Order a salad as your first course and when dinner order arrives, serve the lowest calorie foods on your plate.

(v) Go for balance. If you really want a high fat or high calorie item, balance it with rest of the meal.

Here are some healthy choices you can make at different types of restaurants:

At a pizzeria, choose plain pizza with vegetable toppings. Avoid meat pizza. Ask for bread sticks, instead of bread. Order pasta with red sauce such as marnara instead of choosing chicken dishes instead of meat and sausage. choose steamed rice instead of fried rice and include a number of different vegetables. In a food buffet restaurant, fill your plate with plain vegetables. Don't go for meat. Look for grilled, broiled or flame cooked chicken, fish and lean meat, avoid anything breaded, butter-dipped or fried. If there is a salad bar, concentrate on crunchy vegetable and bean mixtures; leave the potato, macaroni and tuna salads. While on Indian foods, first of all don't fill your plate with food, take plenty of salad. Eat less of paranthas, purees or samosa. Take small quantity of fat free dishes. Do not over eat. Stop eating when some hunger is still left. You can skip sweat dishes or take only a spoon or two.

DELIGHTFUL ASIAN FOODs

When you imagine Asian food, you think of soya sauces, seasame oil, dried noodles and exotic spices, from ground ginger to Piaz (onion) and Khatti Lassi (Chachh). Indian cuisine bring forth lots of fats and frying and Masalas. Japanese and Chinese foods presents many vegetables and fishes. A native of southern China, a researcher works in a lab that grinds fruits and veggies to study potential disease fighters called phytochemicals. In test-tube studies of 22 vegetables, antioxidants in kale, spinach and galic proved strongest at disarming free-radical molecules that can damage cells.

The objective of study is to find out the health benefits of Asian Cuisines in most troublesome health problems, plaguing us—heart disease, diabetes, obesity and cancers of the breast, colon and prostate. Strangely, the Incidence of these ailments is far less common in places like China and Japan. For every five American women who die of heart trouble, only one Chinese woman suffers. The disease kills 17 times more middle aged men in the United States than in China. And China has the lowest rate of breast cancer in the world. The rigors of farming life in China no doubt help to keep the body trim and hale, and even city office workers pedal their bicycles everywhere. But if activity and lean-ness help keep the Chinese healthy, diet plays a crucial role as well. The Chinese style of eating is known as fan tsai. The heart of each meal is the fan, typically rice or wheat noodles, but sometimes millet or corn meal. Savoury side dishes of steamed or stir-fried tsai (vegetables) liven up the repast. Because meat has been, until recently, a rare commodity in most of China, it is used sparingly. In the early 80s, scientists at Cornell University, USA, wondered whether fan tsai dinning, with its almost-vegetarian emphasis, could explain China's lower rates of certain cancers.

The right mix is vital to good health. In recent years, scientists have found that some classic Asian foods and spices are loaded with chemicals that fight disease.

(a) *Soya.* Experts believe that generous servings of soya may partly explain why breast and prostate cancer rates are so low in China. The focus is on isoflavones, plant oestrogens with antioxidant and other tumour blocking powers. Isoflavones also seen to bolster bone density and may ease menopausal symptoms.

(b) *Tea.* Tea compounds called polyphenols may ward off cancer and heart disease. In a study, precancerous mouth sores shrank inpatients treated with tea. Meanwhile, a Netherland's survey found that drinking one to two cups of black tea daily nearly halved the odds of developing severe antherosclerosis.

(c) *Chillies.* Capsaicin, which gives chillies their fire, is used in creams to relieve cluster headaches or resistant pain of neuropathies. Capasaicin is also an antioxidant that can impede the growth of cancer cells.

(d) *Garlic.* Galic juice kills various micro-organisms and may protect the heart by lowering cholesterol and easing blood pressure. There is growing evidence it may nip cancer in the bud thanks to pungent sulphur compounds. One Chinese study found that the stomach cancer death rate was lowest in northern provinces, where garlic is eaten regularly.

(e) *Ginger.* In some studies, ginger powder lessened nausea and vomiting after surgery and during pregnancy. Gingerol, a major ingredient, soothes inflammation and alleviates fever in animal studies. In one South Korean study, rubbing gingerol on shaved mice protected them from developing skin cancer.

(f) *Mushrooms.* An ingredient of mushrooms, called lentinan, appears to rev up the body's production of immune cells. Japanese doctors have reported that some stomach and colorectal cancer patients survived longer when they took purified lentinan with chemotherapy. Eritadenine, also from shiitake muschrooms, may lower cholesterol.

(g) *Cabbage.* In China, cooked cabbage is a remedy for stomach aches; cabbage soup with honey, a cure for cough and sore throats. Honey sweetened bok choy broth is given for ulcers. The cabbage family is loaded with tumour fighting compounds. Sulphoraphane cranks up the production of enzymes that help rid the body of carcinogens. Indole-3 carbinol appears to slow the abnormal growth of breast cells, a stage in the initiation of cancer.

In a study in China, it was found that more fruits, veggies and grains at the table and the less meat and animal protein—the lower the rates of breast cancer and heart disease. When the intake of vitamin C and beta-carotene went up, the odds of getting lung and stomach cancer went down. While rural residents had an average cholesterol count of 127 was far below the US and Indian levels of around 203 adding even a little meat to the diet raised the levels upwards. And though Chinese women got about half as much calcium as Americans, osteoporosis was fairly uncommon.

There is one aspect of Asian diets you have to be careful about and that's high carbohydrate intake. Couch potatoes in particular are prone to blood glucose surges and a condition called insulin resistance, which raises heart disease and diabetes risk. Moderate quantity of plant based foods and moderate exercises with simple stressful life are the keys to good health and long life.

EXOTIC TURNS TOXIC

While nutritional value and the ingredients of food are important to health, the cook-ware, hygiene, cooking practices, mixing of non-edible food items or elements (inadvertently or otherwise) is a matter of great concern for the safety of food or its nutrition quotient. Whereas unintended mixing of aluminium, while cooking or storing food is known to be toxic, exposure of the food to bacteria or other germs can lead to severe ailments. Similarly, use of tobacco as a food, which is otherwise non-edible, is widely practiced by our people in different forms and with consequent health hazards. On the day following a big dinner for city's elite, a large number of people were admitted to hospitals at Chandigarh with gastro-enteritis and dehydration. What went wrong? Probably it was a glaring lapse of hygienic practices, leading to food poisoning.

Food poisoning or toxicity cases usually increase in the summer and rainy seasons. Many people are sensitive to certain foods and suffer a food allergy. Food poisoning is caused by bacteria that grow in food that is not handled properly. Bacteria can grow rapidly when certain foods, especially meat and dairy products, are not prepared carefully or left at high temperatures.

(a) GENERAL MEASURES

(a) Wash your hands after handling raw meat. Wash your hands and utensils before preparing other foods. Do not eat meat, dressing salads or other foods that have been kept for more than two hours between 34°C and 40°C.
(b) Keep party foods on ice. Do not eat raw eggs or preparations made with raw eggs.
(c) Discard any cans or jars with bulging lids or leaks.
(d) When you eat out, avoid rare and uncooked meat. Eat salad bar and other items before they get warm.

(b) ALUMINIUM COOKWARE

In India, aluminium pots and pans are widely used in cooking: being cheaper, lighter and easily available, they are preferred by a majority of the population. Aluminium is highly prone to corrosion, that occurs due to small impurities in the metal. Even anodized aluminum vessels, i.e. those coated with protective layers wears off with time. The greatest amount of leaching of aluminum into the food occurs when acidic food is cooked in aluminum vessels or stored in them. Nor is Teflon-coated cookware so safe, since the coating layer wears off and the underlying aluminum layer is exposed. Also there is the Alzheimer disease (a derangement of brain function) scare. Many researchers now believe there is enough evidence to conclude that aluminum is probably a significant co-factor in the development of Alzheimer's disease. Scientific studies support the hypothesis but have not conclusively proved it. Some Dos and donts are:

(i) Only new anodized aluminum vessel may be used for cooking
(ii) Never use a high flame when cooking in aluminum.
(iii) As far as possible use a wooden spoon to stir food being cooked in aluminum vessels.
(iv) Don't cook acidic food in aluminum
(v) Salt and vinegar also react with aluminum
(vi) Avoid boiling tea or coffee for long hours in aluminum kettles
(vii) Avoid storing cooked food in aluminum vessels or in aluminum foil, especially acidic food
(viii) Avoid scouring soiled aluminium vessels with an abrasive sponge. Instead, use a soft sponge and warm soapy water. It is best to discard very badly burnt vessels. Use cast iron sizzler pans, made out of an iron-zinc alloy, these pans retain heat and like non-stick pans, require very little oil.

(c) DISEASE CAUSING GERMS

It is not uncommon for the germs to gain access to raw or cooked food, especially under Indian conditions, where hygiene is given a back seat. Even in the United States, which has one of the safest food supplies in the world, there are still millions of cases of foodborne illness each year. You can reduce your risk for food borne illness by:

- Improving food handling practices
- Knowing how food becomes contaminated
- Knowing what encourages bacteria to grow.

The following are a few common diseases caused by microorganisms:

Botulism, E.Coli, Salmonella, Staphylococci, Toxoplasma, Hepatitis virus, cholera, Amoebiasis, etc.

Bolulism occurs with a bang within 12-36 hours of ingestion of toxins, generally from canned foods, especially meat or fish. A good cooking and proper canning can prevent this infection. Other bacteria and virus can also cause infection if contaminated water or food is taken and cause symptoms from a variable period. Common symptoms are vomiting, diarrhea, pain abdomen, weakness, dehydration, acute kidney failure, etc. Keep your sanitary practice above board.

(d) TOBACCO AS FOOD

Tobacco is freely used by Indians as food in Pann, Khaini or smoked as Biris or cigarettes. Such food practices sadly cause 11,000 deaths every day-worldwide. The health impact of tobacco use are among the most often described,. Much of the stress has been placed on the increased risks of cancer and heart disease. Nevertheless, tobacco can have many of the same effects when consumed in various smokeless tobacco forms, e.g. mixed with food, chewed or swallowed for kick. It is the use of tobacco, rather than how it is used, that is harmful to health.

What it may cause to tobacco user?

(i) Cancer;
(ii) Heart disease;
(iii) Chronic obstructive pulmonary disease.
(iv) Stroke;
(v) Peripheral vascular disease;
(vi) Osteoporosis;
(vii) Diabetes;
(viii) Green tobacco sickness (GTS).

Details of these ailments or how tobacco causes them, may be beyond the scope of this piece

Regular exercises; panacea!

Exercise as a part of healthy living to comes on the top. Nature intended us to move for health in search of food and work. Now more people die due to eating excess of food coupled with no exercise. In India 3 out of 4 people are said to be completely inactive. Burning as few as 150 calories a day (mild exercise) can reduce the risk of heart disease, high blood pressure, cancer and diabetes considerably, according to a report. When you select an exercise activity, it is important to choose something that you enjoy doing. Otherwise, you will not make it a part of your lifestyle.

Children and adults alike should set a goal of accumulating at least 30 minutes of moderate-intensity physical activity on most, and preferably all, days of the week, e.g. swimming, brisk walk, riding a bicycle, washing and waxing car, climbing stairs, and cleaning up the yard. You don't need to join an expensive gym or a health club to safeguard your health. If you have a history of cardiovascular disease or if you are male over 40 years of age or a female over 50 years, you should consult your doctor before starting any vigorous exercise. If you do most of your personal work yourselves and do not depend to be served by servants and vehicles, many problems on health front can be prevented.

As we have become more civilised, we prefer a way of life that is making us avoid physical movements and exercises, which are so essential to healthy lifestyle. Civilised people have developed sedentary habits and we have been tempted to give up even the minimum physical exercises that would allow us to develop into a healthy human being. Even while sitting in the office, we remain glued to our chairs with no movement of limbs or torso, lest excess movement may be considered uncivilised. We avoid even going to the bathroom often—since we pretend that we are very busy. Here you are, the couch potato—the fat, lazy and sick being. This is bound to curtail your continuance of life. Obesity, diabetes, hypertension, cardiovascular diseases, strokes, the top killers and many other non-communicable diseases are known to have been caused by defective style of living—lazy living and not liking to engage in the minimum amount of physical exercises that could keep us fit and active. Sedentary lifestyle is known today as one of the top ten global causes of death and disability. We must keep ourselves fighting fit and to do that sedentary/comfortable modern lifestyle should be given up. Walk to market, to your office, wash the car, play with the kids, biking, hiking, gardening, working, sports—play games and remain vibrant and healthy. So far we have won the war against most of the infectious diseases—but we may fail in the realm of self-created diseases if we cannot give up our sedentary habits.

I. Beware of lethargy: Indulge in regular physical activity

Regular physical activity reduces the risk of dying from heart disease (1/3 of global deaths) type II diabetes (90% of world diabetes cases) and colon cancer. Evidence may also suggest that physical activity may provide protection against breast cancer, help control weight and prevent/ reduce hypertension (affecting 20% of the adult world population), helps reduce osteoporosis, reduces stress, anxiety and feeling of depression, enhances functional capacity and independent living in older persons, promotes social interaction and contribute to social integration. Appropriate regular moderate physical activity is a simple, enjoyable, cost effective and accessible-multipurpose medicine for all. So if you believe in indulgence, indulge in regular physical exercise.

(a) Higher levels of physical activity

The non communicable diseases which are emerging as major group of causes of death, morbidity and disability worldwide, share a relatively small number of common and preventable risk factors: specially, lack of physical activity, tobacco use and an unhealthy diet. Physical activity interacts positively with strategies to improve diet and discourage tobacco use or facilitate its cessation.

(b) Social and economic benefits

While the burden of non-communicable diseases (NCDs) is growing silently worldwide, there is a vast body of knowledge, experience and scientific evidence which shows that appropriate regular physical activity provides people of all ages, male and female, with substantial physical, social and mental health gains and general well being. It reduces the risk of premature mortality in general and, to a large extent, protects against the development of the major NCDs.

How it offers social and economic benefits?

(i) Reduces the risk of dying prematurely.
(ii) Reduces the risk of dying from heart disease.
(iii) Reduces the risk (upto 50%) of developing heart disease, diabetes (type II), colon cancer, and lower back pain.
(iv) Helps prevent/reduce hypertension.

(v) Reduces stress, anxiety and feelings of depression and loneliness.
(vi) Helps control weight.
(vii) Helps build and maintain healthy bones, muscles, and joints.
(viii) Helps reduce osteoporosis and fractures.
(ix) Helps older adults become stronger and better able to move without falling.
(x) Enhances functional capacity and independent living.
(xi) Promotes psychological well-being, better cognition, social interaction and social integration.
(xii) Helps minimize the consequences of certain disabilities and can help in the management of painful conditions.
(xiii) Helps control risk behaviors, especially among children and youth (e.g. tobacco use and other substances, unhealthy diet, violence).

The appropriate physical activity can bring economic benefits in terms of reduced health care costs, increased productivity, healthier physical and social environments, better performing schools and work sites, stronger participation in sports and recreation and increased sporting achievements.

(c) Strategy for Health and Well-being

Along with ban on tobacco use and promotion of healthy diet, physical activity is recognized as a significant strategy to curb risk factors for NCD. Presently this accounts for almost 77% deaths in developing countries and 85% burden of disease in low and middle income countries. Despite the benefits of physical activity and its potential accessibility to all, it is estimated that over 60% of the world population is not physically active enough to gain health benefits, especially among girls and women. The overall inactivity trend is prevalent in urban areas of both developed and developing countries among poor and rich communities alike.

(d) What efforts may work?

(i) Putting special focus on young people.
(ii) Working with the sport community.
(iii) Making linkages with healthy diet and no tobacco use.
(iv) Ensuring equity in accessibility and practice of physical activity/sport for all (e.g. gender issues, activity for persons with disability).
(v) Promoting physical activity in key settings; communities, schools, workplaces and health institutions.
(vi) Making use of major sport, youth, health, education and cultural events.

(e) The lesson to be learnt

(i) Promote broader understanding of physical activity.
(ii) Promote Public health perspective.
(iii) Promote effective advocacy and dissemination of knowledge.
(iv) Promote use of life settings (e.g. school, workplace, health and social settings).
(v) Involvement of family, peers, communities, mohallas and concerned sectors.
(vi) Let physical activity provide enjoyment, feedback and variety.

(f) How WHO can participate

(i) Set-up a database on physical activity benefits, trends, determinants, best practices, policy and programme quidelines.
(ii) To produce advocacy/communication materials on physical activity role in promoting health and preventive NCDs.
(iii) To support the assessment of physical activity levels, practices and determinants within countries.
(iv) To develop initiatives to increase young people involvement in physical activity and sport, in and out of school.
(v) Mobilize existing and new networks on physical activity and sport for all.

2. Essentials before exercise

Don't be in haste when planning an exercise. Be prepared for work-up mentally and physically, else you may get an injury. Be careful and prepared. Persons from well to do families viz. housewives, company executives, youths, children all throng to gyms. They can minimize the risk of getting injured while doing exercise by taking a few simple precautions.

(a) Use proper shoes and other protectives

Use equipment appropriate to the sport you are playing. Cricketers should wear gloves, pads and a box and should consider a helmet, thigh pads and an arm guard. People playing contact sports like rugby should wear mouthguards, and runners and basketball players should wear specially designed impact absorbing shoes. Shin guards and ankle supports which are inexpensive and can prevent bruises, fractures and sprains, should be used in football and hockey. Do not play games on hard courts, wearing thin soled canvas shoes.

(b) Warm-up before you exercise

Gentle warm-up exercises include arm circling, leg swing, forward and side bends and jogging on the spot. Perform muscle stretches by extending gently until you feel a pull, then holding the position for ten seconds. Indeed, the stress is not only on the importance of warming up beforehand, but also on cooling down afterwards. The worst thing you could do after you have exercised is to just stop or take a cold shower. Your muscles need time to return to their original condition. So gently stretch them. This will promote circulation and allow your body to rid itself of the pain producing lactic acid which accumulates during exercise. If your muscles are still tight when you stop, you will be less flexible next time you play, increasing the risks of strains.

(c) Take help of an instructor

Before joining a gym, find out whether the instructors are adequately qualified. Also make sure it's the right level for you. If in any doubt, consult your doctor before doing anything physically strenuous.

(d) Don't overstrain: Listen to your body

Athletes often fall prey to injuries as the demands of their sport drive them harder. Overstraining can lead to many kinds of serious problems. It can lead to chronic fatigue syndrome and even susceptibility to frequent infections. In women, overstrain can be associated with the syndrome known as the Female Athlete Triad, which consists of disordered eating patterns, weight loss, and missed periods. Estrogen levels can fall dangerously low, causing demineralisation of bones or osteoporosis, often leading to stress fractures. To avoid problems caused by overtraining, follow these guidelines. Cut down training if you experience reduced appetite, difficulty in sleeping, constant exhaustion or weight loss. Exercising should be a happy and beneficial experience. Sport and exercise prevent heart problems, delay the early onset of arthritis and joint disorders and above all, help you relax and enjoy life more.

(e) Food has a role in fitness

Adequate carbohydrate intake is vital for those who take part in vigorous physical activity. It provides the calories an exercising body needs. Two hours before vigorous exercise, eat a meal of dal and vegetables with rice or chapatis. And drink more water than your thirst calls for, during exercise. Afterwards, replenish burnt calories with potatoes, rice or vegetables and reduce fat intake. To ensure bones don't lose vital calcium supplies in the long-term, experts advice you to add dairy products, leafy green vegetables like spinach, curd, beans and dried fruits to your diet.

Two myths need to be mentioned here. One, abstaining from food can be helpful in giving spiritual strength and second that fasting cleanses your system. In fact while fasting you are depriving your body of nutrients which are essential. Instead eat a variety of foods. Don't use fasting for weight loss either. Eat less, eat proper, don't overeat.

3. How exercise makes you happy?

It is common to see youngsters from well to do families complaining of lethargy, fatigue, body aches and depression. There is hardly any work, they do in their homes. Every work is done by the servants. They lead an inactive life. A person who walks or takes exercise daily, remains cheerful and happy the whole day. Scientists have concluded that lethargy and depression go hand in hand.

(a) Where is happiness?

Exercise releases a number of chemicals in the body called endorphins, which stimulate brain cells. These mentally stimulating chemicals impart a feeling of cheerfulness to the mind. Regular exercise tones up our muscles and keeps the brain alert. It burns away unnecessary calories in the body and saves one from obesity. One looks smart and active and radiates energy. A positive attitude develops towards life. Regular exercise is good for diabetics and those who suffer from hypertension. Under the guidance of their specialist, heart patients can also do regular exercises. The exercises bring fitness and happiness even to the disabled, though the range may be limited.

(b) The 20 minute formula

If you devote 20 to 30 minutes of your time to exercise and do not let anything come in the way, then you can easily turn your life around. Many give excuses to avoid exercising. Many say they have no time. What is more important? The feeling of lethargy, weakness, indigestion, body aches, constant cold and coughs, depression and stress, all are symptoms of sedentary life. So if you want to ward these evils away—exercise. Start your day with 1000 steps, i.e. spot marching for 10 minutes with music. The whole family should participate, the elderly and kids also, but each to their own pace. This should be followed by yoga exercises as per your capacity. The following three asanas, help to stretch and shape the body when performed in the warmth of your partner:

(i) *Upavishtakonasan*: Sit with legs apart opposite your partner. Now hold each other's elbow and bend forward and down aiming your abdomen on the floor;

(ii) *Pashchimottanasân*: Sit with your legs together and feet against each other. Keep your back straight, chest out and eyes on your feet. Hold each other's elbow and pull. This posture helps abdomen, hamstring, quardriceps and calves;

(iii) *Utthita Trikonasan (variation)*: Stand with your legs apart, bend on your side, hold each others arms and pull for maximum stretch. Your arm should be above your head and behind your ear. Lock your elbow (keep it straight). Repeat on the other side. This exercise is for waist and arms.

Some other asanas are described elsewhere in this chapter, for better posture and good health.

(c) Walk your way to health

Besides burning calories and reducing body fat, brisk walking helps relieve stress, strengthen your heart and lowers blood pressure. People who walk regularly also reduce their risk of heart disease and diabetes. It is well known that walking 3 kms. A day at any pace reduces your risk of coronary heart disease. Moderate walking will also lower the bad cholesterol in your blood and help build strong bones, protecting women (as well as men) against osteoporosis. It is also a great way of letting off steam and boosting your energy levels. The rhythmic, repetitive movement can be calming and soothing and may even stimulate creative thinking. While walking at a gentle pace is good, but power walking is best. Start by walking on flat ground until you are ready to progress to more strenuous terrain, e.g. climbing mountains.

(d) Technique

Start with posture check, i.e. Relax your shoulders. Keep your neck long and chin parallel to the ground try focusing on a point 4.5 m (15 ft) in front. Lift and open your chest. Don't arch your back. Keep your stomach tight and hips square. Warm up slowly, Gently increase your speed. Three kilometers per hour may be enough to increase your heart rate so that you are in your training zone. As you get fitter, pick up the pace to 6-8 km/h.

Don't forget to stretch after your workout. Stretch all your major muscle groups calves are especially important, otherwise they will tighten up and make your shine sore: While running, lengthen your stride as you speed up. Keep your arms bend at 90 degrees and swing them in time with your step. (*Fitness Times,* June 2002, Chandigarh).

4. Take a vow to move: Strengthen your heart and bones and beat the stress

What is the best way to strengthen your heart, shape your muscles and build up your bones? exercising of course. We said so in the paragraph above also, about the benefits of walking.

(i) Heart

Just walking 3 km in half an hour four times a week improves or maintains heart and lung fitness enough incase your chances of living healthier and longer. Walking is an aerobic exercise. All that means is; it's a rhythmic, whole-body activity that uses the big muscles of your body (those in the legs, buttocks, back, shoulders) in a repetitive fashion. You can walk, jog, cycle, dance, swim, stair-climb or bench step. It doesn't matter. Any kind of aerobic exercise make your heart and circulatory system more efficient, so more oxygen and nutrients get to your muscles, allowing them to work longer and harder and giving you more energy while upping your longevity odds.

For 30 minutes workouts a week is all you need for basic fitness. If you want more fitness than that, make workouts longer, more frequent or more intense (For instance, you could start out with brisk walking, slow jogging or cycling. When you are ready for a little more push, try jogging, stair climbing or a low impact aerobic dance class. As a beginner you can be slow. Stepping can be hard on knees. To avoid problems, place your foot flat on the bench with each step; don't bend knees more than you would climbing stairs; and don't step back so far that you can't easily get your whole foot down.

(ii) Bones

You need three components to ensure strong bones; exercise to stimulate strong bone formation; calcium to mineralize that new bone; and estrogen to improve the absorption of calcium and to protect against bone loss.

Traditional wisdom had it that bones could be strengthened only through weight bearing exercise in which the body is supported by the feet, funning, walking, jogging. But today we know that strength-training exercise, such as working with weights—while it doesn't cause direct impact, stimulates bone growth by pulling on the muscles attached to the bone.

The following chart rates various activities according to how beneficial they are as bone strengtheners.

Most Beneficial

Aerobic, weight bearing moderate impact activities: Walking, climbing stairs, hiking, dancing, jogging, aerobic dance, rope skipping. Non-aerobic weight bearing activities that work against gravity; weight training with machines or free weights.

Somewhat beneficial

Aerobic, weight-bearing, low impact activities: Stair-climbing, aqua aerobics, rowing, non-aerobic, weight bearing, moderate impact activities: Racquet and court sports.

Least beneficial

Aerobic, non-weight bearing, non-impact activities: Cycling, swimming, deep water running.

Unknown Benefits

Non-aerobic, non-impact activities: Abdominal crunches, isometric exercises (like leg lifts) without added resistance.

Best workouts for back and tricky joints

Aerobic exercise often helps make achy backs and joint feel better because it increases blood flow and relaxes tense muscles. If you are suffering from a bad back, no one but your doctor can tell you exactly which workouts to do (or not), or how soon to start them after a serious problem. Still, there are some basic and helpful guidelines:

1. *Avoid impact*: That means running, high impact aerobic dance, even too fast walking, anything that causes you to pound.
2. *Avoid fast, twisting motions*: These almost inevitably stress your back. This can mean some moves in aerobic dance or bench stepping classes.
3. *Watch your form*: Don't arch your back when you are dancing, running, weight lifting or doing anything except an exercise specifically for the back. (In fact, regular exercises to keep the back strong and flexible are a good idea.
4. *Keep weight down*: Excess pounds put pressure on back and knees.

So what should you do? Smartest choices are moderate walking or swimming.

The following back-specific exercises are time tested:

1. *Pelvic tilt*: Lie on the floor with knees raised and arms extended. Press lower back down against the floor by tightening the abdominal muscles, squeezing the buttocks and rolling the top of the pelvis backward. Hold for a few seconds and repeat.
2. *Partial curl (or crunch)*: Lie on your back with knees bent. Extend hands between thighs. Slowly curl upper torso until shoulder blades leave the floor. Hold a few seconds; go down and repeat. Exhale as you rise.
3. *Advanced curl*: Lie on your back, knees bent, fingers lightly touching ears. Slowly curl upper torso until shoulders leave the floor. Hold a few seconds, inhale as you go back down.
4. *Twist curl*: Lie on the floor, knees bent. Fold arms across chest. Slowly curl right shoulder off the floor toward the left knee until left shoulder leaves floor. Hold for a few seconds, breathing deeply. Repeat, but with left shoulder toward right knee.

Two easy leg exercises are enough to help you become steadier on your feet. All you need is a pair of strap on ankle weights available in most sporting goods stores. A report on nine elderly, frail men and women who did knee extension exercises for eight weeks, using a simple cable and pulley weight machine, say. They more than doubled their leg strength, and their walking speed and balance improved by almost 50 percent. The movements used in this study can be done at home, using ankle weights, anywhere from one to five pounds, and add weight as your exercise one leg at a time. Each repetition should take six seconds—three going up and three going down.

For leg extension: Sit on a sturdy, hard backed chair and slide back so that edge of the chair fits into the crook of your knee. Straighten your leg until it is parallel to the floor. Do 10 repetitions for each leg.

Hip Extension: Stand upright while holding on to the back of a chair with one hand. Lift the opposite leg slowly backward and upward from the hip as far as possible, keeping the knee straight. Do 10 repetitions for each leg.

(iii) Brain

The active lifestyle does as much for the brain, as it does for the heart. Regular exercise improves blood flow to the brain, checking the risk of stroke and some kinds of dementia. How important it is to exercise in avoiding strokes and neurological deterioration? Walking, tennis, swimming, golf, gardening or any other daily exercise is a good idea at my age: to fine tune your brain and mind both. It seems the entire nervous system, from taste buds right upto a taste for intellectual pleasures, does better when we exercise. That's something inspiring indeed.

(iv) Stress

The most effective place to intervene is at the physical level. Learning effective coping skills, can make the physiological reaction of the system less intense and more automatic. While meditation may be good supplement to beat the stress you have to indulge in vigorous exercises. Get tough in body to beat the stress.

5. Perfect posture: The yoga way

The traditional Indian exercises grouped under yoga, have been considered useful to maintenance and promotion of health. Yoga requires little in the way of apparatus. A thin mat, a small wool blanket, some pillow perhaps. It demands no special clothing or spectacular time allotments. It does not dictate we join a crowded gym or hire a costly personal trainer. It can be practiced in a space as small as a foyer in as little time as it takes to wash and dry our hair. And yet it is a complete workout, one that balances every part of us, incorporating the muscles, bones and breath in a symphony of movements that frees the body from stress and fatigue. Numerous studies show that yoga strengthens the spine and boosts lymphatic activity which is at the core of our immunity system.

The asanas, fall under five basic types—standing, inversions, back-bends, forward bends, twists plus the meditational postures.

(a) Standing postures

These strengthening postures are the most demanding.

The Triangle (Utthica Trikonasana)

Strengthens and stretches the legs, waist and buttocks. If you wish, stand against a wall, feet set wide apart, for alignment. Left foot points left, right foot slightly left. Inhale and raise your arms. Exhaling, bend left, contracting the buttocks and outer thighs. Stretch the left arm to grasp your toes, or as far down as you can, while raising the right arm, palm out. Imagine a straight line from your right wrist across your heart to your left wrist. Look up, feeling the stretch across the pelvis. Breathe slowly for upto 30 seconds. Come up slowly on the inhale, and repeat on the other side.

(b) Inversions

These send blood to the brain, increasing circulation.

The shoulder stand/plough (Halasana). It flexes the spine; strengthens, neck and arms.

(a) Sitting, feet on the floor, back straight, tighten your abdominals and raise your arms above your head, palms in. Slowly roll back, until you are lying on your back.
(b) Inhale as you push down on the floor, and bring your legs straight up into the air, lifting your hips. Exhale and move your hands to support your back. Elbows are securely braced on the floor, as close together as possible. Try to make your legs vertical and spine straight. Your chin is pressed into the base of your throat. Breathe deeply, and work your elbows close together and hands nearer your shoulder blades, maintaining balance. (It is your shoulders, not your neck, bearing your weight).
(c) Exhale, and slowly let your feet fall behind your head towards the floor, using your abdominals as your body folds backward, lace your fingers, arms on the floor behind your back if you can. Chin is pressed to the chest. This is the Plough.
(d) Breathe, and come back into the shoulder stand, one leg at a time, Roll down.

(c) Backward-bending postures

This asana is said to exhilarate by opening the chest, heart and lungs.

The bridge (Sethubundasana): Flexes the spine; strengthens the abdominals and lower back muscles. Lying down with your knees bent, raise your hips and back, keeping feet flat on the floor, while arching your back. If you have back problems, lift your back only as far of the floor, as you comfortably can. Lace your fingers together. Take several deep breaths. Keep your chest lifted and, if possible, walk your legs out as far as you can with your feet flat on the floor. Hold the pose for several deep breaths, then walk your feet back in toward the body. Inhale, and lower your hips to the floor. Always be mindful of the breath.

(d) Forward bending postures

These postures are said to energize the body. The forward bend (Paschimottanasana). Lengthens calf, hamstring and back muscles; tones the abdomen. Sit back lengthened, legs extended and arms outstretched above your head, fingers open. A. Exhale and bend forward at the waist, reaching out with your hands and chest, chin towards your shins. B. Inhale and grasp whatever part of your legs you can without bending your knees or curling your back. Feel the stretch in your spine and legs. Breathe deeply.

(e) Twists

Twisting postures are thought to cleanse the body.

Half spinal twist (Ardha Matsyendrasana): It strengthens and stretches the back. From a sealed position with your legs extended in front of you, bend your left knee and bring your left foot to the inside of your right thigh. Inhale as you lift up through the spinal column. Exhale into the twist as you rotate your trunk to the left. Balance yourself by placing your left hand on the floor behind you. Wrap your right arm around your left knee so your hand is against your outer left thigh. With your next exhale, twist farther to the left, looking over your left shoulder. Keep your spine straight but relaxed. Breathe and hold for 20 to 30 seconds, switch legs and repeat the sequence, twisting to the right (Modified from *Health and Nutrition*, August, 2001).

6. Let exercise make their arteries elastic

Exercises not only loosen the muscles and clear the mind—it also makes the arteries more stretchy and less prone to hardening. Most people don't understand that arterial stiffness is something distinct from the building up of plaque in the arteries. The building up of plaque clearly is related to cholesterol and other lipids (fats) in the blood. But the people who report the most activity have the stretchiest arteries. This is confirmed by some hard scientific measures—waist circumference, blood glucose levels and resting heart rate. People with bigger waists tend to be overweight and have more heart disease, as do people with higher glucose levels, which can progress to diabetes. And the higher someone's resting heart rate, usually, the worse physical shape he or she is in and again, the higher the risk of heart disease. Although heart rate goes up temporarily during activity, people who are frequently active have a lower overall heart rate. Athletes have the lowest heart rates of all. And exercise lowers glucose levels. Glucose, or blood sugar, can chemically interact with the walls of the blood vessels, damaging them and causing them to stiffen. This also explains why slender people can have heart disease, if they have sedentary habits and end up with diabetes and stiff arteries.

7. Exercise can enhance sex life

If the promise of better health, a trimmer physique, smart look and a longer life haven't been enough to convince you to exercise regularly now hold your breath. More you exercise, the more sex you will have and the better it will be.

How does the exercise work?

(a) Exercise produces a higher level of endorphins, natural pain relievers believed to produce the runner's high—a feeling of well-being that can extend to sexual desire.

(b) At the sensual level, exercise is a way of heightening basic body awareness that can spill over into the bed room.

(c) Men can look forward to better erections. One of the effects of exercise is to improve circulation—including enlarging the smaller vessels that distribute blood to the peripheral organs. If you increase the flow, the penile balloon fills faster and more completely

(d) In the long-term you will look better and you will feel better about yourself. As you loose fat and gain muscle, your cloths will fit better and your wardrobe including your lingerie will begin to look more exciting and add to your sex appeal.

To get the most out of the exercise stimulant, work out with your partner as a two some. Intimate relationships may suffer when just one partner exercises. The one who doesn't may feel bad about his or her body image because of not working to improve it. Plus, exercise done at the expense of time spent together isn't going to help your sex life.

8. Lead a high energy life: Avoid fatigue

Who would not like to have more energy and also avoid fatigue? It is easier to enhance your energy than to inflate your bank balance.

(a) Hasya-mudra

Don't start your day rushed and tired. Start your exercise with Hasya-mudra in cheerfull mood and with gusto. This will give you a new enthusiasm and energy to disarm the robbers of health e.g stress of days' work, family problem, job-related challenges, etc. Let the exercise programme be long enough, not tiring and not over straining. This should be the beginning of the day with exercise and not end of exercise programme. Exercise is not for one block time—Do it several times a day—all day long. Get up and move at least every couple of hours.

(b) All day activity

Besides exercising as a all day activity, breathe deeply when you are free or in stress and feel each breath going in and going out. It is relaxing and energizing

(c) Direct your strong emotions

Don't fall prey to strong emotions like anger; redirect them to your advantage, work harder, take more exercise to rid the ill effects. So no to unwelcome situations, persons, commitments.

(d) Let not be your life colourless

Nobody like darkness, have variety and colours around you in physical sense, e.g. red, green, purple or any other. Love music, don't over react to any unwanted happening. You are more important, so is your mood. Take a break from the monotony, holidays are important. Avoid exposure to drugs, medicines, nicotine, alcohol, etc.

How Exercise may help?

Muscle fibres, like all the other cells in the human body, run on a molecular fuel called ATP, which the body makes naturally from nutrients in the foods you eat. When we talk about burning calories during exercise, we are really talking about burning ATP.

(a) Oxygen supply

During workout, maintaining supply of oxygen in your body is the main concern. A working muscle burns about 70 times more oxygen during moderate exercise than it does at rest. The first time you can be around the track, your body did its best to increase the oxygen supply. Neuro-chemical signals instructed your heart to beat faster, increased your breathing rate to get more oxygen into blood stream and dilated your arteries and capillaries to get the oxygen rich blood to your muscles faster. Even so, your heart was unprepared for the new demands. By the end of the run, you were gasping for breath to try to correct the oxygen imbalance, and your legs were tired because lactic acid, which is the residue of a chemical reaction that has too little oxygen, had built up in your muscles. While you continued diligently sticking to your exercise schedule, your body has been steadily upgrading its infrastructure. Some of the biggest changes have taken place inside the individual muscle fibres you have been exercising. Studies indicate that regular aerobic exercise may increase levels of a muscle compound called myoglobin, which helps speed the transfer of oxygen from the blood stream into the muscle fibre. Increase in blood flow and enzyme activity also improve the muscle fibres ability to oxidize fats and carbohydrates carried in the blood, especially fats. That's one reason exercise is so effective for losing weight.

(b) Heart beats forcefully

Most important, your blood supply system has been responding to the increased demand for oxygen. Because your heart beats more forcefully during workouts, it has become stronger and slightly larger—reflecting changes in its muscle fibres and blood flow. The result is that your heart is pumping significantly more blood with each stroke than it did before you started training. Other improvements also occur in the cardiovascular system. The number of capillaries, the tiny vessels that feed blood to the muscle fibres, tends to increase with endurance training, and because the muscles use the blood more effectively, they no longer need to draw it away from organs like the skin, liver and kidneys during strenuous workouts.

Interestingly, the long muscles get more efficient from exercise, allowing you to breathe more deeply and less frequently. Another change you may see is in your body composition. Aerobic exercise encourages fat loss if you are overweight. The result is that you retain muscles mass as you are dieting. The ratio of good HDL to bad LDL cholesterol also improves with aerobic endurance, a major reason, alongwith improved circulation. That is why exercise helps ward off heart disease.

(c) Playing Tennis

What about exercises that involve short, intense bursts of strength, such as lifting weights or sprinting or playing squash or tennis with their quick start and stop action? In these activities, your primary fule comes from your muscles energy reserves. CP and glycogen. The supply is replenished during rest breaks through the process of producing fuel by combining nutrients with oxygen in the muscle. This sudden increase in demand for oxygen is why you will be short of breath playing squash or basketball but you won't during a five mile run.

(d) Muscle strength

To increase the strength of a muscle instead of its endurance, you need to train it to use these short-term energy supplies more effectively. This means you have got to try to exhaust the muscle in less than 90 seconds; any longer than that and the muscle fibres aerobic ATP supply will start kicking in. Examples of an aerobic training include 100 yard wind sprints, a fast lap in the pool and lifting a heavy weight eight to 12 times. If you do this kind of training twice a week for three months, the appropriate muscle fibres will start to generate more power with each contraction. The working muscles become stronger. In reality, every muscle fibres relies on aerobic and anaerobic energy sources at the same time during any one exercise; it's just the proportion that changes, depending on the intensity of the effort. Likewise, many activities require a blend of aerobic conditioning and quick muscle strength movements. Even a distance runner can benefit from some strong contractions at the end of the race, and a power tennis player needs some aerobic endurance to keep it at for an hour or two.

Smoking, drugs and alcohol

There is little doubt about the devastating effects of smoking and other intoxicants on health. The World Health Organisation (WHO) estimates that on a global scale, smoking claims three million lives annually. Besides an increased risk of cancer and heart disease, smokers suffer more frequently from colds, gastric ulcers, chronic bronchitis, and higher blood pressure than non-smokers.

Drug abuse, of course, is becoming a common problem in India, like other countries. Every year anywhere from 160,000 to 210,000 people worldwide die from injecting drugs. In addition, millions use other types of harmful drugs, such as khat (a green-leaflet stimulant), betal-nut and cocaine. While hard drugs like cocaine and heroin capture public attention, the abuse of alcohol inflicts even greater damage in volume terms. Besides severe damage to liver and consequent fatal outcome at prime of age, alcoholics contributes immensely to indirect causes of death and disability. While Indian figures are not available, it is estimated that in United States, alcohol is contributing factor in 50 percent of fatal automobile accidents and fires, 45 percent of drowning, and 36 percent of pedestrian accidents. Alcohol abuse is also implicated in many violent crimes. Those committing murder, assault, rape, child abuse, or suicide often have alcohol as a silent partner.

Obesity as a curse

Obesity shortens a large number of lives, afflicting its victims with diabetes, hypertension, heart disease, and certain types of cancer. More than a third of adults and more than 20 percent of children and youths in this country are significantly overweight. And the situation is getting steadily worse. The situation calls upon us to adopt a low fat, low-sugar, vegetarian food with more fruits and vegetables, and to exercise more. True and lasting weight loss means a permanent change of lifestyle. Low fat, low sugar, high fiber diet is not a temporary measure to be discarded when body weight reaches the desired level. It is a permanent new way of eating and must be coupled with exercise. The care and planning against the hazards of obesity has to start in early childhood and continue through youth and middle age to old age. The concept that children must eat voraciously and put on weight, giving a 'plum or chubby' look need to undergo change. An overweight child is more likely to end an obese adult with consequent health problems. Health studies have repeatedly shown that exercising for 30 minutes, three times a week in concert with a low-fat diet will trim off that deadly cargo; the extra weight and more importantly, strengthen the heart, circulatory system, and respiration. This, in turn, goes a long way towards avoiding the illnesses associated with obesity. All you need to invest is a pair of good walking shoes and a visit to your doctor, who can recommend a diet and exercise plan tailored to your state of health, and then monitor your progress.

Punjabi lifestyle; *Rujj ke Kha and Dubb ke Vah*?

The Tribune dated March, 3, 2002 focused on perils of modern Punjabi lifestyle. It was observed that favorite pastime of Punjabis is eating. We eat when we are hungry, we eat even when we are not hungry, we dine when we are happy, we hog when we are sad or upset. In short, every time is eating time, come day, come night unlike other living beings, we not only eat more than what we should, we eat what we shouldn't and we eat the way we should not. The digestive system has to struggle hard to deal with the overload that we thrust upon it.

(a) The Death Warrant

What is so delicious for the tongue is a death warrant for the system.

If you are over-weight, you are more likely to develop health problems, such as heart disease, stroke, diabetes, certain types of cancer, gout (joint pain caused by excess uric acid), and gallbladder disease. Being overweight can also cause problems such as sleep apnea (interrupted breathing during sleep) and osteoarthritis (wearing away of the joints). The more over weight you are, the more likely you are to have health problems.

(b) Food-cum-obesity epidemic

Punjab is particularly caught in this obesity epidemic. In the good olden days Punjab advocated *Rujj Ke Kha* (eat to your satisfaction), and *Dabb Ke Vah* (Plough your fields with the gratest effort and vigour). Modern Punjabi youth has metamorphosed to his own disadvantage. He uses a vehicle to travel even a small distance, may be to flaunt his status, he does not plough his fields (which has become mechanized anyway), and he does not put in labor of any kind. He does not allow even a drop of sweat to flow, enjoying the comfort of chill of A.C. Mostly unemployed, after getting a primary or secondary education, he leans to drugs and alcohol, besides generous intake of chicken, mutton and paranthas with Masala.

(c) Hobby and Past-time

This has become his hobby, as well as past time. This has also become his way of socializing and showing off his father's prosperity. Living in the stress of longings for easy and unearned money his good senses have been overtaken by lust and greed for food, besides three 'Ws' (wine, woman, wealth). He takes comfort in the pleasures of palate but allows his bones, muscles and vital systems to rust in limbo, with the potential of suffering discomforts unlimited. Lack of exercise, overeating, excessive intake of fats and salts with stressful lifestyle, laden with smoking and other toxic elements presents lethal combination. Food addiction starts early in life and is made worse by lack of exercise and constant stress. Keeping up with friends makes every school or college student go in for junk food. Hogging on junk food regularly makes one's body a junkyard.

(d) Few engage in any physical activity

Barely one out of four young persons participates in light to moderate activity (e.g. walking, cycling, etc.) on a daily basis. Even fewer engage in vigorous physical activity, while the vast majority shuns exercise like the plague. The only exercise most get is while moving their hands from the plate to the palate. Mahatma Gandhi had warned about the perils of pleasure of the palate without hard work many years ago.

(e) Can Obesity be reversed?

The obesity epidemic is already beyond controllable limits, yet not many are concerned about it. Most victims are convinced that they are not really fat, a bit plump may be. Nobody sees the co-relation between wrong food habits and several serious diseases. What we eat, how we respond to stress, whether we smoke, how much we exercise, and how well our social relationships support us can make powerful differences in our health and well-being, even to our survival. A series of scientific studies conducted during the past 25 years demonstrated that the progression of even severe coronary heart disease can be stopped or reversed by making comprehensive changes in one's diet and lifestyle. These include adopting a low-fat, plant-based, whole foods diet, stress management techniques (including yoga and meditation), moderate exercise; smoking cessation, and psychological group support.

(f) High cholesterol

High blood cholesterol level is the single greatest risk factor for heart disease and the single most important factor in raising blood cholesterol level is the consumption of saturated fat (Meat, Desi Ghee, hydrogenated oils, egg, etc.). Weight loss can help improve the harmful effects of being overweight. However, many overweight people have difficulty reaching anywhere near their healthy body weight. Studies show that you can improve your health by losing as little as 5 to 10 kg. A senior doctor lamented that whenever he told his well heeled patients that all their problems were because of unhealthy lifestyle, they simply shifted to other specialists.

(g) Cranky Elders

Every youth lectured on this topic thinks that his elders are becoming cranky. By the time he is mature enough to take heed, it is too late. As George Bernard Shaw had rightly said, "Youth is a wonderful thing; it is a shame to waste it on young people." Rich greasy, non-vegetarian foods that we have come to prefer, require (for production) excessive use of pesticides, insecticides, antibiotics and other chemicals and misuse of land, i.e. water and air resources (it takes 23 gallons of water to produce one pound of potatoes but 1,630 gallons of water to produce one pound of pork); untold cruelty to animals; outbreak of diseases like Mad-Cow, and proliferation of unsafe, genetically engineered crops. There are millions of human beings in less developed countries, who are going hungry while their land, labor, and resources are being used to feed livestock so that wealthy people can eat meat. The consequences of this is obviously malnutrition to both segments of people, i.e. one segment dying of starvation related deaths and other due to being overfed.

Obesity as a mother of serious diseases

Obesity is a major risk factor for the development of diabetes, hypertension and cardiovascular diseases. In a recent study, it was found in Haryana that urban population had greater obesity and greater girth of waist and a higher rate of coronary heart disease. Haryana is becoming a California of India in this regard. The rate of heart disease is much lower in Japan and China, because the incidence of obesity is much lower in these countries. Also the fatal heart disease is coming to Indians at a much younger age. The prevention will include prevention of obesity, in addition to a regimen of no smoking and 'regular exercises' The prevention of obesity should begin in childhood.

A newer more useful measure of overweight is the so-called Body Mass Index (BMI). The BMI is obtained by dividing the weight in kilograms by height measured in meters and then squared (W/H^2). The lowest morbidity and mortality, for both sexes occur in persons with a BMI of 22-25 kg/m^2. Mortality rate begin to substantially rise at weights 20% greater than desirable, this corresponds to a BMI of 27 kg/m^2. Individuals with a BMI of 30 kg/m^2 or greater have clearly increased mortality. However if the higher weight is due to developed muscles and not due to fat deposit in the body, the harmful effects will not occur. Those with higher than desirable weight will suffer from killer diseases like coronary heart disease, stroke, diabetes, cancers and increase in gall bladder disease. In men aged 15 to 39 years, whose relative body weight when initially measured is 125% to 135% of normal, there is an aggregate mortality of 170% of usual in a 15-22 year follow up. In men 40% above desirable weight, there is a 55% increase in mortality from all causes, 70% increase from coronary artery disease, 75% increase from stroke, and 400% increased mortality from diabetes.

Malignant obesity is a term now used to define persons 60% above desirable weight; this corresponds to an absolute excess of a minimum of 100 pounds. With this degree of obesity, there is a minimum doubling of the prevalence of all causes of morbidity and mortality. Weight reduction should be recommended for patients with BMIs equal to or above 27. Weight gain in young adult life is a potent risk factor for the later development of hypertension, central or upper body fat being more likely to raise blood pressure than lower body fat in the gluteal or thigh region. It is calculated that, in men, for each 10% increase in body weight there is approximately a 20% increase in the incidence of coronary artery disease. In men, the risk of cardiovascular disease increases sharply when waist/hip ratio (WHR) is above 1.0, and in women above 0.8.

The association of abdominal fat with metabolic abnormalities is additive to the effects of generalised body obesity. The abdominal obesity can increase the risk of diabetes mellitus ten fold. Even mild to moderate obesity should be treated if excess adipose tissue is found mainly in the abdominal region. Overweight men have a significantly higher mortality rate from colorectal and prostate cancer. Men whose weight is 130% or more above average are 2.5 times more likely to die of prostate cancer. Menopausal women with upper body fat localisation have an increased risk of developing breast cancer. Overweight women also have higher rates of cancer of uterus and ovaries. Thus cancer creeps in as the prosperity is the form of obesity is acquired. Obese women, especially those with upper body obesity, show more irregularity in menstrual cycles as well as greater frequency of other menstrual abnormalities than normal weight women.

They also have more problems during pregnancy with an increased frequency of toxemia and hypertension. In obese girls, the onset of menarche occurs at a younger age than in normal weight girls. Menstruation is probably initiated when body weight reaches a critical mass. Obese women in the 20-30 years age range have a six fold increase in the risk of developing gall bladder disease compared to normal-weight women. By age 60, nearly one-third of these women can be expected to have developed gall bladder disease. There are several abnormalities in pulmonary function in obese individuals. High body weight adds trauma to weight bearing joints, which is a major predictor of osteoarthritis of the knee. Weight loss will markedly decrease the chance of developing osteoarthritis and other problems.

The Quality of Life

The obese individual has functional impairment in the activities of daily living. This dysfunction is related to sleep, recreation, work and social interactions. Obese persons have physical incapacity due to back and joint problems and shortness of breath. This contributes to their proneness to fatal accidents. Emotional disturbances are often likely to be a consequence of obesity rather than the cause. In some studies, obese persons were found to be significantly more anxious and depressed than normal weight persons.

What to do?

Prevent obesity in your children and youth. Do not allow them to eat rich food and in excess of need, even if you are rich and affluent. Set a good example yourself, by avoiding excess eating. Do not show your love and affection to your children through food. Encourage them to remain active and slim and let them be small to moderate eaters. Let them not feel proud of overeating or overweight. Encourage them to excel in games and sports and not to let them be passive or lazy-watchers of T.V. or play computer games till late night and then getting up at mid-day, instead of next morning. Bicycle ride is far better for him than using a car to go to school or to a play ground. Let him understand health, through just adequate food and vigorous exercises, leading to sweat on his brow.

While diet control is important, modification of lifestyle, behavior and regular exercises are equally important. Not all cases of severe obesity will respond—hence prevention of obesity is the thrust area. Where obesity has come and is not responding to above mentioned measures, use of medicines in the treatment of obesity becomes imperative by decreasing appetite, impaired energy absorption and enhanced thermogenesis. Sibutramine is the latest effective drug in this category. However the medicine should be used under medical supervision only.

I. Whether or not your weight is Healthy?

Being too thin or too fat is unhealthy, but good health is about much more than just your weight. It depends on many things—including your family history, your genes, whether you smoke, the type of food you eat, and how active you are. It is therefore difficult to set an exact healthy weight that applies to everyone. We are surrounded by images of glamorous people, many of whom are in fact underweight. Looking at yourself in the mirror is not a very useful way to assess whether or not you are a healthy weight.

Doctors check your body size by measuring your weight and height. This calculation is known as the Body Mass Index (BMI). Research has shown that people within a certain range of body size tend to live the longest, and enjoy the best health during their lives.

Another method is to take a tape measure and put it around your waist. For a man, a waist measurement greater than 94 cm (37 inches) and, for a woman, greater than 80 cm (32 inches), suggests you should try not to gain any more weight. Try to lose 1-2 inches at the waist. If your BMI or your waist is above the healthy range, you are at increased risk of heart disease and diabetes. You are also more likely to suffer from joint problems and back pain. You may find you become breathless and may have difficulty sleeping.

2. Medical problems

In the foregoing chapters, we have repeatedly mentioned a number of medical problems, which overweight brings with it. The more weight you gain, the more severe these problems may become. The good news is that losing weight will alleviate many of these conditions. Your health can also suffer if you weigh too little. Some people are constitutionally lighter than others and may be fit and well. But if you have recently lost weight unintentionally you should consult your doctor to check, if there is no underlying problem. Other people who voluntarily restrict their food in order to lose weight may also find they have reached a stage of underweight. This may be an indication of an eating disorder and should also consult your doctor. Being underweight is unhealthy. You may develop a number of nutritional deficiencies. Young women especially are at risk of anaemia and insufficient calcium may lay the foundation for osteoporosis later in life. Amenhorrhoea (missing menstrual periods) is common, and leads to infertility.

3. What causes overweight?

Some people have a tendency to gain weight easily, whereas others seem to stay the same weight for many years without any effort. These differences may be due to genetic factors. People who tend to choose foods, which are high in fat or which contain a lot of energy (calories) in just a small portion are more likely to gain weight than people who tend to fill their plates with bulky, low energy foods such as bread, potatoes and vegetables. Eating too much fat can also increase your risk of heart disease. Many people find themselves turning to food when they are tired, bored or emotional. Using food as a quick 'pick-me-up' even when we are not really hungry can often lead to a weight problem. At difficult times try to find ways other than food, of improving your mood. Phoning a friend, taking a short walk or tackling an outstanding chore can all be useful distractions from food.

People who lead an active life are much less likely to gain weight than those who spend most of their day sitting down in front of a computer or TV, or in the car. Regular exercise can help to control your weight and improves fitness too, reducing your risk of heart disease and diabetes. Obesity does not develop overnight. It takes around 3500 excess calories to gain just 0.5 kg(about 1 lb). Few people gain more than one or two kilograms each year. Weight fluctuates from day to day, but you should aim to stay about the same weight from week to week. If you notice a consistent increase in your weight, you should try to stabilize your weight before it develops into a serious weight problem. Begin by reducing the amount of fat in your diet and incorporate 20-30 minutes of activity into your day.

4. Losing Weight

Losing weight is about reducing the number of calories you eat to less than the calories you burn off in your everyday life. Try to make small but permanent changes in your lifestyle, rather than opting for a dramatic new diet. You may lose weight more slowly—but you will reduce the changes of regaining weight later. Most 'diets' do help you to lose weight, by reducing the number of foods you are allowed to eat, or by making eating very complicated. This helps to cut the number of calories you consume. But they are hard to stick to in the long-term and when the novelty wears off most people find themselves moving onto the next 'wonder diet'. Some diets, especially those which exclude some of the major food groups, e.g. dairy products, may not provide all the nutrients your body needs. You may lose weight, but your general health may also suffer.

Use the following guide to help plan your own personal eating plan to lose weight:

(i) Plan three meals a day. Skipping breakfast does not help you to loose weight because you are more likely to snack during the morning.

(ii) If you are a confirmed snacker, plan your snacks in advance and reduce the amount you eat at meal times accordingly. Save dessert as a snack for later or ensure you have other suitable snacks available. For example, fruit, low fat yogurt, or a slice of toast with a thin scrapping of low fat spread.

(iii) At each meal aim to fill about half your plate with vegetables, one quarter with bread, potatoes, pasta, rice or other starchy foods and the remaining quarter with lean meat, fish or poultry.

(iv) Choose low fat foods wherever possible. For example, skimmed or semi=skimmed milk, low fat spreads, extra lean meat, tomato-based rather than creamy pasta sauces, and salad dressings such as lemon juice or vinegar instead of mayonnaise.

(v) Bake, steam or grill rather than frying or sauteeing.

(vi) Dont add extra fat during cooking or when serving food. Indian practice of pouring spoons of Desi Ghee on your Dal, Sabzi or Kheer while serving, as a matter of additional love or respect to the guest, to win his favour is avoidable. It adds to your calories, unmistakably. For example, cook onions in stock rather than frying in fat for stews, use yogurt or low fat cheese with baked potatoes instead of butter, use jam or marmalade instead of butter on toast, and avoid buttering vegetables.

(vii) Eat high fat/high sugar calorie-rich foods only very occasionally and in small portions.

(viii) Watch out for products labeled as 'low fat' but which are still packed with calories—especially cakes, biscuits and desserts.

(ix) Drink alcohol in strict moderation, aiming for no more than one unit per day. Alcohol is high in calories and after a few drinks most people find it very hard to stick to their eating plan.

(x) If you are not losing weight, stick with the same types of food but choose smaller portions.

Most doctors recommend that on average, you should aim to lose no more than 1 kg (2 lbs) per week. Some weeks you may lose more weights than others.

As long as your weight is continuing to decrease overall, there is no need to worry. If your weight stays the same for a week or two, don't abandon all that you have achieved; instead, focus again on the amount and type of foods you are eating and try to be a little more active. Losing 5% of your initial body weight in 3 months, or 10% in 6-12 months, is an excellent start.

5. Weight maintenance

For most people, weight maintenance is a greater challenge than losing weight. Research shows that regular exercise is one of the most effective ways to keep the weight off.

A few tips:

(i) Cut down the amount of time you spend watching television.

(ii) Get out of your chair whenever you can at home and at work. Stand up whilst on the telephone, hid the remote controls for the TV and hi-fi.

(iii) Seek out rather than avoiding the opportunity to be active during your day. Use the upstairs bathroom, park the car at the edge of the car park rather than at the supermarket door, walk to the local postbox/news-agent, etc.

(iv) Use household chores as an exercise class. Turn on some music and tackle the work with vigour.

(v) Plan a 20-30 minute period of specific activity on most days of the week; for example, walking, swimming, or gardening.

(vi) Encourage the whole family to be active by making a part of your social activities. Take a family trip to the park or swimming baths instead of the cinema, play badminton or go dancing with friends rather than a night in the pub.

(vii) Take part in a specific sporting activity. Consider resuming a sport you enjoyed at school, learn how to play a sport you enjoy watching or join a local club. Managing your weight is difficult and at times you may feel frustrated and disheartened. It helps if your family and friends support and encourage you. Many people find that attending a commercial weight loss group can be a very effective method to maintain their motivation in the longer-term.

Some major and minor Ailments:

Cancer

While the causes of all cancers aren't fully understood, the key to surviving almost any type is to catch it early, before it can spread throughout the body. Breast, colon, prostate and testicular cancer, for example, are easily detected by examination and tests and are highly treatable in the initial stage. Lung cancer, on the other hand, is hard to spot early and is among the biggest killers. A cure for lung cancer has not been found, but an almost fool proof preventive technique has: Don't smoke cigarettes. A few news items and tips are given below:

(i) The world's most promising anti-cancer drug, Taxol, is now barely a few steps away from commercial production. Derived from the bark of yew trees, Taxol works by interfering with cells' ability to replicate themselves—in turn, halting the spread of malignant growths. In several trials so far, the drug has caused tumours to shrink in about 30 percent of women with incurable ovarian cancer, and in some 60 percent of women with breast cancer. Doctors are also testing it inpatients with lung cancer and leukemia.

(ii) Special fats fight Cancer ! A recent study in France adds to the evidence that omega-6 polyunsaturated fats (vegetable oils) may have anti-viral powers that can fight some types of cancers. Mice were injected with a virus that causes lymphoma, a form of cancer that is usually fatal. Then they were fed diets rich in fatty acids—either omega-3 (eicosapentaenoic acid, from fish oil) or omega-6 (linoleic acid, from safflower oil). The fish oil fed mice died very quickly but most of the mice who got the safflower oil were still alive at the end of the study. The researchers speculate that omega-6 fats could be used to bolster the effects of drugs that fight lymphoma. Those medicines have toxic side effects, but adding safflower oil could allow doctors to lower the dosage they use.

(iii) A protein may battle the crab. Havard Medical School researchers have found that Interleukin-4, one of the immune system's helper proteins, may battle cancer by stimulating white blood cells known as eosinophils. These cells also help cause allergic reactions, but if those side effects can be controlled, doctors could use interleukin-4 to treat a wide range of cancers, including breast, lung, brain and lymphoma.

Cancer has always sounded as a warrant of death for the patient. It has been viewed as inevitable, incurable, and unpreventable and may be proverbial—Divine death sentence. However not long ago it was stated by American Cancer Institute that 1/3 of all cancers are related to our food and another 30% result due to smoking of tobacco. The inference is clear—cancer is not inevitable and that it is preventable to a great extent..

1. Food

If we eat carefully (and quit smoking), we can fight/prevent some cancers. Improvement in hygiene and restraining our sexual habits may further prevent some percentage of cancer. What does it mean? Cancer can be prevented to a great extent. Our concern here is about the food we eat and occurrence or prevention of cancer. The culprits again are fats and meats and the savious are vegetable juices, vegetables, fruits, grains, etc.

2. Exercises

Similarly, exercise is good for health, since it makes you fit, reduces your obesity and enhances your immune response. Hence it can help in preventing cancer as well as to fight the miseries of cancer to some extent. So bank on healthful food and fitness exercise to beat the cancer. Let not the deadly cargo, overload you.

3. Fats

It is widely believed that all fats saturated and unsaturated are involved in the growth of certain kinds of cancer cells. In the United States where high fat diet is consumed, colorectal cancer is the second most common cancer. According to the American Cancer Society, groups of people who relocate to a country with high incidences of cancer eventually develop the cancer rate of that land, depending on the length of time it takes for them to switch to the new lifestyle and diet. "Japanes immigrants are developing a Western cancer pattern: high for colon and breast cancer, low for stomach cancer—the reverse of the Japanese pattern." Evidently, cancer is linked to diet and not to race or genes or environment of the country of origin.

If your diet is high in total fat, saturated fat, cholesterol and calories, you need to reduce them drastically. A good diet can lead to good health and can even reverse many ill effects of a bad diet. In view of such options as painful cancer surgery or byepass surgery, which often costs heavily, this is surely desirable. By sensibly choosing what you eat, you can lose weight, improve how you feel, and help yourself avoid or reverse some diseases. A total fat intake of no more than 20 percent of daily calories and reducing saturated fat to less than 10 percent of calories is recommended. A 1-percent decrease in caloric intake of saturated fats ordinarily leads to a drop of 3 milligrams per deciliter in the blood-cholesterol level..

4. Fibre diet

Populations that eat fibre-rich diets suffer less cancer. That's the reason why nutritionists recommend a fibre intake of 20 to 30 grams a day. The insoluble fibre—the indigestible stalks and peels of fruits and vegetables and husks of whole grains, called roughage, bulk up stool and speeds it through the colon. It is said that cancer-causing agents are swept quickly away with the stool. And it is also the bulking action of insoluble fibre that may also help relieve constipation, hemorrhoids and diverticular disease. If your fibre intake is low, build it up gradually. Start by adding only a few extra grams of fibre per week. Drink plenty of water, since fibre soaks up fluids. Also limit the intake to 35 grams of fibre a day. Too much fibre may interfere with nutrient absorption and cause intestinal upset.

The chart below shows the amount of fibre, you can get from a particular food items:

Item	*Service size*	*Dietary fibre (Grams)*
Fruit		
Figs, dried	5 fruits	8.7
Pear	1 large	6.2
Dates	5 fruit	3.2
Orange	1 fruit	3.1
Raspberries	½ cup	3.1
Prunes	5 fruit	3.0
Apple, with skin	1 fruit	3.0
Strawberries	¾ cup	2.9
Apricots,dried	10 halves	2.7
Raisins	¼ cups	1.9
Banana	1 fruit	1.8
Plums	3 small	1.8
Apricots	2 fruit	1.5
Cherry**	100 gms	1.24
Peaches	100 gms	2.28

**Skin included in edible portion

5. Haldi

Turmeric plays an important role in our food since ancient times. It is used as aromatic flavour to various dishes, as flavour colouring agent, digestive properties, condiment, dye, drug, cosmetic, wool silk, textile and oil industries. It is a rich source of vitamin ABC and Niacin which is also used in food preparations. It is used as stomach tonic and as a blood purifier. Its efficacy in asthma is documented. It is also used in cosmetics, in making perfumes. Turmeric contains oleoresins such as volatile oils, non-volatile fatty acids and curcuminoids. The advantages of plant based dietary interventions in combating certain chronic diseases like diabetes, cancer is well known. The benefits are: 1. Turmeric is an inhibitor of the process of carcinogenesis; 2. Curcumin are potent antimutagens which can probably used to prevent neoplasia; 3. It has a role in dietary fibre as non-starch polysaccharides (NSP), consists of complex polysaccharides such as cellulose and lignins with different chemicals; 4. It is used in prevention of diseases such as cancer, diabetes, cardiovascular diseases and elephantiasis, etc.; 5. Warm milk with pinch of turmeric powder can control cold and asthma; 6. It is good for skin disease and has got an antiseptic properties. Also using 5 grams a day with jaggery balls at the time of menstruation period (MC) or after delivery period is a good generator and blood purifier. Take Haldi regularly.

6. Vitamin E may prevent prostate cancer

Nutritional supplements such as Vitamin E may be able to stop prostate cancer before it starts, according to health researchers. The point to a major new trial involving 3,00,000 men to study the potential of Vitamin E and also of a mineral selenium, to help prevent onset of prostate cancer, which strikes about one in six men during their lifetimes. One professor of clinical cancer prevention in Texas said the new trial is 'tremendously significant'.

The Wall Street Journal recently reported on the trial citing "compelling evidence" that nutritional supplements including Vitamin E may be able to "stop prostate cancer before it starts."

7. Pleasurable floods

Most cancers excluding those from heredity or environmental hazards- are preventable. To start with, quit smoking, start exercising and reduce your fat and alcohol intake. Then quit worrying and arm yourself with these tips that experts have come up with to fight cancer, i.e. eat pleasurable foods and prevent cancer.

(a) Fruits: Lower your risk 50 percent

Next time you bring a big sack of fruits and vegetables (the more colours the better), resist the urge to run to the sink and start splashing them around. Cut and wash fruits and vegetables just before cooking or eating them. That keeps vitamin levels at their max imam. And don't cut them into tiny pieces. The more surface area exposed to oxygen, the faster vitamins lose their potency. Vitamins are important because they are excellent cancer fighters, but popping a multivitamin won't do the trick, say researchers. It is the fibre, roughage and protective chemicals in fruits and vegetables that rid your body of carcinogens. According to a study of more than 2,000 Welsh men, those who ate the most fruit had half the risk of dying from cancer.

(b) Water: Drink more

In a study, who drank more than four glasses of water daily had a 32 percent lower risk of colon cancer. It is just one more reason to drink up. And don't wait until you are thirsty.

(c) Tomato: Pour the ketchup

A Havard study of 48,000 men showed that those who consumed the most lycopene, a powerful antioxidant abundant in tomato products, had a 21 percent lower risk of prostate cancer and those who had two to 4 servings reduced their risk by 34 percent.

(d) Onion

Onion, best known for their antibacterial (and aromatic) properties also contain strong class of anti cancer compounds. These tough guys seem to activate enzymes that neutralize cancer causing substances.

(e) Exercise: Maintain perfect form

You already know that exercise is the best way to improve your life. In a study on the same, those who exercised the most cut their risk of colon cancer in half. Not only does exercise boost your immune system, but it may also speed food through the colon, so there is less contact between carcinogens and your gut. The same study found that men who gained 18-20 kgs since age 21 had nearly double the risk of colon cancer. Shed your "deadly cargo" through regular exercises.

(f) Plenty of "Ghas Phoos" (vegetarian)

Eat brassica vegetable, including broccoli, cabbage, Brussels sprous, khol-khol, turnip greens, mustard greens and cauliflower. Subjects who consumed the most brassicas had a 40 percent lower risk of cancers.

These vegetables, which were used for medicinal purposes in ancient times (also for torturing ancient youths at supper time), contain sulforphane, which may be the most powerful anti-cancer compound of all. Sulforaphane seems to boost natural defenses and lower cancer risk.

(g) Victory over stress

One theory is that feeling helpless lowers immune response. As soon as stress hits, do whatever puts you in a good frame of mind. If you can't think of anything, go for a walk.

(h) Soya lowers your risk

Soya products contain phytoestrogens which may ward off prostate and breast cancer.

(i) Avoid alcohol and smoking

Be moderate, if you must. Plenty of green black tea is advised to prevent cancer. No place for smoking at all.

(j) Mix up your whole grain flour cereals.

Those who ate the most fibre had half the risk of colorectal cancer and that an additional 13 grams of fibre a daycould reduce colorectal cancer risk by 31 percent. For the most benefit, mix and match wheat bran and oat bran, the best fibre source of all. Variety is key

(k) Aspirin: Can it reduce your risk?

Preliminary studies suggest that aspirin may reduce the risk of colorectal cancer by 60 percent and oesophagal cancer by 90 percent. However, aspirin can cause internal bleeding in some people. But if you are already taking it for heart disease, you will get the added benefit.

(l) I am sorry

With the diagnosis of cancer, the patient is condemned with the words "I am sorry." In fact he needs much more information and guidance about his ailment and continuous counseling on the ways, he can live comfortably as long as possible, saying "I am sorry" doesn't help.

(a) More and more cancer

Every year around 800,000 Indians are told that they have contracted the disease. One in nine of us will have cancer at some time in our lives. More and more of us will be living with cancer. Thanks to better screening, more effective drugs and improved surgical procedures, more men, women and children are surviving cancer, or atleast having their cancer controlled and lifespan extended by several years. Today a third of all cancer patients are cured. If the cancers are detected early enough, the figure could rise to two out of three. Most cancer patients would like to be told about the possible side effects of treatment and their chances of surviving. However, many doctors have very heavy workloads and may not be able to spend as much time as they would like to, with their patients.

Cancer support groups urge doctors to be more responsive to their patients' needs. The disclosure should be done in privacy and that doctors should allow time for the grim facts to sink in. "They should have all test results ready before they break the news to the patient and use only terms that the patient can readily understand.

(b) What questions arise?

- What are the treatment options?
- Where, and by whom, will treatment be carried out?
- What are the side effects of the treatment?
- What are the chances of cancer being cured? If it cannot be cured could you give a rough idea of life expectancy?

(c) Positive outlook

Fear, anger, guilt, resentment, confusion and defeat are just a few of the emotional stops on cancer's roller coaster, which is why many people turn to support groups. Doctors and counselors keep advising patients to have a positive outlook. But when you don't know how long you are going to live or what the quality of your life is going to be like, it can be very difficult to be positive. Don't keep brooding about cancer. Lead as normal a life as you can. Don't ever give up. And think positively—it is very helpful. Gene therapy, immunotherapy, blocker drugs and other developments all promise much more in the war against cancer over the next two decades. Most important of all, improved information is helping destroy myths about a disease that 10 years ago was barely referred by name.

CANCER NEWS

(a) Cancer Gene

London (AP)—Scientists have determined that a spontaneous change in a certain gene is involved in 70 percent of cases of melanoma, the deadliest form of skin cancer, which kills nearly 40,000 people a year worldwide. Experts say the finding might lead to more effective drugs for melanoma, which accounts for just 11 percent of skin cancer, but is hard to treat once it has spread and accounts for almost all deaths from cancer skin.

Cancer is the disease that lends itself best to an analysis of the human genome because all cancers are a disease of DNA, said Mike Stratton, head of the Cancer Genome Project, which aims to identify which of the 30,000 human genes are involved in cancer and how. Maturation can be acquired in two ways: either when DNA is damaged by such toxins as radiation, chemicals or viruses, or when mistakes are made before cell division. Most of the mutations are harmless. However, sometimes a mutation will occur in a particular cell in a key gene and the result will be that the gene will be either switched on or switched off. That cell will then start to behave abnormally. It will divide when it should stop dividing. It will move out of its usual position in a tissue and may even float off into the bloodstream and deposit in another organ. That is how cancer evolves. Experts estimate, it takes about 25 years from the first gene mutation for a tumour to appear in an adult. Meltzer, who was not involved with the research, said the melanoma finding raises great hopes that the ambitious cancer genom project will span out. The first abnormality they have found in the gene called B-RAF, which is one of a chain of genes that must all be switched to the "on" position for a cell to grow and divide. Normally, it switches on and off, but the scientists found that the mutation makes the gene stay switched on all the time and ignore prompts to run itself on. The cells with the mutation keep multiplying unchecked, leading to cancer.

The scientists also found that about 10 percent of colon cancers had mutations in the B-RAF gene and less frequently in a variety of other cancer types. Stratton said that because the B-RAF mutation was found in 70 percent of melanoma cases and because the fault in the gene is so specific, it is promising target for a new melanoma drug, which would be designed to switch off the gene only in cells with a mutated version. We are very excited, but we have to temper that with a certain amount of caution. Cancers are devious beasts, they are unpredictable beasts. "They don't always respond in the way we would like them to", Stratton said. We should be optimistic but we should recognize that the path will take several years.

(b) Putting Cancer Risk in Perspective

Hanover, N.H., June 4, 2002 (United Press International via Comtex)-A set of simple risk charts could help people put in perspective their risk of dying from cancer, smoking and other diseases and conditions. Each chart contains a row for age alongwith columns including two types of vascular disease, five types of cancer, three types of infections, accidents and all causes of death combined. To use the chart, an individual simply finds his or her age and then reads across to the condition. The number found there represents the number of women or men per 1000 who are projected to die of that condition in the next 10 years.

In addition to overall risks, the charts points out some strong connections between smoking and other conditions. For example, Woloshin notes smoking increases a number of risk factors. "A smoker who is 40 years old has an all-cause mortality risk of (a non-smoker), who is 50. It's like they are ten years older. Smokers also face a much greater risk of dying of prostate cancer. I think that's pretty dramatic, Woloshin said. The charts appear in the June 5 issue of the Journal of the National Cancer Institute (Reported by Jim Kling, UPI Science News, in Washington).

(c) Nation-wide survey suggests kids ignore sun-safety advice

Chicago—Sun-worshiping kids are still seeking tans—and not using sunscreen—despite warnings about the dangers of skin cancer, a survey of preteens and adolescents found. Only a third of the 10,079 youngsters surveyed said they routinely used sunscreen during the previous summer, and nearly 10 percent said they had used a tanning bed. Most reported having atleast one sunburn during the previous summer, and half with multiple sunburns said it was worth it to get the tan that followed.

Research has shown that severe sunburns in childhood can significantly increase the risk later in life of developing melanoma, the most serious type of skin cancer, while the use of tanning beds has been linked to other skin cancers. Studies have suggested that using sunscreen in childhood could reduce the risk of developing skin cancers other than melanoma in adulthood by as much as 78 percent, the researchers said. More than 1 million Americans are diagnosed each year with skin cancer, and excess sun exposure is the leading cause. With rates rising nationwide, public health messages from the Centers for Disease Control and Prevention and the American Cancer Society have urged sun-protection measures for all ages, including using sunscreen and avoiding tanning beds.

(d) Cancer and childbirth: Mutually Exclusive No Longer

Marybeth Zea of Little Falls, Minn., was only 28, married but childless, when breast cancer struck in 1988. The surgeon who performed her mastectomy told her that because her cancer was not hormone-sensitive, pregnancy would probably not make much difference to her chances of a recurrence. He told her that pregnancy was a personal choice. When Randi Gaier, a 34 year old mother of two preschoolers in Wynnewood, Pa., was treated for Hodgkin's disease 15 years ago, surgeons first moved her ovaries out of the radiation field before administering the radiation therapy that cured her. Still, she worried enough about the possibility of a recurrence and whether her body could sustain a pregnancy. Today, as millions of men and women of childbearing age and younger are surviving cancer, the question of reproduction is arising as a paramount consideration in planning treatment. Among the issues are the ability to preserve fertility while curing the disease and the safety of pregnancy for both mothers with cancer and their future children.

While some cancer treatments—drugs as well as radiation—can cause sterility or reduced fertility in men and women, preliminary evidence suggests that cancer therapy, in general, affects the ability to reproduce and to produce healthy children less than previously thought. All the same time, new ways are being devised to reduce the effects cancer treatments on fertility and on pregnancies already in progress when a cancer is discovered. Dr. Giuseppe Del Priore, director of gynecologic oncology at Bellevue Hospital in New York, and his colleages at the New York University School of Medicine noted in the January issue of Contemporary Ob/Gyn: "Less than a generation ago, reproductive-aged women with cancer generally had little to hope for and even less to look forward to. But things have changed. Many cancers are no longer a death sentence. More and more women with cancer are now becoming pregnant and raising legitimate fertility concerns. Today a doctor could tell Ms. Zea of Minnesota and other women like her that pregnancy is no longer ill-advised. Even women whose breast cancers are discovered during pregnancy should no longer be advised to terminate the pregnancy, because there are no data indicating a therapeutic benefit from such as abortion, the New York experts said.

Today, even cancers directly involving the reproductive organs—ovaries, uterus and cervix—can sometimes be treated in ways that permit future pregnancies and the births of healthy babies. Many of the modern chemotherapeutic agents are less damaging to ovarian function than the older drugs and do not induce permanent early menopause. Thus, a women's fertility may return months or even years after treatment ends. Fears that potent anticancer drugs will damage the DNA of a women's eggs or a man's sperm and result in birth defects have not been borne out by experience.

There are, however, cancers that run in families, and susceptibility to these cancers could be transmitted to patients' children, but the treatment itself is not now considered a factor influencing genetic risk. While men and adolescent boys with cancer who wish to preserve their fertility can easily bank sperm for future insemination before starting treatment, only about a quarter of childless men do so, the survey indicated. The reproductive issues for women with cancer are far more complex and less certain to succeed. It takes weeks to stimulate the development and release of mature eggs, and during that time, cancer treatments must be delayed. Then, the eggs must be fertilised and grown into early embryos before they can be frozen for future impregnation. For some cancers, like breast cancer, the potent hormonal stimulation needs to harvest eggs, could further endanger a women's health. Even if cancer treatment leaves a woman's reproductive organs intact, some lifesaving cancer drugs, for example, adriamycin and bleomycin, can damage the heart or lungs, making it difficult to go through pregnancy. But it is possible to assess in advance, with various tests, a woman's ability to withstand the biological and physical demand of pregnancy. Also refinements in radiation therapy often makes it possible to protect reproductive organs from radiation damage without compromising the success of treatment. Modern diagnostic tools, like magnetic resonance imaging, may permit an accurate assessment of the extent of a tumour without exposing the patient to radiation and high dose radiation used in treatment can now be delivered to a more circumscribed area. It is recommended that decisions about future pregnancies be dictated in part by the time period during which a cancer is mot likely to recur, if ever. Since most recurrences of breast cancer and melanoma occur within two years of diagnosis, a women may delay pregnancy until that high risk period ends to increase the likelihood that the child will have a healthy parent.

Heart disease

One of the world's leading killers, most deaths caused by heart disease come as the result of heart attacks. Because heart disease is often undetected until it is too late, doctors now recommend that all men over age 30, and women over age 50, get a cholesterol screen every five years. The top 5 risk factors are; a family history of heart disease, cigarette smoking, high blood pressure, elevated cholesterol and obesity. The incidence of heart disease is lower in women than in men, but the fatality rate is higher in those women who do have heart attacks. Some news and tips to save heart attacks is given below:

(i) Switching to a vegetarian lifestyle may not only prevent heart attacks; it may actually unclog arteries. Dr. Dean Ornish's trail-blazing studies in the US (which emphasized a strict, very low fat vegetarian diet, besides moderate exercise and stress reduction training) have now been successfully endorsed by the results of other studies. One of the latest was a 12 month investigation by researchers in Moradabad, India, which was reported in the *British Medical Journal*. The findings indicate that a diet heavy on fruits, grains, nuts, fish and vegetables protects the heart better than does a more conventional heart healthy eating plan that involves cutting back on high fat meats and dairy products. The researchers speculate that the experimental regimen is beneficial because it provides large amounts of soluble fibre, antioxidant vitamins (C, E, A and beta carotene), and minerals such as magnesium and potassium.

(ii) Take an aspirin at the first warning sign of a heart attack. That's what leading-edge cardiologists are suggesting to help ease the heartache of a coronary event and may be even save your life. Taken immediately, at the first sign of a heart attack, aspirin begins to act on the blood clot that may be forming in the artery and prevent it from becoming complete. It could tilt the balance from a serious heart attack to one with no muscle damage by delaying the complete blockage of the artery.

High blood pressure or hypertension is hitting more people today than ever before. Many don't even know that they have it. The disease runs in families, but it is also linked to cigarette smoking, stress, a high fat diet and high salt diet and being overweight. Left untreated hypertension can damage arteries and lead to heart attack or stroke.

(i) Eating high potassium foods may help to regular your blood pressure. Men with normal blood pressure were placed on two different kinds of diet for nine days each: One diet had adequate amounts of potassium; the other was low in the nutrient. On the normal diet, the men showed no significant blood pressure change. But on the low-potassium diet, their blood pressure rose significantly. One of the researchers speculates that not getting enough potassium may cause sodium retention and that, over a time, it can lead to high blood pressure. So include these high potassium foods in your diet; bananas, potatoes, tomatoes, milk, orange juice, tuna, sardines, apricots, figs, prunes, raisins, etc.

(ii) Regular, moderate exercise can not only lower blood pressure in moderate hypertensive, but may also prevent potential candidates from ever getting hypertension in the first place. The key word is moderate: while evidence mounts that aerobic exercise as well as mild to moderate strength training can do the trick, heavy duty resistance training can heighten not only physical stress but also blood pressure.

Don't lose heart

The following points are important:

(a) *Balance and consistency*: This is the key to healthy weight loss. Your diet to cut the extra intake of calories and be consistent in your exercise programme. With time this will help you achieve the desired results:better health, increased muscle mass and less fat percentage.

(b) *Patience pays*: You cannot lose weight in a day nor is there any short cut for this. A good weight loss programme takes time and you must accept and follow it. Don't hurry otherwise you may regain the lost weight in even lesser time.

(c) *Maintain a timetable*: A daily schedule will help you keep track of your activities. Keep your daily schedule realistic and doable, give enough time to your weight loss plan and stick to it.

(d) *Customize your approach*: There is no hard and fast rule for losing weight. If your friend lost a whole lot in six months, you may do it in four and someone else in eight months with the same workout schedule. So customize your approach and have a clear idea of what exactly you need to do.

(e) *Don't lose heart*: If you have tried to lose weight before without much success, do not lose heart. Learn from your past mistakes and restructure your programme again.

(f) *Find a partner*: It 's a good idea to have a partner in your weight loss journey who can empathize with you and support you in a positive way. This will help you more than it sounds.

(g) *Incorporate your plan into your everyday life*: Walk as much as you can. Park your vehicle at some distance from your destination and enjoy walking. Similarly, play as much as you can. Join in with the neighborhood children as they play soccer or badminton.

How one may be exposed to heart disease?

1. High Fat Diet

A high fat diet is, in fact, linked to five of the ten leading causes of death. At the top of the list is heart disease. The connection between diet and heart disease is seen in a study conducted in seven countries on some 12,000 men. The extremes are particularly revealing. The study showed that men eating 20 percent or more of their calories as saturated fat-had elevated blood cholesterol levels, while those eating only 5 percent of their calories as saturated fat-had low blood cholesterol levels. And the men who ate more fat, had a rate of heart attack six times greater than the control group of men.

Coronary heart disease is common in India now. In the past several years, as Western style fast food have become popular here, the consumption of animal fats has gone up 800 percent. Now, Punjabi boys have even higher blood cholesterol levels than Amercian boys of the same age ! Clearly, dietary fats are implicated in life threatening conditions, particularly heart disease.

2. The Cholesterol

Cholesterol is found in varying amounts in food we eat. The two types of lipoproteins that carry most of the blood cholesterol are low-density lipoproteins (LDL) and high density lipoproteins (HDL). LDLs are rich in cholesterol. Most cells in the body have LDL receptors, and they take up some LDL. But the liver is so designed that 70 percent of the removal of LDL from the blood stream by LDL receptors occurs here. HDLs, on the other hand, are cholesterol thirsty molecules, they soak up surplus cholesterol and transport it to the liver. The liver breaks down cholesterol and eliminates it from the body. The problem occurs when there is excessive LDL in the blood. This increases the possibility of a build up of plaque on artery walls. When plaque buildup occurs, the arteries become narrow and the amount of oxygen-carrying blood that can pass through them, decreases. This condition is called atherosclerosis. The process continues slowly and silently, talking decades to cause symptoms. One symptom is angina or chest pain, like the one Gurpreet experienced.

3. The Heart attack

When a heart artery is completely blocked, often by a blood clot, the part of the heart that receives blood from that artery, dies. The result is sudden, often deadly, myocardial infarction—better known as a heart attack. Even partial blockage of a coronary artery can lead to death of heart tissue. Blockage of arteries in other parts of the body can cause strokes, gangrene of the legs, and even loss of kidney function.

4. The Blood Tests

LDL is called bad cholesterol, and HDL good cholesterol. If LDL is high or HDL is low, the risk of heart disease is high. A simple blood test will often indicate impending danger long before a person experiences noticeable symptoms, such as angina; the pain in the chest behind breast bone. It is important, then, to keep your blood cholesterol level in check. Let us now see how your food can affect this level.

5. The food

Meat, eggs, fish, poultry, and dairy products all contain cholesterol. Foods from plants, on the other hand, have less of cholesterol. The body produces its own cholesterol, so cholesterol consumed in food is extra. Ordinarily, as dietary cholesterol enters the liver, the liver processes it and decreases its own production of cholesterol. This keeps the total amount of cholesterol in the blood regulated. What happens, if the diet is abundant in cholesterol? The likelihood of cholesterol directly entering the cells of the artery wall is increased. When it does, the process of atherosclerosis occurs. Cutting down on your intake of food cholesterol, then, is a course of wisdom.

6. The Fats

Fats fall into two categories—saturated and unsaturated. Unsaturated fats can be either monounsaturated (e.g. olive oil) or polysaturated. (safflower or fish oil). Unsaturated fats are better for you, than saturated, since consuming saturated fat raises the level of cholesterol in the blood. Saturated fats suppress LDL receptor of livers cells, reducing the speed of removal of LDL from the blood. Saturated fats are primarily found in foods of animal origin, such as butter, egg-yolks, lard, milk, ice cream, meat, and poultary.. They are also prevalent in chocolate, coconut and its oils, and palm oil. Saturated fats are solid at room temperature. Unsaturated fats, on the other hand, are liquid at room temperature. Foods that contain monounsaturated fats and polyunsaturated fats may help to lower blood-cholesterol. While polyunsaturated fats, common in corn oil and sunflower-seed oil, reduce both good and bad cholesterol, monounsaturated fats, plentiful in olive oil and canola oil, reduce only the bad cholesterol. The fat requirements of the body, however, are very small. They are easily met through the consumption of vegetables, beans, grains, and fruits. So minimizing the intake of saturated fats. Offers protection to heart.

7. The regulation

The intake of fats in general and cholesterol in particular has to be regulated. However, even if your blood cholesterol is normal, you have to reduce food cholesterol intake, since increase in dietary cholesterol may increase the risk of coronary heart disease independently of its effect on blood cholesterol. Cholesterol-rich foods promote heart disease even in people with low blood cholesterol. And that's why eating less cholesterol must be of concern to all people, irrespective of their blood cholesterol level. Too much fat in the blood, be it from saturated or unsaturated fat in the food, causes red blood cells to clump together. Such thickened blood does not pass through the narrow capillaries, causing the tissues to be deprived of nutrients. Clumped cells moving along the arteries also disrupt the oxygen distribution to artery walls, causing surface damage, where plaque can easily begin to form.

8. The Salt: A pinch of it can be too much

More than a teaspoon of salt a day can increase risk of heart attacks, strokes, osteoporosis and stomach cancer, warn experts. Medical specialists in the UK and USA are calling on manufacturers to cut down on the amount of salt they add to ready meals and other processed foods. A reduction of salt intake by three grams is predicted to reduce the incidence of stroke by 25 percent and heart attacks by 16 percent. In India there is no such guidance available. A lot of salt is being consumed in meals in the restaurants and in processed foods, with consequent stress on heart, brain, kidney, etc. In adults, when the level of sodium is too high, the body retains excessive water and the volume of bodily fluids increases. Scientists believe that with high levels of fluid circulating through the brain, there is a greater chance of weaknesses in the brain's blood vessels being exposed and consequently bursting, causing a stroke.

Similarly, a greater volume of fluid passing through the heart can place additional strain on the organ, increasing the possibility of coronary artery disease (CAD). It has now been found that excess of salt in the diet can lead to calcium loss and thereby increase the risk of osteoporosis. High intake of salt can also significantly increase the risk of stomach cancer. Salt is present in almost all the food items that we take these days. And today, the kind of work and work environment we are in, we hardly require more than 5-6 grams of salt a day to replenish our daily salt excretion. People who do very little physical work and spend most of their day in an air-conditioned office actually don't need any additional salt, either at the table or in cooking. By the time we attain 60 years of age, our kidneys become 50 percent less efficient. Instead of throwing out excess sodium through urine, the kidneys start retaining it in the body, leading to diseases such as hypertension, oedema, stroke and cardiovascular diseases. So it is advisable that people who don't do much physical work should cut on their salt consumption in cooking.

We require to consume salt daily because we lose it from our body every day. There are two ways of losing salt from the body, first, through excretion in faeces, and second through secretion via skin and kidneys. The retention of excess salt may be reflected by hypertension or swelling or puffiness in the face, legs and hands. There are four main ways of reducing salt intake

- Don't add salt to food once it is served. Also add minimum salt in the food as you are cooking it.
- Choose food articles with a reduced sodium content.
- Carefully monitor the salt or sodium content of processed foods by reading the ingredient labels.
- Eat more fruit and vegetables. They contain potassium, which balances the effect of salt on the body.

The rapid increase in the incidence of cardiovascular disease (CVDs), the second most deadly category of non communicable diseases after diabetes, also lends support to the fact that while our daily salt intake on the table in cooking has remained at constant levels, our lifestyle has become more sedentary. This, coupled with our growing predilection for manufactured and processed foods, has led to the growth of CVD incidence in India. The incidence of CVDs is higher among the upper income groups.

In case of corporate executives, they move in air conditioned cars, work in air-conditioned offices—a climatic condition that doesn't trigger sweating. So, for them, the sodium and water remain retained within their bodies. If they consume excess salt, it may lead to hypertension or kidney diseases at a later stage. They should stick to the lower limit of the minimum salt requirement—six grams or less a day.

Recognize heart attack

If you are obese, eat a lot of fat, smoke, don't do any exercise-always beware of heart attack. This can manifest as a dull pain in the shoulder or neck or jaw and not necessarily crushing pain under the breast bone, going to the left upper arm. There can be associated tiredness or it may be the only symptom. It may manifest as discomfort in upper abdomen or indigestion.

Other symptoms can be breathlessness or exhaustion. There can be sudden death during sleep. Don't delay treatment even if the symptoms are mild. Sometimes a major heart attack produces only mild symptoms. It is important to take note of the following: Attach due importance if the symptoms has never occurred before or atleast never with the same severity and you feel uneasy. Second, when the symptom persists. And third, when the problem jolts you out of sleep and doesn't go away after a few minutes. Pain originating from the heart usually doesn't go away—or worsen—with rest or changes of position. Nor does it respond to pain relievers, hot pads and message. The pain may suddenly start even when you are resting. Such cases are especially worrying. At this stage don't conclude that this can't be a heart attack. Smokers, tobacco chewers, diabetics, people over 50, and patients with high cholesterol, high blood pressure or a family history of heart disease should be especially alert to unusual symptoms. Nearly 15 percent of heart attack victims in India are below 40. In addition, studies have shown that women become more vulnerable to heart attacks after menopause.

Heavy sweating, shortness of breath and extreme exhaustion, sometimes accompanied by fainting, nausea, lightheadedness or intense anxiety should not be taken lightly. A silent heart attack is well known among diabetics, since the disease destroys the nerve, which carries the pain signals.

Lowering your risk of heart disease

The following steps are useful to help you lower your risk of heart disease:

(i) *Stop smoking*: Quitting today can cut your risk of heart disease within a year.
(ii) *Lose weight*: If you are overweight, losing as few as five kgs can make a difference.
(iii) *Exercise*: Regular exercise helps to lower bad cholesterol (LDL), keep blood pressure from rising, and keep off excess weight.
(iv) *Eat less saturated fat*: If your LDL is high, switch to leaner cuts of meat and try 1-percent (low fat) milk or skim (fat-free) milk instead of 2 percent milk.
(v) Limit or quit alcohol consumption.
(vi) Eat more fruits, vegetables and other plant foods rich in soluble fiber.

Heart Health News

(i) Tea may prevent heart attacks

Drinking lot of tea (no milk, no sugar) may provide some protection against heart attacks. The study looked at 1900 people who were considered after having heart attacks, moderate tea drinkers had a 28 percent lower death rate than those who drank no tea, and the heavy tea drinkers had a death rate about 44 percent lower. It was found that tea drinkers generally had lower death rates regardless of age, gender, smoking status, obesity, hypertension, diabetes or previous heart attack.

(ii) Ban on Tobacco advertising and Public smoking

The control of tobacco use is a matter of survival. There is simply won't be enough resources to treat the complex and costly chronic problems resulting from tobacco addiction. The advertising restrictions will go into effect on January 1 and the cigarette package warnings will be effective as on June 1, 2003, in Mexico. The Government already has banned smoking in all federal buildings, a major step in a country where the habit is still widely practiced in public places, including shopping malls, airports and restaurants. In India also, there is a ban on smoking in public places, but compliance is limited.

(iii) Nuts can lessen heart risk: Study

Eating a handful of nuts twice or more a week may cut one's risk of deadly heart disease, says a study. Nuts and fish are plentiful in the Mediterranean diet, which is known to be heart friendly, and many types of nuts are also a healthy source of unsaturated fats, magnesium and vitamin E. They found a 47% lower risk of sudden cardiac death among those who consumed an ounce of nuts at least twice a week compared to those who did not eat nuts at all. They also found a 30% lower risk of coronary heart disease death among the nut eaters.

(iv) Doctors warn against use of drug coated stents

A leading cardiologist has warned against the indiscriminate use of drug coated stents, just introduced in India, as an answer to open heart surgery. More research and data is needed before we jump to any conclusion. There are studies which prove the efficacy and safety of these devices and say that there has not been a single case of stent thrombosis, which has been a problem with brachytherapy (another method to prevent restenosis), he said. To come to any conclusive answer we will have to closely monitor patients for a minimum of 10 years, and this is not possible because we cannot wait for 10 years before treating patients, who can benefit from the technology. That is why, it is important for doctors to have cautions optimism.

(v) A cholsesterol drug good for heart

Cholesterol lowering drugs called statins help prevent heart attacks and stroke. They observed in a study, a 56% lower risk of cardiovascular events and a 44% lower all cause mortality associated with the use of statins among people whose average age was 72. The study does contribute to the growing evidence that cholesterol lowering therapy is effective for reducing risk for coronary heart disease events in older persons.

Constipation: mother of all diseases?

It has been hammered into the mind of each Indian since childhood that clearing the bowl is absolutely essential and one should go to the commode several times a day, until you are satisfied. It is also true that our population do not feel satisfied until the commode is full to the brim. It has been customary for the village doctor or the bare foot doctors on visiting spree to hold the pulse of anyone and blurt, you have a serious health problem, i.e. you seem to be suffering from constipation; unless you take remedial measures—you will lose all your health. With such pronouncements by self-styled doctors, with great confidence and style, the vulnerable and ignorant mind of the prospective patient accepts it as a gospel truth and bags the 'Doctor' to be relieved of his constipation. And with that starts the next ordeal.

I. Excreta, the residual waste

There is no doubt that foods you consume are not fully digested and a good part of it, subject to the quantity of roughage consumed, is spared as 'residual waste' by the intestine, to be voided at periodic intervals. The interval can be over a day or twice a day or even every two days. Much depends on the habit, facilities of toilet, convenience of time, etc. Besides the food intake, it also depends on the stress, to which person was subjected. In turn non voidance of faecal matter due to lack of bowel movement or inadequate toilet facilities or minimal waste available for removal—can lead to enhanced stress to the gullible mind. Besides this feeling of not being free/italics from excreta, scientifically constipation is not known to cause any tangible ailments, on the day of occurrence or in the long run. So the old concept, which is still being exploited among ignorant populace, is subject to scrutiny.

2. What is constipation?

As mentioned above, it is non-voidance or unsatisfactory voidance of excreta. It leads to a hard stool which is difficult to expel, or motions which occur at intervals of several days. In most cases, it is harmless but it can be a symptom of an underlying disease. If a person over 40 years old develops persistent constipation (or any other change in bowel habits) then a doctor should be consulted to obtain an accurate diagnosis.

3. Symptoms

There may not be any symptoms of not passing stool or there may be many symptoms of anxiety. If stool is hard, there may be pain associated with bowel movements, a feeling of incomplete emptying of the bowel, or a feeling of bloatedness in the stomach region. There can be symptoms of underlying disease, which has caused constipation.

4. Causes

Constipation can be caused by several factors, but most important are—intake of food with less residue, i.e. low fibre diet and stresses of various kinds. Other factors may be:

- Certain medicines, e.g. codeine-containing pain killers, morphine-like pain killers, calcium channel blockers, beta blockers, antidepressants and antacids.
- Insufficient fluid intake
- Lowered metabolism
- Irritable bowel syndrome
- Back pain
- Chronic kidney failure
- Colon or rectal cancer
- An inactive lifestyle
- Too much calcium in the blood, etc.

5. How to prevent constipation?

A well balanced diet high in fibre, including bran, fruits and vegetables is often helpful. Do not discard the peelings of vegetables and fruits, they have insoluble fibre, which is so important to prevent constipation and render other healthful benefits. As mentioned above most of the complaints of constipation are due to unhealthy lifestyle and not due to any real ailment. When it starts suddenly, it can be due to a serious disease. In most cases of chronic and habitual constipation, the intestine has to be re-educated.

(i) Also drink at least 8-10 glasses of water a day.
(ii) Hot beverages, such as coffee, tea or hot water may stimulate bowel movements.
(iii) Prunes and plum juice can also be beneficial, also take plenty of fruits.
(iv) Reduction in intake of white bread, cakes and sugar. Add bran to your diet.
(v) Regular exercise improves digestion, and reduces stress.
(vi) Get used to a regular bowel habit. The best time is usually the first hour after breakfast. Do not be in a hurry. Sit for at least 10 minutes, regardless of whether you manage to expel any stool or not.
(vii) Take adequate quantity of foods and do not miss a meal.
(viii) Do not get worried about constipation. It is the faulty weight loss programme, which can cause constipation.

6. Complications

- Heamorrhoids
- Dependency on laxatives
- Hernia (bulging of the abdominal contents through a weak point in the abdominal wall). This is made worse by too much straining when trying to get rid of hard stools.
- A prolapse of the uterus or the rectum.

7. Role of medicines

Do not take medicines as far as possible, at least do not make it a habit. If absolutely necessary you take stool softeners (such as lactulose), occasionally. Stimulant laxatives which help the bowel muscles to work (such as senna) may also have to be given. There are many different combination laxatives available both on prescription and across the counter. Depend on adequate and fiber rich food, plenty of fluids, regular exercise and cheerful mood.

8. Capsicum may help

It is one of the best carminative and appetizer agent and removes gas from intestine. Its regular intake as a part of Indian cuisine, ensures better appetite and better digestion. Resultantly the food is more palatable and its intake is adequate. Hence it helps to prevent constipation.

Skin; a mirror of health and appearance

You can't expect skin to be glowing in health or look beautiful, if you are in poor health and suffer from multiple deficiencies of foods, foods—supplements or water. The emphasis would be again on proper and adequate nutrients and exercises of body on a regular basis.

As said elsewhere, excess of fat and sugar is not good for health of your blood vessels, heart, bones, skin, etc. If being fat, affects your circulation in the body—it can do the same to the small blood vessels of your skin. Be restrained on fatty and sugary foods.

1. It is not just pretty

Healthy skin does a lot more than look pretty; It maintains moisture throughout your body and sweat out bacterial and other toxins. But even healthy skin needs constant protection from free radicals. (Cellular bye products of sun exposure—regularly pummel your collagen, the spongy network of fibres that keeps skin line free). Antioxidants may help figh that rusting, while antioxidant-infused lotions will improve the appearance of your skin because it is an external organ, the health of your skin comes from within.

2. Food and Skin

The relationship between food and skin is not clearly defined though vital. However, some foods are skin unfriendly, saturated fats that clogs arteries may also gum up the capillaries that whist nutrients to, and waste from, skin cells. And overdosing on sugar may mess with collagen, contributing to saggy, inflexible skin and brown spots.

3. What should you eat?

What is good for general health is also good for skin health. Most of the foods and nutrients are listed elsewhere also. Let us count some of them here.

(a) Water

Though not a food, yet it is the best skin reviler. Hydrated skin looks moist and plump, which makes wrinkles less obvious. Make sure to down about ten 200 ml glasses daily—more if you exercise. In summer plenty of water is essential. Drink water in winter as well, old people must take plenty of water.

(b) Green leafy vegetables

Leafy greens like methi, spinach, amaranth (chowli), drumstick leaves are full of antioxidants. Plus, they are a great source of iron when eaten with vitamin C rich foods. (Women who don't get enough iron are especially prone to dark circles under their eyes). Greens also contain zinc. In one Swedish study, acne prone patients who added a zinc supplement to their diets saw 85 percent of acne clear up after three months. Zinc also helps break down damaged collagen, allowing new collagen to form. Replace one meal with green salads or cooked vegetables.

(c) Unsaturated oils

Intake of some fat is key to smooth, supple skin. Individuals with persistently dry, flaky skin may not be getting enough good fats found in poly and monounsaturated oils like sesame, mustard, peanut and olive in their diet. When they add them, the condition usually clears up in a few weeks. Just a tablespoon daily may make a huge difference to dry skin. If clogged pores are a problem, the essential fatty acids in these vegetable oils can help keep them clear by thinning the oils they secrete. Be discrete, don't overeat.

(d) Fish

A fatty fish like Salmon or sardine have plenty of face friendly omega-3 fatty acids, which do everything from attack acne to help deflate inflamed areas. Also found in mackerel, shark, etc. are essential fatty acids which battle collagen damaging free radicals and help smooth out fine lines. Eat fish three times a week. If you cant stand sea food, a fish oil supplement may offer the same benefits.

(e) Alsi (flax seed)

Add flaxseed (alsi) oil and nuts to your diet. Alsi also contain essential fatty acids and zinc, which helps quell acne flare ups and increase cell growth.

(f) Tomato

Tomato packs high levels of the antioxidant vitamin A and C as well as skin cancer fighting chemicals. Vitamin C helps keep skin elastic and prevents bruising. Vitamin A aids in healing acne from the inside out by boosting resistance to infection. Find these antioxidants in other dark red, green, orange and yellow fruits and veggies, too.

(g) Fruits

They are a great source of polyphenols, powerful antioxidants that are currently being studied for their anti-aging capabilities. In recent studies, blueberries packed three times the antioxidant punch of an orange. A hefty handful of jamuns, strawberries or just 2 to 3 amlas has all the antioxidant vitamin C your body requires each day to reconstruct your collagen, the scaffolding that keeps skin from drooping. MELON: is a colourful fruit, which is full of carotene like compounds such as lycopene, which reduces the deep down collagen damage that promotes wrinkles. The orange orb is also a great source of beta-carotene, which is converted to vitamin A. This nutrient prevents keratonic plugs, the rough patches that are often found on the backs of the arms.

(h) Soyabean

This bean is a skin saver. It is full of chemicals that act like estrogen, and may help prevent acne. It is also loaded with vitamin E, which boosts new cell growth and keeps skin moist. Try eating atleast half a cup of soya beans 3 times a week.

(i) Carrots et al.

Crunch all you want—carrots are bursting with the beta-carotene (vitamin A), a key to keeping dry, flaky skin at bay. You will also find this nutrient in orange fruits and vegetables, such as apricots, papaya, pumpkin, mango and sweet potatoes. Take plenty of fresh vegetables and fruits.

(j) Breakfast cereals

Oat meal and other breakfast cereals supply a rich dose of fibre. If oatmeal is too expensive, go for ragi (nachni) or barley. These cereals are also rich in B vitamins, which aid new skin cell growth.

(k) White rice, white bread and white sugar

Refined carbohydrates and excess sugar present in the above mentioned foods, allegedly binds collagen fibres into inflexible bundles. This causes skin ageing and hence avoid these white looking foods and instead choose brown rice, brown bread and humble Gur.

4. What not to eat?

(a) Alcohol
(b) Caffeine
(c) Saturated fats

Red meat, ice cream, butter, trans-fatty acids, found in the hydrogenated oils that inhabit chips, cookies, biscuits and cakes.

Diabetes

Diabetes is the body's inability to use sugar as fuel in a normal way. Unlike type I diabetes (insulin-dependent), which usually strikes men in their teens, type II diabetes, the most common type, generally hits overweight men after age 40 (nearly 9 out of 10 diabetes are overweight). Typical symptoms include an insatiable thirst, frequent urination, slow healing wounds, blurred vision, recurring gum infections, intense itching, and pain or tingling in the legs or feet. Diabetes can also lead to blindness, heart disease, and stroke and kidney failure. Some tips and news are given below:

(i) Lifting weights may improve sugar metabolism. In a study on type II diabetes, the joggers and weight-lifters saw improvements in their ability to metabolize sugar. Strength training helps by building muscles, which use up more from sugar from the blood stream.
(ii) Anti-histamines may help prevent blindness among diabetics. Diabetes causes blood vessels in the back of the eye to expand and lose tone, allowing blood and other substances to leak

through the vessel walls into the retina/fundus of the eye; leading down a path toward blindness. It is possible that advances in genetic engineering may make this possible, in which case doctors would have an unlimited supply of insulin producing cells, from tumor cells (which produce insulin).

What is diabetes?

To a layman diabetes mellitus means simply passing sugar in urine. He doesn't know from where the sugar comes and how it causes any health problems for the sufferers. First of all he doesn't understand if faulty food or lack of exercise was the causative factor? Incidently, most of the people also do not know what are the warning of diabetes, which will take him to a doctor for consultation. He is unaware of the hazards and complication, which will occur to him, if he does not care adequately and at an early stage. While neglect of diabetes will definitely lead to serious complications in most of diabetics, the diagnosis itself should not sound a 'Life Sentence" of ill-health and misery. Most of the diabetics respond to management with diet control, weight reduction and physical activity with or without medicine. Such well controlled diabetics lead a near normal life in forms of quality of health, performance and longevity. Hence the information "Are you a diabetic?" should neither be startling to the listener, nor a stigma to the sufferer.

I. Diabetes on the rise

Millions of Indians don't know they have the disease. So look out for simple warning signs. Most of the time it is silent and no warning symptoms may be present. It is only urine and blood test, done routinely or for a medical examination for LIC, that the bitter truth of the presence of sugary disease is revealed. So it would be prudent to get periodic medical assessment of your health, especially for diabetes, after the age of 40 years or earlier (May be 30), if any of the warning symptoms are present.

- Abnormal, intense diet
- Frequent urination
- Extreme hunger
- Sudden, unexplained weight loss
- Slow-healing cuts, bruises or skin infections
- Recurrent infections
- Blurred vision
- Unexplained weakness and extreme exhaustion
- Genital itching or impotence.
- Sweet-smelling breath
- Obesity
- Irritability
- Nausea or vomiting
- Tingling or numbness in feet/hands
- Drowsiness

2. Indian Scenario

Experts estimate that over 50 percent of India's 33 million diabetics don't know they have the disease. And what's more, it is becoming more prevalent. The World Health Organisation predicts that by 2025, India will have more than 57 million diabetics. By then one out of every four of the world's diabetics will be an. Nearly 20 percent of our hospital beds are occupied by diabetics, and although there are no figures for how much is spent on diabetes care, it is enormous. Some studies in urban rich population have revealed an incidence as high as 13% of the causes and implications are not too far to seek. This can have disastrous consequences to the health care delivery system of the nation. The rich have to use their money for a better cause than pleasure of palate or comfort of limbs.

3. How diabetes is caused?

Normally, insulin, a hormone produced in the pancreas, enables the body to turn blood glucose into immediate energy or to store it in cells. But if insufficient insulin is produced, or if it does not work properly (insulin resistance) the glucose remains trapped in the blood causing damage to blood vessels, nerves and tissues.

In less than five percent of Indian diabetics, mostly children and teenagers, the insulin producing cells in the pancreas are destroyed. Sufferers of this form, Type 1 diabetes, will die unless they get daily injections of insulin. However, majority of diabetics, have Type 2 diabetes, where they produce some insulin, but not enough to use and store glucose satisfactorily. Type 2 diabetes, formerly known as late-onset diabetes, generally affects Indians early, i.e. soon after the age of 40, may be genetically predisposed to developing the disease. In India, diabetes was recognized as a disease more than a thousand years ago. "All the three classic treatises Charaka Samhita, Ashtanga-hridaya Samhita and Sushruta Sahmita—deal with diabetes." Uncontrolled blood glucose leads to several ailments, including heart attacks and strokes, which kill upto 70 percent of diabetics. As a result of nerve damage, known as peripheral neuropathy, wounds and infections are harder to heal, and chronic foot ulcers and amputations more likely. Indeed, diabetes is one of the most common reasons for amputations in India. In some diabetic men, especially those who have had the disease for several years, nerve and vascular damage leads to impotence. Diabetes may also affect the small blood vessels of the retina of the eye, which is the leading cause of blindness among urban Indians. Although this visual loss is largely preventable by good control of blood sugar and laser treatment, around 20 percent of newly diagnosed diabetics already have damaged retinas (since they report late). Nearly half patients with diabetes in its early stages have none of the typical symptoms. Both husband and wife have diabetes, there is a 60 percent chance that their children will develop it—there are a number of other risk factors too. Lack of exercise is a major one. Sedentary men aged 42 to 60 are twice as likely to get Type 2 diabetes as men, who took vigorous exercise for atleast

40 minutes a week. Another risk factor is obesity. The fatter you are, the more insulin your body needs to maintain the right level of blood glucose, and the more insulin your body needs to maintain the right level of blood glucose, and the more likely your pancreas is found inadequate.

A high fat diet is another risk factor for developing Type 2 diabetes. For women, pregnancy can provide an early warning sign: raised blood glucose in pregnancy indicates an increased risk of type 2 diabetes later. By the time they are diagnosed, atleast 30 percent of diabetics have developed one or the other kind of complications-hypertension, serious infections and tissue damage that suggests that they have had the disease undetected for many years. Don't hesitate if anyone in your family has diabetes or the other risk factors or symptoms seem to apply to you, go to your doctor right away. Everyone over 30 should get themselves tested for diabetes annually. Don't get the urine test only, it is unreliable. A blood test is accurate. Once diagnosed, a diabetic should have a regular test for protein in the urine as per the requirement. Type 2 diabetes can cause kidney damage In a quarter of patients, but there is evidence that good blood pressure, glucose control and a low protein diet can delay the progress of kidney disease. What can you do? Avoid junk food. A low-fat, low sugar, largely vegetarian diet, which includes complex carbohydrates may be the answer. Combine proper food with regular, moderate exercise. This combination can prevent type 2 diabetes.

4. Longstanding diabetes

People who have had diabetes for a few years develop other health problems. These are called complications. Complications include damage to the nerves, eyes, kidneys and heart and blood vessels. Light glucose control can prevent or stop eye damage, nerve damage and kidney damage. However, the prevention complications with control of DM is not absolute. Despite a good control of blood sugar, some complications can still occur.

5. Nerves

The damage diabetes causes to nerves is called diabetic neuropathy. There are several types. They vary in what part of the body the damaged nerves are in damaged nerves—no longer carry messages properly. Several symptoms can develop, e.g. prickling, tingling, burning or jabbing feelings, loss of feeling, weak muscles, fainting, vomiting, bladder infections, diarrhea, sexual problems.

To prevent nerve damage

Keep your glucose levels well controlled, don't smoke, drink little or no alcohol, eat a healthful diet rich in vitamins and minerals, exercise regularly. Treatment, improving blood glucose control can help nerve damage. Nerve pain can be treated with antidepressant drugs, exercises, or special skin creams. Surgery can sometimes help.

6. Kidney

Diabetes can lead to the kidney disease called diabetic nephropathy. The job of the kidney is to filter wastes from the blood, diabetes may cause the kidneys to lose their ability to filter properly. As a result, protein that the body needs is lost in the urine, and wastes that the body doesn't need build up in the blood. Several symptoms can arise, so your doctor should test your urine for protein each year. You may also have blood test done. Kidney damage cannot be reversed. So it is important to prevent it. There are two treatments for when kidneys no longer work:

(i) Dialysis, a machine cleans the blood.
(ii) Kidney transplant, the person gets a new kidney from someone else.

7. Eye

In non-proliferative diabetic retinopathy, the milder form, blood vessels leak blood and fluid into the eye. In the more severe but rarer form, proliferative diabetic retinopathy, new blood vessels sprout and grow out of control. They can bleed or cause scarring, which pulls on the retina. Retinopathy may not cause any symptoms in all or when it causes, it may be quite late. So you should see an eye doctor each year after you are 30 years old (or, if you are younger than 30, each year after you have had diabetes for 5 years). You should get a special exam with eye drops to look for retinopathy. You should also see your eye doctor if—

(i) Your vision is blurry;
(ii) You see double;
(iii) You see spots or floaters
(iv) One or both eyes hurt;
(v) You feel pressure in your eye;
(vi) You lose the ability to see things at the side;
(vii) You have trouble reading;
(viii) Prevention to head off eye damage;
(ix) Keep your glucose levels well controlled.

The two main treatments are:

— Photocoagulation, in which a laser seals leaky blood vessels.
— Vitrectomy, a surgery that removes blood and scar tissue from the eye.

8. Blood vessels and Heart

Diabetes makes you more likely to get hardening of the blood vessels or have a stroke. You can also have peripheral vascular disease, in which not enough blood reaches the areas farthest from your heart. When you have diabetes, your body chemistry changes. As a result, your blood may clot too easily. Your blood vessels may narrow. And fat may build up in your blood vessels faster. If you have poor circulation, you may have many infections, your skin may itch, or your legs may become shiny and lose their hair. Your calves may hurt when you exercise. If you are a man, you may trouble having an erection. Your doctor can do tests for these problems. If your blood pressure or cholesterol level is high, it signal that you are at risk of heart or blood vessel damage.

You can lower your risk of heart and blood vessel disease. These steps make your body chemistry more normal. And they keep your blood vessels more open. Keep your glucose levels well controlled; don't smoke, eat a low fat diet that does not contain a lot of salt, keep your blood pressure down. Lower your cholesterol if it is over 200 mg/dL, exercise often, lose weight if you need to.

9. Skin

Damaged nerves and narrowed blood vessels both can lead to dry, itchy skin. Poor circulation also makes infections more likely and longer lasting. Other skin problems include spots of various colours, bilsters, yellow bumps, and rashes. Also skin on the hands and toes may become waxy and tight. To keep your skin in good shape, keep your diabetes well controlled. Keep your skin clean. Moisturize your skin. Wash cuts carefully, but do not use harsh cleaners like alcohol on them.

10. Impotence

Impotence is the inability to get or keep an erection long enough for satisfactory sex in at least one out of four tries, according to an expert. It's estimated that one out of every three men over age 40 has potency problems. Clogged arteries may be to blame for nearly half of these problems. It is quite common among diabetics. Some news and tips are given below:

(i) A patch that delivers an erection-causing drug into the penis through the skin, instead of by injection, is now in clinical trials. The patient just applies a patch when he wants an erection. More natural erections have been noted with a new penile injection. A Danish Urologist has completed clinical trials of a new injection that achieves more natural erections in impotent men than those in current use—papaverine or prostaglandin.

(ii) A dose of nitric oxide might help to keep it up. Nitric oxideis involved in the relaxation of smooth muscles in the spongy portion of the penis. When these muscles relax, blood can flow in, causing the penis to expand. Research at this point is directed at determining nitric oxide's precise role in erections. Then it might be possible to develop therapies based on this simple compound.

11. Mouth problems

High glucose levels provide an inviting home for germs. So people with diabetes are more likely to get gum infections. Poor circulation slows down healing. To protect your teeth, have them cleaned every 6 months. Make sure your dentist knows you have diabetes. Brush teeth with a soft brush at least twice a day. Floss every day.

12. Foot problems

Nerve damage and reduced blood flow affects your feet. When you can't feel your feet well, it is easy to bump and scrape them. And you may not even be able to tell you'have injured them. Poor blood flow then keeps the sore from healing. How to care them?

(i) Washing feet each day, then drying them carefully;
(ii) Checking your feet for injuries each day;
(iii) Flaying your shoes fit by a trained fitter.
(iv) Buying and wearing only comfortable, supportive shoes with a low heel and plenty of wiggle room for your toes. Checking your shoes before putting them on for stones, paper clips, nails, and other things that could rub your feet.
(v) Wearing stocks without seams or mended areas; and
(vi) Not going barefoot even to the bathroom at night.

13. Women and diabetes

Women of child bearing may have several problems, e.g. still birth, large baby with poor survival, pre education, etc. and accelerated complications of DM in mother as mentioned above in this chapter. Congenital abnormality of baby, fatal growth restriction, hydromonios, premature delivery, antenatal asphyxia, pre-eclampsia, etc. The women may have higher incidence of bacterial and fungal infections of genital organs and urinary tract and which require specialised treatment, besides the control of DM.

How to prevent diabetes?

It is well known that frequent check ups can catch diabetes early. Also with a careful diet, regular exercise and if necessary, drugs, also you can control type 2 diabetes. But do you know, you may save yourself from ever getting diabetes?

Until about a decade ago, people were pretty fatalistic about getting diabetes. It was looked on as one of the signs of getting old-like wrinkles and a sagging gut. There was nothing you could do about it. Doctors found that there was nothing inevitable about it. Now there is evidence that losing weight with a combination of diet and exercise helps people not only to control Type 2 diabetes but even prevent diabetes.

Can you cure diabetes?

Several studies give reason to hope last year, a group of Swedish doctors released a study that shows diet and exercise can not only prevent diabetes, they can actually reverse it once started. The men in were given advice on limiting fats and cholesterol in their diets and put on a regular aerobic exercise programme. For the first two years of the study, the men were given blood and fitness tests every six months, then the interval was lengthened to a year for three more years. The results were so encouraging that almost none of the men dropped out of the study. And the benefits lasted the whole five years, as long as they kept exercising and eating right. Over half of the glucose intolerant men regained normal sugar sensitivity and none of them progressed to diabetes.

In another study they found that the most active men (burning atleast 3500 calories in activity per week) were half as likely to develop diabetes as the most sedentary (expending less than 500 calories in activity). Those who participated in strenuous sports, such as swimming, running or tennis had the lowest risk of developing diabetes. And, those people at highest risk for developing diabetes were found to benefit the most from exercise. Women, who exercised vigorously at least once a week were significantly less likely to develop diabetes. The protective effect of exercise was due only in part of its effect on weight control. The researchers found an independent beneficial effect of exercise among obese and non-obese women, older and younger women, as well as among those with a family history of diabetes and those without. Keeping your weight down, avoiding high fat and cholesterol in your diet and exercising regularly, may keep you away from developing diabetes.

Glycemic index

Now some health experts say that the glycemic index may offer dramatic health benefits. The glycemic index (GI) assigned carbohydrate-containing foods a number based on how they affect your blood sugar. Foods with a GI less than 55 cause only a little rise in blood sugar; those in the 55 to 70 range raise it a little higher; and rose with GIs more than 70 send blood sugar level.

What makes a GI number high or low is how quickly the food breaks down during digestion. The longer your body has to wrestle with the carb to break it down into glucose, the shower the rise in blood glucose and the lower the GI. Often, fibre-rich foods have lower GIs. Fibre, especially the soluble type in oats and beans, creates a web in the intestines that traps carb particles. Not surprisingly, beans have low GI numbers. When fibre is ground finely, as it often is in whole what floor, it doesn't present enough of a digestive challenge to lower the GI of these foods. That explains why whole wheat bread has a GI number nearly identical to white bread.

Surprisingly, table sugar has a lower GI (59) than potatoes (70). That's because it is made of two sugars, glucose and fructose; the glucose half sails right into the blood stream, but the fructose segment has to detour through the liver, where it slowly gets converted into glucose. But the starch molecules in potatoes are strings of glucose.

The problem with eating lots of high GI foods in this; when your blood sugar soars, so does the hormone insulin. Insulin's main duty is to scoop up excess blood sugar and sore it safely in a muscle tissue. In moderation, insulin is a good guy, but it becomes a killer when its levels spike repeatedly and causes the fatty tissue to stop responding to it. Ordinarily insulin should signal the body to stop eating, but if a person has chronically elevated glucose levels due to inefficient insulin, he may eat more. Worst case scenario; diabetes, heart disease, and possibly cancer. Excess insulin can also lead to increased salt and water retention, sleep disorders, increased LDL cholesterol, and showed metabolism.

The glycemic index not only helps diabetes to control blood sugar and insulin, but provides appetite suppressing effects that help them lose weight. (In many people weight loss alone can reverse type 2 diabetes). A Swedish study of type 2 diabetes found that 4 weeks on a low GI diet lowered blood glucose and insulin by 30 percent compared to a high GI diet.

Secrets to make work for you—

1. *One per meal*: Try to choose one third to one-half of your daily starches from the low GI list.
2. *Go whole grain*: Whole grain-based foods such as barley and wheat have a low GI, mainly because their high fibre content slows digesion.
3. *Rough it up*: The least processed and rougher the grain or flour, the lower the GI.
4. Preparation can also rob foods of their natural fibres, increasing their glycemic response. Bake them and eat the skins, or boil potatoes and eat with foods high in protein. Also, the longer you cook rice, the higher you push their index rates.
5. *Fresh wins over frozen*: Dried peas and beans have substantially lower numbers than their canned or frozen brothers.
6. *Watch for added sugar*: Cold cereals tend to be sugar culpable. Exceptions are oatmeal and most bran brands.
7. *Bring down low*: Chinese food has low glycemic response if you skip the rice.

   Add some beans: Throwing in low GI foods brings down the GI rating of the entire meal. Adding some fat or protein also lowers the GI level.
8. *Be savvy about snacks*: That's fine if you are having a local snack, whether the GI is high or not. But if you are having a high GI bun, which is also high in calories, the glucose won't get blunted by other foods. So avoid starchy, high GI foods as snacks.
9. *Load up on fruits, vegetables, and legumes*: The higher the fibre, the lower (and better) the glycemic ranking.

References

Agarwal AK, Yunus M and Ahmed J. A clinical-Epidemiological study of hypertension in rural population of Jawan Block, District Aligarh (U.P) India. *J Roy. Soc. Health.* 1994.

Ahlawat SK, Singh, MM, Kumar, R *et al.* Time trends in the prevalence of hypertension and associated risk factors in Chandigarh. *J Indian Med Assoc* 2002 Sep; 100(9): 547-52, 554-5, 572.

Anand K, Chowdhury D, Singh KB, *et al.* Estimation of mortality and morbidity due to stroke in India. *Neuroepidemiology.* 2001; Vol. 20: 208-211.

Antani JA. A comparative clinical study of ischaemic heart disease in the yough and the elderly. *Indian Heart J.* 1973 Jul; 25(3): 157-60.

Arvind K, Pradepa,R,Deepa R. *et al.* Diabetes and coronary artery disease. *Indian J Med Res.* 2002 Nov; 116: 163-76.

Ashok S *et al.* Prevalence of Neuropathy in Type 2 Diabetic patients attending a Diabetes centre in South India. *J Assoc. Phy. India.* Vol. 50: 546-550.

Bahl AL. Incidence and complications of coronary heart disease. *J Indian Med Assoc.* 1968 Feb 1; 50(3): 110 passim.

Bahl VK, Prabhakaran D, Karthikeyan G. Coronary artery disease in Indians. *Indian Heart J* 2001 Nov-Dec; 53(6): 707-13.

Banerjee R. *et al.* Association of hemorheological parameters and risk of stroke in hypertensives of Indian origin. *Clin. and Exp. Hypertension.* 2000; 22: 687-694.

Banerjee TK, Mukherjee CS and Sarkhel A. Stroke in the urban population of Calcutta- An Epidemiological study. *Neuroepidemiology.* 2001; Vol. 20: 201-207-62

Beegom Raheena, Beegom Razia, Niaz MA, *et al.* Diet, Central obesity and prevalence of hypertension in the urban population of south India. *International J Cardiology.* 1995; Vol. 51: 183-191.

Begom R,Singh RB. Prevalence of coronary artery disease and its risk factors in the urban population of South and North India. *Acta Cardiol.* 1995; 50(3): 227-40.

Bhalla A, Gupta OP and Gupta SB. Predicting mortality in stroke. *Neurology India.* 2002; Vol. 50: 279-281.

Bharucha NE and Thomas Kuruvilla. Epidemiology of stroke. *NIMHANS Journal,* Vol. 17(4): Oct 1999.

Bhatia ML. Prevalence of coronary heart disease in India: a contemporary view. *Indian Heart J.* 1995 Jul-Aug; 47(4): 339-42.

Bhatnagar D, Anand, IS, Durrington PN *et al.* Coronary risk factors in people from the Indian subcontinent living in west London and their siblings in India. *Lancet.* 1995 Feb 18; 345(8947): 405-9.

Bhopal R, Unwin N, White M *et al.* Heterogencity of coronary heart disease risk factors in Indan, Pakistani, Bangladeshi, and European origin populations: cross sectional study. *BMJ* 1999 Jul 24; 319(7204):215-20.

Bhopal R. Hayes L. White M *et al.* Ethnic and socio-economic inequalities in coronary eart disease, diabetes and risk factors in Europeans and South Asians. *J Public Health Med* 2002 Jun; 24(2): 95-105.

Bhopal R. What is the risk of coronaryheart disease in South Asians? A review of UK research. *J Public Health Med* 2000 Sep; 22(3): 375-85.

Bhopal RS. Heterogencity among Indians, Pakistanis, and Bangladeshis is key to racial inequities. *BMJ* 2002 Oct 19; 325 (7369): 903.63

British Heart Foundation Statistics Website: www.heartstats.org. Chadha SL, Gopinath N, Krishnan SR, *et al.* Epidemiological study of coronary heart disease in rural population of Gurgaon Distt. (Haryana State). Indian *J Comm. Med.* 1989; Vol. 14: 141-147.

Chadha SL, Gopinath N, Ramachandran K. Epidemiological study of coronary heart disease in Gujaratis in Delhi (India). *Indian J Med Res* 1992 Apr; 96:115-21

Chadha SL, Gopinath N, Shekhawat S. Urban-rural differences in the prevalence of coronary heart disease and its risk factors in Delhi. *Bull World Health Organ.* 1997; 75(1):31-8.

Chadha SL, Radhakrishnan S, Ramachandran K *et al.* Epidemiological study of coronary heart disease in urban population of Delhi. *Indian J Med Res.* 1990 Dec; 92:424-30

Chadha SL. Problems of population based epidemiological surveys. *J Commun Dis.* 1995 Dec; 27(4): 267-71

Chakrabarti KC. Prevalence of tobacco use in Karnataka and Uttar Pradesh in India, 2001. Report of an ICMR-WHO study. W3.whosea/EN/section 1174.

Chakrabarti RN, Dutta K, Sikdar S *et al.* Smokeless tobacco and premalignant lesions of the oral cavity. *Indian J. of Med. Sci.* 1991; 45(10): 273-75

Chandalia M, Deedwania PC. Coronary heart disease and risk factors in Asian Indians. *Adv Exp Med Biol.* 2001; 498:27-34.

Chaturvedi HK, Phukan RK, Zoramtharga K *et al.* Tobacco use in Mizoram, India: sociodemographic differences in pattern. *Southeast Asian J Trop Med Public Health* 1998: 29(1); 66-70.

Compendium of India's Fertility and Mortality indicators 1971-1997 based on the Sample Registration System (SRS), Registrar General India, New Delhi 1999.

CS Ray, Gupta PC and Beyer J. Data base on tobacco control research in India (Including Betel Quid and Areca Nut), 2003, Action Council against tobacco-India. http://www.actindia.org/home.html.

Dalal PM, Dalal KP, Vyas AC, *et al.* Stroke in the young population in westcentral India- some observations on changing trends in morbidity and mortality. *Neuroepidemiology.* 1989; Vol. 8: 160-164.

Das S, Mishra RK, Jena BB *et al.* Mortality events amongst non-insulin dependent diabetes mellitus patients in Orissa. *J Assoc Physicians India* 1991 Jul; 39(7): 519-20.

Derry CW, Bourne DE, Sayed AR *et al.* Variations in mortality of the coloured, white and Asian population group in the RSA, 1978-1982. Part VI. *Ischaemic heart Disease S Afr Med J.* 1987 Nov 21; 72(10): 698-700.

Dewan BD, Malhotra KC, Gupta SP. Epidemiological study of coronary heart disease in rural community in Haryana. *Indian Heart J.* 1974 Apr; 26(2): 68-78.

Dhamija RK and Dhamija SB. Prevalence of stroke in rural community –An overview of Indian experience. *J Assoc. Phy. India.* 1998; Vol. 46. No. 4: 351-354.

Dhawan J. Coronary heart disease risks in Asian Indians. Curr Opin Lipidol 1996 Aug; 7(4): 196-8.

DhawanJ, Bray CL. Asian Indians, coronary artery disease, and physical exercise. Heart. 1997 Dec; 78(6): 550-4.

Enas EA, Garg A, Davidson MA *et al.* Coronary heart disease and its risk factors in first-generation immigrant Asian Indians to the United States of America. *Indian Heart J.* 1996 Jul-Aug; 48(4): 343-53.

Enas EA, Senthikumar, A, Juturu, V *et al.* Coronary artery disease in women. *Indian Heart J.* 2001 May-June; 53(3): 282-92.

Enas EA, Yusuf S, Mehta JL. Prevalence of coronary artery disease in Asian Indians. *Am J Cardiol* 1992 Oct 1; 70(9): 945-9.

Enas EA, Yusuf S, Sharma S. Coronary artery disease in South Asians. Second meeting of the International Working Group. 16 March 1997, Anaheim, California. *Indian Heart J.* 1998 Jan-Feb; 50(1): 105-13.

Enas EA. Coronary artery disease epidemic in Indians: a cause for alarm and call for action. *J Indian Med Assoc* 2000 Nov; 98(11): 694-5, 697-702.

Gajalakshmi CK, Ravichandran K, Shanta V. Tobacco related cancers in Madras, *India. Eur. J Cancer Prev.* 1996, 5(1): 63-68.

George A, Varghese C, Sankaranarayanan R *et al.* Use of tobacco and and alcoholic beverages by children and teenagers in a low-income coastal community in south India. *J Cancer Educ* 1994: 9(2); 111-113.

Ghosh P, Khan SA. Coronary heart disease in Indian Asians. *Lancet*. 2000 May13; 355 (9216): 1727.

Gopal Premlatha *et al.* Prevalence and risk factors of Peripheral Vascular Disease in a selected south Indian population. *Diabetes Care*. 2000; 23:1295-1300.

Gopalan C. Rising incidence of obesity, coronary heart disease and diabetes in the Indian urban middle class. Possible role of genetic and environmental factors. *World Rev Nutr Diet*. 2001; 90:127-43.

Gopinath N, Chadha S L, Jain P, *et al.* An epidemiological study of obesity in adults in the urban population of Delhi. *J Assoc. Physicians India*. 1994; Vol. 42. No. 3: 212-215.

Gopinath N, Chadha SL, Jain P *et al.* An epidemiological study of coronaryheart disease in different ethnic groups in Delhi urban population. *J Assoc Physicians India*. 1995 Jan43 (1): 30-3.

Gopinath N, Chadha SN, Sood AK, *et al.* Epidemiological Study of hypertension in young (15-24 years) Delhi urban population. *Indian J Med. Res.* 1994; Vol. 99: 32-37.

Gouri-Devi M, Rao VN, Prakash R. Neuroepidemiological study in semi urban and rural areas in South India: Pattern of neurological disorders including motor neurone disease: in Gouri-Devi M(ed): Motor Neurone disease—Global clinical patterns and international research, New Delhi, Oxford and IBH Publishing, 1987, pp 11-22.

Gupta PC and Ray CS. Tobacco and youth in the South East Asian region. *Indian Journal of Cancer*, March 2002; 39: 5-34.

Gupta PC, Mehta HC. Cohort study of all cause mortality among tobacco users in Mumbai, India. *Bull. World Health Org*. 2000; 78(7): 877-83.

Gupta PC. Health consequences of tobacco use in India. World smoking and health, Spring 1988: 5-10.

Gupta PC. Mouth cancer in India: A new epidemic? *J Indian Med Assoc* 1999; 97(9): 370-73.

Gupta PC. Survey of sociodemographic characteristics of tobacco use among 99,598 individuals in Bombay, India using hand held computers (1996); Cited in Data 67 Base on Tobacco Control Research in India. Action council against Tobacco-India, 2003. www.actindia.org,

Gupta R, Gupta VP, Ahluwalia NS, *et al.* Educational status, coronary heart disease and coronary risk factor prevalence in a rural population of India. *Brit. Med. Journal*. 1994; Vol. 39: 1332-1336.

Gupta R, Gupta VP, Prakash H *et al.* Hindu-Muslim differences in the prevalence of coronary heart disease and risk factors. *J Indian Med Assoc* 2002 Apr; 100(4): 227-30

Gupta R, Gupta VP, Sarna M *et al.* Prevalence of coronary heart disease and risk factors in an urban Indian population: Jaipur Heart Watch-2. *Indian Heart J.* 2002 Jan-Feb; 54(1): 59-66.

Gupta R, Gupta VP. Meta-analysis of coronary heart disease prevalence in India. *Indian Heart J.* 1996 May-Jun; 48(3): 241-5.

Gupta R, Gupta, HP, Keswani P. *et al.* Coronary heart disease and coronary risk factor prevalence in rural Rajasthan. *J Assoc Physicians India*. 1994 Jan; 42(1):24-.

Gupta R, Prakash H, Gupta VP, *et al.* Prevalence and Determinants of coronary heart disease in a rural population of India. *J Clini. Epi.* 1997; Vol. 50: 203-.

Gupta R, Prakash H, Gupta,VP *et al.* Prevalence and determinants of coronary heart disease in a rural population of India. *J Clin Epidemiol.* 1997 Feb; 50(2): 203-9.

Gupta R, Prakash H, Majumdar S. *et al.* Prevalence of coronary heart disease and coronary risk factors in an urban population of Rajasthan. *Indian Heart J.* 1995 Jul-Aug; 47(4): 331-8.

Gupta R, Sharma S, Gupta VP. Etal. Smoking and alcohol intake in a rural Indian population and correlation with hypertension and coronary heart disease prevalence. *J Assoc Physicians India*. 1995 Apr; 43(4): 253-8.

Gupta R, Singhal S. Coronary heart disease in India. *Circulation*. 1997 Nov 18; 96(10): 3785.

Gupta R. Lifestyle risk factors and coronary heart disease prevalence in Indian men. *J Assoc Physicians India*. 1996 Oct; 44(10): 689-93.

Gupta R. Recent trends in hypertension epidemiology in India. *South Asian J Prev. Cardi.* 2003; Vol. 7.No. 2: 90-100.

Gupta SP, Khetrapaul NK. Incidence of acute myocardial infarction and sudden coronary death in Rohtak city. *J Assoc Physicians India* 1981 May; 29(5): 365-72.

Gupta SP, Malhotra KC. Urban-rural trends in the epidemiology of coronary heart disease. *J Assoc Physicians India* 1975 Dec; 23(12): 885-92.

Gupta SR, Gupta SK, Reddy KN *et al.* Coronary artery disease in young Indian subjects. *Indian Heart J* 1987 Jul-Aug; 39(4): 284-7.

Gururaj G, Satishchandra P and Subbakrishna DK. Epidemiological correlates of stroke mortality: Observations from a tertiary institution. *Neurology India*. 1995; Vol. 43: 29-34.

Health Information of India-1999, Central Bureau of Health Intelligence, Directorate General of Health Services, Ministry of Health and Family Welfare, Government of India, New Delhi.

Heng DM, Kee Hm Chew,SK *et al.* Incidence of ischaemic heart disease and stroke in Chinese, Malays and Indians in Singapore: Singapore Cardiovascular Cohort Study. *Ann Acad Med Singapore*. 2000 Mar; 29(2): 231-6.

Hughes K, Lun KC, Yeo PP. Cardiovascular diseases in Chinese, Malays, and Indians in Singapore. I. Differences in mortality. *J Epidemiol Community Health*, 1990 Mar; 44(1): 24-8.

Hughes K. Mortality from cardiovascular diseases in Chinese, Malays and Indians in Singapore, in comparison with England and Wales, USA and Japan. Ann Acad Med Singapore 1989 Nov;18(6):642-5 Jain S and Maheshwari MC. Cerebrovascular diseases: A review of the indianexperience in the last 35 years. *Neuroepidemiology*. 1986; Vol. 5: 1-16.

Jajoo UN, Kalantri SP, Gupta OP *et al.* The prevalence of coronary heart disease in rural population from central India. *J Assoc Physicians India*, 1988 Dec; 36(12): 689-93.

Kannel WB. Framingham study insights in to hypertensive risk of cardiovascular disease. *Hypertens Res*. 1995; 18(3): 181-96.

Kaul R, Motta A and Razdan S. Epidemiology of young strokes in rural Kashmir, India. *Acta. Neuro. Scand*. 1990; Vol. 82: 1-3.

Kollapan C and Gopi PG. Tobacco smoking and pulmonary tuberculosis. *Thorak* 2002. 57: 964-66.

Krishnamurthy S, Ramaswamy R, Trivedi U *et al.*: Tobacco use in rural Indian children. *Indian Pediatr* 1997: 34(10); 923-927.

Krishnaswami S, Richard J, Prasad NK eta. Association between cigarette smoking and coronary arterial disease inpatients in India: how quantitative is? An assessment by selective coronary arteriography. *Int J Cardiol* 1991 Jun; 31(3): 305-.

Krishnaswami S, Richard J, Sathyamurthy I. Etal. Multivariate analysis of risk factors in coronary artery disease—predictive value in case detection in cardio vascular epidemiology. *Indian J Med Res*. 1984 Mar; 79:439-44.

Krishnaswami V, Radhakrishnan T. John BM. Pattern of ischaemic heart disease: a clinical study. *J Indian Med Assoc*. 1970 Sep 1; 55(5): 153-7.

Krishnaswamy S. Prevalence of coronary artery disease in India. *Indian Heart J* 2002 Jan-Feb; 54(1): 103.

Kumar S. Changing scenario of coronary artery disease. *J Indian Med Assoc*. 2000 Nov; 98(11): 682-3.

Kutty VR, Balakrishnan KG, Jayasree AK *et al.* Prevalence of coronary heart disease in the rural population of Thiruvananthapuram district, Kerala, *India. Int J Cardiol* 1993 Apr; 39(1): 59-70.

Kutty VR, Soman CR, Joseph A *et al.* Random capillary blood sugar and coronary risk factors in a south Kerala population. *J Cardiovasc Risk* 2002 Dec; 9(6): 361-7.

Lee J, Heng D, Chia KS *et al.* Risk factors and incident coronary heart disease in Chinese, Malay and Asian Indian males:;the Singapore Cardiovascular Cohort Study. *Int J Epidemiol.* 2001 Oct; 30(5): 983-8.

Malhotra KK, Behl AL. Diabetes and coronary heart disease. *J. Assoc Physicians India* 1968 Feb; 16(2): 145-50.

Malhotra P, Singh MM, Kumar R. *et al.* Coronary heart disease and its risk factors in first-generation immigrant Asian Indians to the United States of America. *Indian Heart J.* 1996 Nov-Dec; 48(6): 737-8.

Malhotra SL. Epidemiology of ischaemic heart disease in India with special reference to causation. *Br Heart J.* 1967 Nov; 29(6): 895-905.

Mammi MV, Pavithran K, Abdu Rahiman P *et al.* Acute myocardial infarction in north Kerala-a 20 year hospital based study. *Indian Heart J* 1991 Mar-Apr; 43(2): 93-6.

Masironi R, Rothwell K. Trends in and effects of smoking in the world. *World Health Stat Q.* 1988; 41(3-4): 228-41.

Mathers CD, Bernard C, Isburg KM *et al.* Global Burden of Disease in 2002: data sources methods and results. www.who.int/evidence.

Mathur KS, Wahi PN, Srivastava SK, *et al.* Prevalence of coronary heart disease in general population at Agra. *Indian J Med. Res.* 1961; Vol. 49. No: 605-610.

Medical Certification of Cause of Death 1998, Office of Registrar General India, Ministry of Home Affairs (New Delhi).

Mehta HC, Gupta PC, Sarkar S. A survey of medical college students. Action Council against Tobacco, Mumbai, 1998 (Unpublished).

Mishra VN, Mansharmani GG. Diabetes mellitus in geriatric females. *J Indian Med Assoc.* 1989 jun; 87(6): 138-9

Misra A, Pandey RM, Ramadevi J, *et al.* High prevalence of diabetes, obesity and dyslipidaemia in urban slum population in northern India. *Int. J Obesity.* 2001; Vol. 25: 1722-1729.

Misra A, Pandey RM, Sharma R. Non-communicable diseases (diabetes, obesity and hyperlipidaemia) in urban slums. *Natl. Med. J India.* 2002 Jul-Aug; 15(4): 242-4.

Mohan V, Deepa R, Rani SS *et al.* Prevalence of coronary artery disease and its relationship to lipids in a selected population in South India: The Chennai Urban Population Study (CUPS No. 5). *J Am Coll Cardiol.* 2001 Sep; 38(3): 682-7.

Mohan V, Vijayaprabha R, Rema M. Vascular complications in long-term south Indian NIDDM of over 25 years' duration. *Diabetes Res Clin Pract.* 1996 Mar; 31(1-3): 133-40.

Mohan V. *et al.* Intra-urban differences in the prevalence of the metabolic syndrome in southern India—the Chennai Urban Population Study (CUPS No. 4). *Diabetic Medicine.* 2001; 18: 280-287.

Mukherjee S. Tobacco use in a village community in Kheda District, Gujarat, Department of Preventive and Social Medicine, PS Medical College, Karamsad, Gujarat, January 1999 (Unpublished).

Mukhtar HT, Littler WA. Survival after acute myocardial infarction in Asian and white patients in Birmingham. *Br Heart J* 1995 Feb; 73(2): 122-4.

Mulay DV. Coronary prognostic index in acute myocardial infarction. *Indian Heart J* 1985 Jan-Feb; 37(1): 32-6.

Murray CJ, Lopez AD. Global mortality, disability and the contribution of risk factors: Global Burden of Disease Study. *Lancet.* 1997 May 17; 349 (9063): 1436-42.

Murray CJ, Lopez AD. Mortality by cause for eight regions of the world: Global Burden of Disease Study. *Lancet.* 1997 May 3; 349(9061): 1269-76.

Murray CJ, Lopez AD. The Global Burden of Disease. Harvard University Press, 1996.

Nadir EB, Bharucha EP, Bharucha EA, *et al.* Prevalence of stroke in the Parsi community of Bombay. *Stroke.* 1988; Vol. 19. No. 1: 60-62.

Nagarajan D. *et al.* Risk Factor for Stroke: Relative Risk in Young and Elderly. *Neurology India.* 1998; 46 183-184.

Naik CH. Incidence and epidemiology oc coronary artery disease in Gujarat. *Indian Heart J.* 1968 Jan; 20(1): 3-10.

Nandkumar A, Anantha N, Pattabhiraman V *et al.* Importance of anatomical subsite in correlating risk factors in cancers of the oesophagus—report of a case control study. *Br. J Cancer.* 1996; 73: 1306-11.

National Cancer Registry Programme, Two-year report of the Population Based Cancer Registries 1997-98. Incidence and Distribution of Cancer, Indian Council of Medical Research (New Delhi).

Nayak Dinesh, Nair M, Radhakrishnan K, *et al.* Ischaemic stroke in the young adult: clinical features, risk factors and outcomes. *The National Med. J India.* 1997; Vol. 10. No. 3: 107-112.

NBD YLD WORKBOOK (version 0.0.), Nov 7,2002. Epidemiology and Burden of Disease Team, Global Program on Evidence for Health Policy, (EBD/GPE/EIP). World Health Organisation, Geneva, Switzerland. http://www.who.int/evidence/bod.

Padmavati S. Is heart disease on the increase in India? *India Heart J.* 1972 Apr; 24(2): 69-71.

Pahlajani DB, Chawla, MH, Kapashi,KA. Coronary artery disease pattern in the young. *J Assoc Physicians India.* 1989 May; 37(5): 312-4.

Pais P, Pogue J, Gerstein H. Risk factors for acute myocardial infarction in Indians: a case control study. *Lancet* 1996 Aug 10; 348 (9024): 358-63.

Park D, Desai P, Aiyengar J *et al.* Geographic differences in the characteristics of coronary artery disease in India. *Int J Cardiol.* 1998 Dec 1; 67(2): 187-9.

Patadin Svati *et al.* Impaired glucose tolerance and diabetes mellitus in a rural population in South India. *Diab. Res. Clin.* Practice.1994; 24: 47-53.

Pearson TA. Cardiovascular disease in developing countries: myths, realities, and opportunities. *Cardiovasc Drugs Ther.* 1999 Apr; 1(2): 95-104.

Pella D, Thomas N, Tomlinson B *et al.* Prevention of coronary artery disease: the south Asian paradox. *Lancet* 2003 Jan 4; 361 (9351): 79.

Population Projections for India and States 1996-2016, Registrar General India, New Delhi 1996.

Pradeepa R and Mohan V. The changing scenario of diabetes epidemic: Implications for India. Indian *J Med. Res.* 2002; Vol. 116: 121-132.

Pradeepa R, Deepa R, Mohan V. Epidemiology of diabetes in India- Current perspective and future projections. *J Indian Med.* Assoc. 2002; Vol. 100. No. 3: 144-

Proceedings of the ICMR-WHO workshop on Burden of Non-Communicable Diseases (6th – 8th October 2003); Indian Council of Medical Research (New Delhi).

Raheja BS, Bhoraskar AS, Narang S. Risk factors for coronary heart disease in Asian Indians. *Lancet.* 1996 Nov 2; 348 (9036): 1241-2.

Rajadurai J,Arokiasamy J, Pasamanickam K *et al.* Coronary artery disease in Asians. *Aust N Z J Med* 1992 Aug; 22(4): 345-8.

Rajmohan L, Deepa R, Mohan V. Risk factors for coronary artery disease in Indians: emerging trends. *Indian Heart J.* 2000 Mar-Apr; 52(2): 221-5.

Ramachandran A, Snehlata C and Vijay V. Burden of type 2 diabetes and its complications- The Indian scenario. *Current Science (Special Section: Diabetes).* 2002; Vol. 83. No. 12: 1471-1476.

Ramachandran *et al.* High prevalence of diabetes and impaired glucose tolerance in India: National Urban Diabetes Survey. *Diabetologia* 2001; 44: 1094-.

Raman Kutty V, Balakrishnan KG, Jayasree AK, *et al.* Prevalence of coronary heart disease in the rural population of Thiruvananthpuram district, Kerla, *India. Int. J Cardi.* 1993; Vol. 39: 59-70.

Raman kutty V, CR Soman, Joseph A, *et al.* Type 2 diabetes in southern Kerla: Variation in prevalence among geographic divisions within a region. *National Med. J India.* 2000; Vol. 13. No. 6: 287-292.

Ramani A, Bilgrami NL, Kumar S. Morbidity and mortality of acute myocardial infarction in and around Aligarh. *J Indian Med Assoc.* 1990 Jul; 88(7): 192-5

Raychaudhuri B. Editorial: Causes of death in diabetes. *J Indian Med Assoc.* 1973 Jul 1; 61(1): 10-1.

Razdan S, Koul RL, Motta A, *et al.* Cerebrovascular diseases: in rural Kashmir, India. *Stroke.* 1989; Vol. 20. No. 12: 1691-1693.

RCP (1962). Royal College of Physicians. Smoking and health. London: Pitman Medical Publishing.

Reddy KK, Rao AP, Reddy TP. Socioeconomic status and the prevalence of coronary heart disease risk factors. *Asia Pac J Clin Nutr* 2002; 11(2): 98-103.

Reddy NK, Kumar DN, Rayudu NV *et al.* Prevalence of risk factors for coronary atherosclerosis in a cross-sectional population of Andhra Pradesh. *Indian Heart J.* 2002 Nov-Dec; 54(6): 697-701.

Report of ICMR Collaborative Study on Coronary Heart Disease (1989-94); Christian Medical College, Vellore.

Report of ICMR Collaborative Study on Coronary Heart Disease (1989-94); All India Institute of Medical Sciences, New Delhi.

Report of the expert committee on the economics of tobacco use. March 2002, Ministry of Health and Family Welfare (New Delhi).

Sainani GS, Bichile SK, Mehta PJ *et al.* Epidemiology of coronary heart disease (CHD). *J Assoc Physicians India.* 1988 Dec; 36(12): 685.

Sample Registration System Statistical Report 1998. Registrar General of India, New Delhi.

Sample Registration System, Statistical Report 2000. Registrar General, India (New Delhi).

Sankarnarayanan R, Verghese C, Duffy SW *et al.* A case control study of diet and lung cancer in Kerala. *Int. J. Cancer* 1994; 58: 644-49.

Sarvotham SG, Berry JN. Prevalence of coronary heart disease in an urban population in northern India. Circulation 1968 Jun; 37(6): 939-53.

Sathe RV. The problem of diabetes mellitus in India. *J Indian Med Assoc.* 1973 Jul 1; 61(1): 12-6.

Sattar NA, Gaw S. Risk of coronary heart disease in Asian women. *BKN.* 1995 Feb 18; 310(6977): 466-7.

Seedat YK. Hypertension and ischaemic heart disease in Indian people living in South Africa and in India. *S Afr Med J* 1982 Jun 19; 61(25): 965-7.

Seedat YK. Hypertension and vascular disease in India and migrant Indian population in the world. *J Hum Hypertens.* 1990 Aug; 4(4); 421-4.

Sen U. A High School Survey. Epidemiology and Biostatistics, Chittaranjan National Cancer Institute, Calcutta, 1999 (Unpublished).

Sewdarsen M, Vythilingum S, Jialal I *et al.* Risk factors in young Indian males with myocardial infarction. *S Aft Med J* 1987 Apr 4; 71(7): 469-70.

Singh AK. Myocardial infarction in the young. *J Assoc Physicians India.* 1992 Aug; 40(8): 553.

Singh RB, Bajaj S, Niaz MA etl. Prevalence of type 2 diabetes mellitus and risk of hypertension and coronary artery disease in rural and urban population with low rates of obesity. *Int J Cardiol.* 1998 Sep 1; 66(1): 65-72.

Singh RB, Beegom R, Mehta AS *et al.* Social class, coronary risk factors and undernutrition, a double burden of diseases, in women during transition, in five Indian cities. *Int J Cardiol.* 1999 May 15; 69(2): 139-47.

Singh RB, Niaz MA, Ghosh S. *et al.* Epidemiological study of coronary artery disease and its risk factors in an elderly urban population of north India. *J Am Coll Nutr.* 1995 Nov 24; 52(2): 95-9.

Singh RB, Niaz MA. An epidemiological study of coronary heart disease (CHD). *J Assoc Physicians India.* 1995 Sep; 43(9): 653-4.

Singh RB, Niaz MA. Coronary risk factors in Indians. *Lancet.* 1995 Sep 16; 346(8977): 778-9.

Singh RB, Niaz MA. Prevention of coronary heart disease in Indians. *J Assoc Physicians India.* 1994 Jul; 42(7): 545-8.

Singh RB, Sharma JP, Rastogi V *et al.* Prevalence of coronary artery disease and coronary risk factors in rural and urban populations of north India. *Eur Heart J.* 1997 Nov; 18(11): 1728-35.

Singh RB, Sharma, JP, Rastogi V. *et al.* Social class and coronary disease in rural population of north India. The Indian Social Class and Heart Survey. *Eur Heart J.* 1997 Apr; 18(4): 588-95.

Singh RB, Verma SP, Niaz MA. Social class and coronary artery disease in India. *Lancet.* 1999 Jan 9; 353(9147): 154.

Singh RN, Niaz MA, Thakur,AS *et al.* Social class and coronary artery disease in a urban population of North India in the Indian Lifestyle and Heart Study. *Int J Cardiol.* 1998 Apr 1; 64(2): 195-203.

Sinha BC. Pattern of ischaemic heart disease in India. *J Indian Med Assoc* 1970 Sep 1; 55(5): 171-3.

Sinha DN, Hai AA. Tobacco menance in Young Students of Patna, Bihar, 1999 (Unpublished).

Sinha PR, Gaur SD, Somani PN, *et al.* Prevalence of coronary heart disease in urban community of Varanasi. *Indian J Comm. Med.* 1990; Vol. 15. No. 2: 182-185.

Sridharan R. Risk factors for ischemic stroke: A case-control analysis. *Neuroepidemiology* 1992; 11: 24-30.

Swami HM, Bhatia V, Gupta M, *et al.* Population based study of hypertension among the elderly in northern India. Public Health. 2002; Vol. 116: 45-49.

Tan AT, Emmanuel SC, Tan BY. Myocardial infarction in Singapore: a nationwide 10-year study of multiethnic differences in incidence and mortality. *Ann Acad Med Singapore* 2002 Jul; 31(4): 479-86.

Taylor SP, Epstein L, Disler PB *et al.* Variations in mortality of the coloured, white and Asian population group in the RSA, 1978-1982. Part V. Hypertensive diseases. *S Afr Med J.* 1987 Nov 21; 72(10): 696-8.

Thomas G. Final report on tobacco risks from a case-control study. *Indian Heart J.* 2002 Jan-Feb; 54(1): 111.

Trivedi DH, Sharma V, Pandya H. *et al.* Longitudinal epidemiological study of coronary heart disease in a rural population of Kheda district, Gujarat, India. *Soz Praventivmed.* 1996; 41(6): 373-9.

Ughade Suresh N. Zodpey Sanjay P. *et al.* Risk factor for Cataract: A Case Control Study. *Indian J Opthalmology* 1998; 46: 221-227.

USDHHS (1964). US Department of Health and Human Services. Smoking and Health. Report of the advisory committee to the Surgeon General. Washington DC: US Government Printing Office (PHS publication No. 1103).

Vaidya SG, Vaidya NS, Naik UD. Epidemiology of tobacco habits in Goa, India. In: Gupta PC, Hamner JE III, Murthi PR,eds Control of Tobacco-Related Cancers and Other Diseases: Proceedings of an International Symposium, January 15- 19, 1990. TIFT. Bombay. Mumbai: Oxford University Press, 1992: 315-329.

Vaidya SG, Vaidya NS, Naik UD. Epidemiology of tobacco habits in Goa, India (1996):

Cited in Data Base on Tobacco Control Research in India. Action Council against Tobacco- India, 2003. www.actindia.org.

Vallapuri S, Gupta D, Talwar KK *et al.* Comparison of atherosclerotic risk factors in Asian Indian and American Caucasian patients with angiographic cronary artery disease. *Am J Cardiol* 2002 Nov 15; 90(10): 1147-50.

Vardan S, Mookherjee S, Vardan S. *et al.* Special features of coronary heart disease in people of the Indian sub-continent. *Indian Heart J.* 1995 Jul-Aug; 47(4): 399-407.

Walker AR. Problems in studying the epidemiology of coronaryheart disease in unsophisticated populations. *Am Heart J.* 1970 Dec; 80(6): 725-8.

Wander GS, Khurana,SB, Gulati R. *et al.* Epidemiology of coronary heart disease in a rural Punjab population—prevalence and correlation with various risk factors. *Indian Heart J.* 1994 Nov-Dec; 46(6): 319-23.

Wiebel FJ. Health effects of passive smoking. In: Bolliger CT and Fagerstrom KO (eds). The tobacco epidemic. Progress in respiratory research, Vol. 28, Karger, Basel, 1997; 107-121.

Wierzbicki AS, Swaminathan R. Coronaryheart disease in Indian Asians. *Lancet.* 2000 May 12; 355(9216): 1727-8.

Wild SH, Laws A, Fortmann SP. Etal. Mortality from coronary heart disease and stroke for six ethnic groups in California, 1985 to 1990. *Ann Epidemiol* 1995 Nov; 5(6): 432-9.

Wilkinson P, Sayer J, Laji K *et al.* Comparison of case fatality in south Asian and white patients after acute myocardial infarction: observational study. *BMJ.* 1996 May 25; 312(7042): 1330-3.

Wong KS. Risk factors for early death in acute ischemic stroke and intracerebral hemorrhage: A prospectivehospital-based study in Asia. Asian Acute Stroke Advisory Panel. *Stroke.* 1999 Nov; 30(11): 2326-30.

Yeolekar ME. Coronary artery disease in Asian Indians. *J Postgrad Med.* 1998 Jan-Mar; 44(1): 26-8.

Yeolekar ME. Epidemiology oc coronary heart disease. *J Assoc Physicians India* 1989 Jul; 37(7): 479-80.

Yudkin JS. Non-insulin-dependent diabetes mellitus (NIDDM) in Asians in the UK. *Diabet Med.* 1996 Sep; 13(9 Suppl 6): S16-8.

Yusuf S, Ounpuu S. Tackling the growing epidemic of cardiovascular disease in South Asia. J Am Coll Cardiol 2001 Sep; 38(3): 688-9. Murray, C. J. L., and Lopez, A.D. *The Global Burden of Disease.* Geneva: World Health Organisation. (2000). *World Health Report 2000—Health Systems: Improving Performance.*

3

Immunisation in Hospitals: Extension Services Essential

For more than 200 years, since Edward Jenner first demonstrated that vaccination offered protection against smallpox, the use of vaccines has continued to reduce the burden of many bacterial and viral diseases. As a result of successful vaccination programmes, deaths from polio, hepatitis, tetanus, diphtheria, *Haemophilus influenzae* type b and measles are now on the decline. Vaccination not only protects individuals, but also others in the community, by increasing the general level of immunity and minimizing the spread of infection. It is vital that hospitals take every available opportunity to vaccinate children and adults. It is also important that the public be made aware of the proven effectiveness of immunisation to save lives and prevent serious illness. Even now 13 millions deaths occur every year among children and young adults due to infectious diseases. In developing countries 45% of all deaths are due to infectious diseases, whereas 63% of all deaths among children are due to infectious diseases. Acute respiratory infections are the commonest cause of deaths. 3-4 lakhs of children die due to infectious diseases every year.

Immunisation; Primary as well as extended duty of every hospital

Immunisation is one of the most cost-effective health interventions known to mankind. In the relatively short time that we have used this tool, small pox has been eradicated and we are at the threshold of eliminating polio. With the availability of many newer .vaccines, it is necessary that some of these should be considered for routine immunisation and the immunisation schedule has to be changed from the recommendations of the government of India or WHO.

Most of the hospitals have provision to administer vaccines to children and some have facilities for adolescents and adults as well.

However awareness about the importance of vaccination is not universal and some resistance is still visible in backward areas. Immunisation is one of the outstanding public health successes of developing countries. Millions of children who would have died of vaccine preventable diseases, like measles, are now able to lead healthy lives, thanks to government and NGO efforts in the past two decades. This heartening success story has been achieved at a remarkably low cost. Immunisation in developing countries is one of the most efficient health interventions, costing less than US$15 to fully immunize a child. Though vaccination has been established as a simple and cost effective mode of ensuring child survival, it has been found in several studies that 'nearly two in five have not had all of the recommended vaccinations by age five'. These findings have been upheld according to an analysis of data from the 1992-1993 National Family Health Survey (Pande, R.P., Selective gender differences in childhood immunisation in rural India: Demography, 2003, 40(3): 395-418). Differences between boys and girls in these associations suggest both that parents value sons much more, over daughters and that they "may discriminate selectively" depending on whether they have achieved the 'son', they had desired in their family.

A representative schedule of vaccination

Baby Name:	Namita
Date of Birth:	Friday, March 08, 2002
Date	**Immunisation Due**
9 March-18 March	BCG OPV - Oral polio vaccine - I dose Hepatitis B - Ist dose
8 April 2002	DPT - Diphtheria/Pertusis/Tetanus - I dose OPV - II dose HiB - Haemophilus Influenza B - I dose Hepatitis B - II dose (if started before)
18 May 2002	DPT - II dose OPV - III dose HiB - II dose (if started before)
18 June 2002	DPT - III dose OPV - IV dose HiB - III dose (if started before) Hep B

3 November 2002	Measles
1 June 2003	MMR Chicken Pox
30 August 2003	DPT - I booster OPV - I booster Typhoid
26 February 2004	Typhoid Hep A
7 March 2007	DPT - II booster OPV - II booster Typhoid (if given before)
5 March 2012	TT
4 March 2017	TT Rubella

This is the schedule followed by most of the doctors in India. There may be small variations in practice in different centres.

Recommendations of the IAP Committee on Immunisation

Age	*Vaccines*	*Note*
Birth	BCG OPV zero Hepatitis B -1	
6 weeks	OPV-1 + IPV-1/OPV -1 DTPw-1/DTPa -1 Hepatitis B -2 Hib -1	OPV alone if IPV cannot be given
10 weeks	OPV-2 + IPV-2/OPV-2 DTPw-2/DTPa -2 Hib -2	OPV alone if IPV cannot be given
14 weeks	OPV-3 + IPV-3/OPV -3 DTPw-3/DTPa -3 Hepatitis B-3 Hib -3	OPV alone if IPV cannot be given Third dose of Hepatitis B can be given at 6 months of age
9 months	Measles	
15-18 months	OPV-4 + IPV-B1/OPV-4 DTPw booster -1 or DTPa booster -1 Hib booster MMR -1	OPV alone if IPV cannot be given

2 years	Typhoid	Revaccination every 3-4 years
5 years	OPV - 5 DTPw booster - 2 or DTPa booster - 2	
	MMR - 2	The second dose of MMR vaccine can be given at any time 8 weeks after the first dose
10 years	Tdap HPV	Only girls, three doses at 0, 1-2 and 6 months

Vaccines that can be given after discussion with parents

More than 6 weeks	Pneumococcal conjugate	3 primary doses at 6, 10, and 14 weeks, followed by a booster at 15-18 months
More than 6 weeks	Rotaviral vaccines	(2/3 doses (depending on brand) at 4-8 weeks interval
After 15 months	Varicella	Age less than 13 years: one dose Age more than 13 years: 2 doses at 4-8 weeks interval
After 18 months	Hepatitis A	2 doses at 6-12 months interval

1. The IAP endorses the continued use of whole cell pertussis vaccine because of its proven efficacy and safety. Acellular pertussis vaccines may undoubtedly have fewer side-effects (like fever, local reactions at injection site and irritability), but this minor advantage does not justify the inordinate cost involved in the routine use of this vaccine.
2. If the mother is known to be HBsAg negative, HB vaccine can be given along with DTP at 6, 10, 14 weeks/6 months. If the mother's HBsAg status is not known, it is advisable to start vaccination soon after birth to prevent perinatal transmission of the disease. If the mother is HBsAg positive (and especially HBeAg positive), the baby should be given Hepatitis B Immune Globulin (HBIG) within 24 hours of birth, along with HB vaccine.
3. Varicella, Hepatitis A and Pneumococcal Conjugate vaccines should be offered only after one to one discussion with parents. Also refer to the individual vaccines notes for recommendations.
4. Combination vaccines can be used to decrease the number of pricks being given to the baby and to decrease the number of clinic visits. The manufacturer's instructions should be followed strictly whenever "mixing" vaccines in the same syringe prior to injection.

5. At present, the only typhoid vaccine available in our country is the Vi polysaccharide vaccine. Revaccination may be carried out every 3-4 years.
6. Under special circumstances (e.g. epidemics), measles vaccine may be given earlier than 9 months followed by MMR at 12-15 months.
7. During pregnancy, the interval between the two doses of TT should be at least one month.
8. We should continue to use OPV till we achieve polio eradication in India. IPV can be used additionally for individual protection.
9. OPV must be given to children less than 5 years of age at the time of each supplementary immunisation activity.

Alternative immunisation schedule:

- At Birth: Hepatitis B #1 (Birth to 2 months)
- 2 months: Hepatitis B #2 (1-4 months), DTaP, Hib, IPV, PCV
- 4 months: DTaP, Hib, IPV, PCV
- 6 months: Hepatitis B #3 (6-18 months), DTaP, Hib, PCV
- 12 months: Varicella, PCV (12-15 months)
- 15-18 months: DTaP/Hib combo, IPV, MMR
- 2-5 years: PCV (Children with chronic illness such as ear infections or a compromised immune system)
- 2-18 years: Hepatitis A (Selected areas. Contact your local health department)
- 4-6 years: DTaP, IPV, MMR
- 11-12 years: Hepatitis B (if not vaccinated in infancy); MMR (if did not receive second dose); Varicella (if lacking a reliable history); Td
- Every 10 years: Td

Hepatitis B is a disease of the liver that can lead to liver failure and/ or liver cancer. Most children do not have any side effects from the vaccine. However some children may experience a mild fever, soreness at the injection site, and fussiness.

DtaP is a vaccine against diphtheria, tetanus, and pertussis (whooping cough). The DTaP vaccine is different from DTP in that is uses acellular pertussis, causing fewer side effects. Diphtheria is a very serious disease that can make a person unable to breathe, cause paralysis, or heart failure. Tetanus (lockjaw) is a disease making a person unable to open his mouth or swallow and causes serious muscle spasms. Pertussis (whooping cough) is a disease causing spells of coughing and choking that make it difficult to eat, drink, or breathe. Most children do not have any side effects from the vaccine. However some children may experience a mild fever, soreness at the injection site for 1-2 days, fussiness, and crying. Hib is a vaccine against Haemophilus influenzae type B that causes many dangerous infections such as meningitis, epiglottitis, pneumonia, and others. It is not the flu. It may be given in a three-dose or a four-dose schedule, depending on the vaccine. Most children do not have any side effects from the vaccine. However some children may experience a mild fever, soreness at the injection site, and fussiness. These side effects can last 1-3 days.

Polio is a disease causing permanent paralysis, difficulty breathing, or death. The vaccine can be given as an injection called inactivated polio vaccine (IPV). The IPV injection is the recommended method in the United States with the exception using Oral Polio Vaccine for controlling outbreaks of paralytic polio; unvaccinated children who will be traveling to endemic or epidemic areas within 4 weeks; children of parents who do not accept the recommended number of vaccine injections. Some side effects of the vaccine are soreness and redness at the injection site. Now the vaccine is available in India as well.

All currently used IPV vaccines are enhanced potency IPV (eIPV) that contains 40, 8 and 32 D antigen units of type 1, 2 and 3 respectively. It is highly immunogenic. Seroconversion rates are 90-95% after two doses given after the age of 2 months at 2 months interval and 99% after three doses when it is started at 6 weeks of age and given at 4 weeks interval. IPV can be used in combination with DTwP and Hib vaccines without compromising seroconversion or increasing side effects. IPV produces excellent systemic/local pharyngeal immunity and some intestinal immunity. Observations from use of the vaccine in the USA and other developed countries indicate that IPV has excellent herd effect. The vaccine is very safe.

IAPCOI Recommendations

The latest recommendations of the polio eradication committee of the IAP have been published. This document highlighted the potential utility of IPV in two key areas (a) to curb wild virus transmission in UP and Bihar (b) switch to IPV DPT combination in polio free states in preparation for the post polio eradication era (in this era OPV use will have to stop but vaccination against polio cannot stop, i.e. switch to IPV is inevitable). Here we discuss the latest recommendations of IAPCOI regarding use of IPV by IAP members in office practice.

In its earlier update (May 2007) IAPCOI had recommended use of IPV in conjunction with OPV in children after one to one discussion with parents. The IAPCOI now recommends offering additional use of IPV with OPV in all children who can afford the vaccine (Category 2) in the schedule discussed below. This change in categorisation of IPV and recommending wider use of IPV is for the following reasons:

- Excellent immunogenicity, efficacy and safety of IPV.
- Switch to IPV is inevitable in post polio eradication era. This switch cannot happen overnight due to large number of doses

that will be required and has to be in a phased manner. IAP-PEC has already recommended that the government gradually introduce IPV in polio free states to facilitate this switch. By promoting use of IPV in the private sector, the committee hopes to create a demand base for the vaccine, increased supply and lower cost of the vaccine.

The committee recommends continuing OPV use for the following reasons:

- In concordance with the government policy of using OPV for polio eradication.
- Mucosal immunity as measured by stool excretion of virus after mOPV1 challenge is superior with combination of OPV and IPV as compared to IPV alone.
- By not giving OPV we might create confusion in the minds of the parents whose children receive only IPV about the efficacy and safety of OPV and interfere with OPV uptake on the national Immunisation Days (NID's) and Sub National Immunisation Days (SNID's). Also as a cascade effect there might be some individuals who might not give immunisation with OPV due to fear of side effects and neither give IPV due to non-affordability.
- The risk of VAPP with this combined OPV and IPV schedule is extremely low as the child receives OPV at the time when he/she is protected against VAPP by maternal anti-bodies(44). Subsequently, he/she is protected from VAPP by IPV. Even if we adopt an all IPV schedule the child may still be at a small risk for VAPP through exposure to the oral polio vaccine virus through contacts/environment before he/she receives his/her first dose of IPV.

The IAPCOI feels that in the current scenario where polio eradication in India is at the cross roads and a highly sensitive issue, the combined OPV and IPV schedule strives to provide the best of protection to an individual child while not deviating from the national immunisation policies.

Some other vaccines

Pneumococcal vaccine is not given routinely, it is only for those on risk. Single dose is given after the age of 2 years. Similarly chicken pox is also given to only those who are at risk, at the age of 12 months to 12 years. The vaccine is given 2 doses at 3 moths apart. MMR is given as a single dose at 12-15 months of age, can be repeated at 5-6 years of age.

Combination Vaccines

Recommendations of the IAP Committee on Immunisation

A combination vaccine consists of two or more separate immunogens that have been physically combined in a single preparation. These immunogens may pertain to the many antigens/serotypes of the given pathogen (e.g. poliovirus vaccines) or of multiple pathogens (e.g. DTP vaccine). This concept differs from that of simultaneous vaccines, which, although administered concurrently, are physically separate.

The combining of multiple related or unrelated antigens into a single vaccine is not a new concept. The first combination vaccine was trivalent influenza vaccine, which was developed as far back as 1945. This was followed by hexavalent pneumococcal vaccine in 1947 and DTP vaccine in 1948. Combination vaccines in common use include diphtheria and tetanus toxoid, available alone (DT, dT) or with pertussis vaccine (DTP); inactivated (IPV) or live oral (OPV) trivalent polio vaccine and MMR vaccine.

The number of vaccines in the immunisation schedule is increasing every year with the result that these schedules are getting increasingly more complex. Many parents opt for one single injection of combination vaccines at a given visit, rather than getting a large number of simultaneous injections. Use of combination vaccines is also likely to result in logistic advantages—reduced burden on the cold chain and reduced storage requirements and syringes/needles apart from easier record keeping. A number of combination vaccines are now available in the Indian market.

The IAP COI endorses the use of combination vaccines, but with the following cautionary statements:

- The manufacturer's recommendations should be adhered to strictly.
- "Mixing" of vaccines in the same syringe (prior to injection) should not be done as far as possible, unless specifically recommended by the manufacturer. In the latter case the manufacturer's instructions should be followed strictly.
- Combination vaccines should not be viewed as being more effective than vaccines given separately.

Current status of new combination vaccines

Already developed

DTPw + Hib
DTPw + Hepatits B
DTPw + IPV
DTPw + IPV + Hib
DTPw + Hib + Hepatits B
DTPw + Hib + IPV

DTPw - hIPV
DTPa + IPV
DTPa + Hib
DTPa + Hib + Hepatits B + IPV
Hepatitis A + Hepatitis B
MMR + Varicella
Under development
DTPa + Hib + IPV + Hepatitis B + Hepatitis A
Available for use in India
DTPw + Hib.
DTPw + HB
DTPw + Hib + HB
DTPa + Hib
HA+HB

MMR

MMR is a vaccine against measles, mumps, and rubella. Measles is a disease causing high fever, cough, rash, and possible brain infection. Mumps is a disease causing fever, headache, and swollen painful glands under the jaw. The disease lasts several days and can lead to meningitis (infection of spinal fluid) and hearing loss. Rubella (German measles) is a mild disease causing mild fever, swollen neck glands, and a rash lasting about 3 days. Rubella is very dangerous to pregnant women because it can severely harm the unborn baby. Children who have had a serous allergic reaction to eggs requiring the attention of a doctor should not receive the measles and mumps part of this vaccine. Some side effects of the vaccine are soreness at the injection site lasting 1-2 days. Some side effects may appear 1-2 weeks after the vaccine was given. They include rash, fever of 103°F, swelling in lymph glands of the neck lasting 1-2 days, and mild pain in the joints lasting 3 days.

Varicella

Varicella is a vaccine against chicken pox. Chicken pox is a disease causing a skin rash over the scalp and body, moving to the face, arms, and legs. The skin rash turns into 250-500 itchy blisters that will dry up and scab 2-4 days later. Mild fever may be present as well. Chicken pox may return as Shingles in adults. This is a very painful disorder involving the nerve roots. It causes numbness, itching, and severe pain. Most children do not have any side effects from the vaccine. However, some children may experience a mild fever, redness and soreness at the injection site, stiffness, nausea and fussiness. Some may also experience a mild rash 1 month after the vaccine was given.

Td is a vaccine against tetanus and diphtheria. Some side effects of the vaccine are mild fever, soreness, swelling, and redness lasting 1-2 days.

Pneumococcal Conjugate Vaccine

Pneumococcal Conjugate Vaccine (PCV) protects against pneumococcal diseases such as bacterial meningitis (an infection of the brain and spinal cord), blood infections and ear infections. Children who have experienced a previous allergic reaction (life-threatening) to this vaccine should not receive it again. If your child is moderately to severely ill, your physician may withhold this vaccine. Children with a cold may receive this vaccine per their physician. Most children do not experience any side effects from this vaccine. Some, however, may develop redness, tenderness or swelling at the injection site and/or a mild fever.

Typhoid Vaccines

Enteric fever is endemic in India and is a major public health problem. Three vaccines were available for clinical use till recently. However now only the Vi typhoid vaccine is available commercially.

The Whole Cell Inactivated Typhoid Vaccine (TA/TAB)

Heat-killed, phenol-preserved or the acetone inactivated lyophilised whole cell Salmonella typhi vaccines were inexpensive products that have been in use in India for a long time. The protective efficacy of acetone inactivated preparation is more than that of the phenol preserved vaccine but the former is more difficult to prepare and is associated with more side-effects. Both vaccines contain Salmonella typhi 1000 million organisms per ml.

Protection begins 4 weeks after vaccination. Use of these vaccines may be associated with fever, local pain and malaise due to the endotoxins in bacterial cell wall. A pure S. typhi vaccine is less reactogenic than the combined TA/TAB vaccines. The vaccine is very safe and is reasonably effective if revaccination can be carried out on a regular basis. The vaccine efficacy has been estimated to be 50-70% in a meta-analysis of the randomized controlled trials available.

The vaccine appears to be protective through the induction of antibodies against cell wall somatic (0) and flagellar (H) antigens. These antibodies can act as a biological marker of the vaccine. It may interfere with the interpretation of the Widal test. It is effective even in children below 2 years of age and can be given to infants over 6 months of age. Primary vaccination requires two doses, 4 or more weeks apart, given subcutaneously. Pediatric dose of the vaccine is 0.25 ml in children aged 6 months-10 years and 0.5 ml in order children. The vaccine should be stored at 2-8°C. It should never be frozen. Revaccination is necessary every 2-3 years to sustain an optimal immune response and should be done preferably before the onset of summer.

Unfortunately, this vaccine is not being manufactured in India at present.

The Vi-Capsular Polysaccharide Vaccine

The vaccine consists of purified Vi-capsular polysaccharide, which during natural infection inhibits phagocytosis and serum bactericidal activity and is responsible for virulence of the bacteria. It has reasonable efficacy of 50-60% in children and low reactogenicity. Protection begins within two weeks of vaccination and the biological marker is anti-Vi antibodies. It is not very effective in children below two years of age because it is an unconjugated polysaccharide vaccine as available in our country at present. The vaccine is now reasonably priced. The vaccine is available as an isotonic phenolated buffer solution. The dose is 0.5 ml, containing 25 mcg of the polysaccharide. It can be given intramuscularly or subcutaneously. The vaccine should be stored at 2-8°C. It should never be frozen. Adverse effects are mild and include pain and swelling at injection site.

Oral Live Attenuated Ty21 a Vaccine

Salmonella typhi Ty21 a is a live attenuated strain with a mutation in gal E gene and lacks the enzyme UDP-gal 4 epimerase. It is genetically stable and is not known to revert to virulence. The efficacy has been shown to be 50-60% with the capsule form and nearly 90% with the liquid form (not available commercially). It provides protection by inducing local gut immunity but there is no biological marker of this vaccine. The vaccine is supplied in an enteric coated formulation as the bacteria are acid labile. It can be given to children six years of age and above as the capsules have to be swallowed intact.

The vaccine is given on an empty stomach in three sittings, on alternate days. The capsule should never be opened before ingestion. Protection begins within a week after completion of the course and the protective efficacy is as good as other available typhoid vaccines. Immunisation needs to be repeated every 3-5 years.

The vaccine should be stored at 2-8"C. Antimicrobials active against S. typhi should not be used 3 days before and 7 days after oral typhoid vaccine administration as these may interfere with the vaccine "take." Unfortunately this vaccine is also not available now in our country.

The efficacy of all typhoid vaccines at best is 50-70%.

Immunisation is not 100% protective

The analyses of immunisation (i.e., whether children had received the full complement of tuberculosis, polio, measles and diphtheria-pertussis-tetanus vaccinations recommended by the World Health Organisation) included more than 25,000 children 12-60 months old. Both samples of children were equally divided between boys and girls. In each, roughly one-quarter of children had no older surviving siblings, one-third had a mix of brothers and sisters, and the rest had only sisters or only brothers; the average family included three children. Mothers were predominantly illiterate, and about one in six had more than a primary education. Half of children lived in a village with no health services, one-third in a village with a hospital and health center, and the remainder in a village with a health center only. One-third of all children (36% of girls and 33% of boys) were severely stunted. Only three in 10 (29% of girls and 31% of boys) were fully immunized, and nearly four in 10 (41% of girls and 35% of boys) had received no vaccinations.

Advantage out girls

Results of analyses suggested that health outcomes were related to the number and gender of older surviving siblings, and that these relationships were tilted against girls and in favor of boys. Girls were less likely than boys to have had a full range of vaccinations. Boys whose older siblings were all girls were more likely and girls were less likely than boys to be fully immunized if they had sisters but no brothers. The analyst characterizes the disadvantage observed for girls as "somewhat surprising" and attributes it to opportunity costs that parents may be unwilling to pay for unwanted children (girls). Overall, the analyst concludes, the results "strongly suggest that parental and societal norms about the values of girls relative to boys and about a desirable family sex composition are key to explaining why certain children fare worse than their siblings and why girls with older sisters fare particularly badly." However, the job of immunizing every child is not yet done. While infectious diseases affect poor children disproportionately, in most communities immunisation coverage is higher in wealthier households. In many cases, children, and girls in particular, living in rural and remote areas have less access to immunisation. Given this inequitable distribution, efforts are required to reach out to each and every child. Support for immunisation must be sustained, since diseases are still rampant and every day sees the birth of new children who require immunisation.

As shown below, improvement in immunisation rates in South Asia resulted in a dramatic reduction in the occurrence of vaccine preventable diseases. For example, during the period 1980 to 1998 the reported number of measles cases has decreased by more than 72 percent, probably an underestimate of the true figures.

TABLE 3.1

Trends in Reported Number of Measles Cases

	1956	*1990*
Pakistan	28,600	2,300
Bangladesh	11,100	6,500
India	114,000	34,000
Total	153,700	42,800

Source: WHO Vacccine Preventable Diseases Monitoring Systems, 1999, Global Summary.

WHO and UNICEF in the fray

In 1976, WHO and UNICEF launched the Expanded Program on Immunisation (EPI) with the aim of controlling six childhood diseases: tuberculosis, diphtheria, pertussis (whooping cough), tetanus, polio and measles. Countries adopted EPI as a central component of their primary health care programme. As part of the EPI framework; the international community launched a global initiative to eradicate polio. Polio has long struck fear into the hearts of parents as they watched their children progress from symptoms of a minor cold to full-blown paralysis of a limb that remains a lifelong disability. This ancient crippler of children is on the verge of being eradicated thanks to the effective and inexpensive Sabin vaccine. Since the mid-1990s polio has disappeared from much of the world. In 1994, the Americas were certified polio free. By the end of 1999, the Western Pacific, including China, appeared free of the poliovirus, and in the European region, there remained only a few isolated areas that were still at risk. At the start of 2000, only 30 countries, largely in South Asia and sub-Saharan Africa continue to harbor polio. South Asia has the largest reservoir of the poliovirus with 60 percent of the global polio cases being reported in India.

Eradication of polio in India is within reach. India has intensified and accelerated the polio eradication programme. Surveillance efforts to track every polio case have been significantly strengthened, and the number of new polio cases has been steadily declining. The number of polio cases in India declined from 1,126 in 1999 to 95 by the end of August 2000. In the 1990s, the World Bank provided support for child immunisation as part of a broad set of activities to improve maternal and child health through the Child Survival and Safe Motherhood Project, the Population Projects VIII and IX, and the more recent Reproductive and Child Health Project in India. In 2000, the Bank financed its first project in India focusing exclusively on immunisation. (The US$ 142.6 million Immunisation Strengthening Project's goal is to eradicate polio and improve the quality of routine immunisation in the country, particularly for poor and vulnerable groups. An important feature of the Immunisation Project is the five to ten year strategy being developed by the Government of India for dealing with other vaccine preventable diseases in the future. Strengthening the vaccine delivery system to ensure that all children are immunized with the basic six vaccines remains the top priority. Introduction of "new" vaccines such as Hepatitis B (HB) is being explored. HB has been in use for almost 20 years in industrialised countries and has proven to be highly effective in combating hepatitis. Haemophilus influenzae type b (Hib) is another vaccine universally used in developed countries, which could have a dramatic impact on pneumonia and meningitis in India.

GAVI

The Global Alliance for Vaccines and Immunisation (GAVI), a unique coalition of public and private institutions, was officially launched in

January 2000 at Davos during the World Economic Forum. GAVI has moved with unprecedented speed toward its shared goal of protecting all children from vaccine preventable diseases. GAVI partners include national governments, bilateral agencies, UNICEF, WHO, the Bill and Melinda Gates Children's Vaccine Program at PATH (Gates CVP), the World Bank, the International Federation of Pharmaceutical Manufacturers Associations (IFPMA), and the Rockefeller Foundation, among others. Less than two decades ago, the crippling disease polio, claimed hundreds of thousands of victims every year. Today, public health officials say they have an unprecedented opportunity to eradicate the disease by 2005. More than $3 billion has been spent so far to drive polio out of every country on Earth but six, including India. Officials say the last few places will be the hardest. India has launched the world's largest public health campaign in an effort to remove itself from the last six. It's the day before the latest round of polio vaccination starts in the northern Indian state of Uttar Pradesh. To get the word out, street musicians in the rural village of Dumraila are singing about the hardships of polio. Here in Dumraila, they have a living example. As the musicians perform, a few villagers lead to the front of the crowd a shy, pretty and reluctant teenage girl on crutches. Mamta is not officially part of the performance, but she is drafted into the show to remind villagers of what can happen to children who are not vaccinated. Ms. Mamta said later that although she was a young child when she had polio, she's still not used to being handicapped. "It's good that these polio campaigns are being done," she said. "Other children will be saved from having this disease." She said that her paralyzed leg makes it hard to get around, especially going long distances. Polio takes a heavy toll on job and marriage prospects. The disease can even be fatal.

India's progress

India has made tremendous progress in saving children from polio. Last year saw the smallest number of cases on record at 225, compared to nearly 5000 cases a decade ago. Massive national immunisation drives are behind that success. Several a year aims to vaccinate the country's 165 million children under five years old. Two years ago, the eradication effort suffered a major setback. Shoddy work plagued the 2001 immunisation drives and the campaign conducted only two major drives. That was a bad idea according to Sanjeev Yadav, campaign leader in seven districts in Uttar Pradesh. "I'll definitely say that the government plus planners, all of us made a mistake that we let off the pressure a little," he recalled. "The number of rounds decreased in 2001 because we thought that we had almost achieved eradication and this mistake cost us dearly and in 2002 we had an outbreak again." The 2002 outbreak claimed 1600 victims, a six-fold increase from the year before. Experts say the experience is a warning to other countries about the hazards of complacency. So India has redoubled its efforts.

The country is planning six major immunisation drives this year. For each drive, that means setting up hundreds of thousands of vaccination booths all across the country, from the biggest cities to the remotest villages. The manpower needed to do the job is staggering. Sanjeev Yadav, campaign leader in seven districts in Uttar Pradesh, said that if you add up all the people in just his seven districts running booths and rallying people to go to them, it is an enormous number. "I think it will come down to, maybe 60,000 or something," he explained. "It's a big operation. It's a very big operation." More than one million people will participate nationwide and to watch that this big operation isn't wasted, there are monitors whose job is to make sure everything is done right. On booth day, teams of monitors are driving around Uttar Pradesh and the whole country checking up on the vaccination booths. There are many things that can go wrong. At this booth, for example, the vaccine arrived two hours late and monitor Jaya Singh finds another problem. Children's fingers are marked with a permanent pen to show they've been vaccinated, but apparently that is not always an accurate indication. "They are marking the child first and then they are giving the drops," she said. "This is the wrong procedure. You can see the mark that this child has taken the drops and that child has not really taken the drops. That is a real problem. I was saying as soon as the child takes the drops, and then you put the mark on his finger." The monitors insist that mistakes like that are rare today and that most booth workers are properly trained. However, there are other potential issues. Vaccine can go bad quickly if it's left in the Indian heat for too long. A color-coded indicator on the side of each vial shows how fresh the vaccine is. Booth day is really just the beginning of the immunisation drive. Only about 50 to 60 percent of the population usually shows up for booth day, but the Indian government's polio programme director, Sobhan Sarkar believes that to eradicate polio that's not enough. "In any other sector you can be satisfied with 60, 70, or 80 percent performance," he explained. "The performance in this sector must be one hundred percent and more importantly, is that it must be uniform all over." So over the next several days, teams of vaccinators will go door to door delivering vaccine to those children who didn't get it on booth day. Once every child in a house has been vaccinated, the team marks the house with a "P." If any child is missed for any reason, the house is marked with an "X." Some X-marked households have refused the vaccine because false rumors have spread that it will make children infertile. Dispelling those myths is part of the vaccinator's job. Vaccinator Rashida Naz said that they're persistent. "If they don't understand the first time, we'll come again a second time, a third time," she said. "After some time, they'll be convinced to give the vaccine." The campaign is convincing more and more reluctant parents that the rumors are false, but officials say vaccinators sometimes just get lazy and mark houses that refused the vaccine with a "P" anyway. So Subodh Kumar, the monitor, checks to be sure that houses marked with a "P" deserve it.

Two children in this X-marked house have already been vaccinated.

After a brief discussion, he finds out why it's still marked "X." "There is another child who has gone to his grandparents," he explained. "So it will be 'X' until that child gets the vaccine." By the end of the door-to-door campaign, every single dwelling in India, from the grandest mansion to the humblest hut, will be marked with either an "X" or a "P." In a nation of more than one billion people, this in itself is a major achievement. The real achievement will come if all that work succeeds and Mamta Berma is part of the last generation of Indians to suffer from polio. Even the top cine stars of silver screen viz. Amitabh Bachan and Aishwarya Rai had been roped in the campaign.

AP Effort

In the Indian state of Andhra Pradesh (AP), health workers and the population at large are well poised to protect the health of newborns from killer diseases. AP has introduced a model system for immunisation that now appears to be having spin-off effects in other states within India and other countries in South Asia. The AP government, in partnership with the Children's Vaccine Program (CVP) at 'Program for Appropriate Technology in Health' (PATH), has over the last three years seen immunisation services significantly strengthened. The effort, known as the Andhra Pradesh Immunisation Strengthening (AP) Project, has received generous support from the Bill and Melinda Gates Foundation. The project set high goals for itself, hoping to build a state-of-the-art immunisation programme. With its population of 75 million people, if Andhra Pradesh were an independent country, it would be the fifteenth largest in the world. The AP effort has led to increased awareness of the value of vaccines, and raised immunisation to a rate of 72 percent coverage of the entire population through adoption of safety features, greater efficiency, and improved management. AP's Top Immunisation Achievements are: (i) Universal coverage of all infants with hepatitis B vaccine for the first time in India. (ii) Widespread adoption of safe injection practices and technologies. (iii) Improved immunisation systems with responsive, supportive management. (iv) Decreased numbers of children infected with Japanese encephalitis, a devastating and debilitating illness.

Introducing New Vaccines

More children in AP are being protected against the traditional six vaccine-preventable diseases (tuberculosis, tetanus, pertussis, diphtheria, polio and measles) than ever before. Now, for the first time, hepatitis B vaccine was added to the routine immunisation schedule. PATH has been a pioneer in forging partnerships to introduce new vaccines where they are most needed. Hepatitis B, a serious disease of the liver, is a major health problem in India, including in Andhra Pradesh. AP adopted use of the hep B vaccine for its newborns and, critically, helped to inspire the government of India to add this vaccine to the schedule for the national immunisation programme. Since its inception in 2001, the AP project has achieved a number of milestones. In 2002, Mr. Bill Gates, co-founder of the Bill and Melinda Gates Foundation, traveled to Hyderabad to view the project's progress. There he joined Mr. Chandrababu Naidu, the then Chief Minister of AP, to launch the second phase of expansion of the project. The project has helped procure 2.55 million doses of hepatitis B vaccine, nearly 14 million safety syringes, and 300,000 safety boxes. Hepatitis B vaccine has prevented over 6,000 cases of hepatitis B-related cancer and chronic liver disease.

Japanese Encephalitis

Japanese encephalitis (JE) is a devastating illness that kills one out of three infected. Most of JE's victims are children under 15 years of age. JE survivors often are left mentally and physically disabled. Each year JE returns to Andhra Pradesh, but faced with limited supplies of vaccine, the government of AP, with assistance from PATH, procured one million doses of JE vaccine from Vietnam. The government also procured additional JE vaccine from the Central Research Institute in Kasauli, India. Use of this vaccine resulted in a 90 percent reduction in cases of JE within the first year of the project, from 300 cases in 2002 to 29 in 2003. PATH is leading a major new initiative to accelerate research and development on JE vaccine. The Japanese encephalitis project (JEP) aims to identify a cost-effective, safe and efficacious vaccine to protect against JE. Activities of this project include improving clinical detection of the disease, and expanding access to a safe and efficacious JE vaccine in Andhra Pradesh.

Immunisation gained widespread attention during AP's self-proclaimed "Year of Immunisation 2003," a communication campaign designed to elevate people's understanding of the importance of immunisation. Immunisation schedules were printed on flipcharts and on school notebooks, and painted on vaccine vans and clinic walls. These messages serve to remind people of when to take their infants for vaccination.

JE infection is more prevalent in the rural area/paddy fields. Vaccination is given at 1-2 years of age. The children are at maximum risk at 1-4 years of age.

Overall AP's Year of Immunisation demonstrated high-level commitment to immunisation, and helped people understand why immunisation is so important. The immunisation programme expanded to protect infants in all 23 districts. An estimated 1.6 million newborns in Andhra Pradesh are now able to receive hepatitis B vaccine. Through information dissemination, education and media coverage, AP's successes became known throughout India. Following the AP example, late in 2003, the Indian state of Kerala announced its own programme of expanding hepatitis B to all of its citizens.

Safety First!

To prevent unsafe injections, AP expanded the use of auto-disable

(AD) syringes that are self-locking after the first use. Injections have historically been a cause for concern in India due to high rates of reuse of syringes and needles. Reuse can transmit life-threatening diseases such as hepatitis B or HIV/AIDS. Preliminary results from an ongoing study show that every third person visiting an outpatient clinic in India receives an injection. Most unsafe injections in India (and globally) are for curative purposes. In Andhra Pradesh, injections for immunisation account for only about one-quarter of all injections. PATH staff led a multi-stakeholder effort to tackle the problem of unsafe injections, leading to wide-scale adoption of AD syringes and other safety devices. AD syringes, free of cost, are now available at more than 12,000 primary health centers and outreach posts. Part of the strategy for building wide-scale interest in injection safety was to involve those most impacted by injection practices. At the national level, an Injection Safety Coalition, composed of several key public and private stakeholders, was established to help guide policy in this area. The coalition meets regularly to monitor activities, is chaired by PATH through its New Delhi staff, and has helped integrate safe approaches to injection as part of the daily routine in India's health systems. Today all 23 districts in AP use auto-disable syringes.

New Technologies Ensure Quality of Vaccine Delivered

The AP project has introduced other quality assurance techniques and innovative technologies designed to protect the health worker and community members. Vaccine vial monitors (VVMs) are used on all polio and hepatitis B vaccines throughout the state. These colored labels, about the size of an aspirin, are printed on every vial of vaccine, and indicate to the health worker if the vaccine has been exposed to too much heat and should not be used. They help to ensure that the vaccine people receive will be effective in preventing disease. Another technology that helps health staff monitor the temperature of vaccines in primary health centers is the Freeze Watch T Indicator. When the project first started, field visits to health centers determined that freeze-sensitive vaccines were being frozen, especially during campaigns. In one instance, 140,000 doses of diphtheria, tetanus, pertussis (DTP) vaccine had to be discarded. Project staff also noted that the stock inventory system was being poorly managed. So they worked with the government to build new cold chain vaccine stores in all districts and to train staff in efficient, effective maintenance of the cold chain.

Better Management and Supportive Supervision

The government and PATH have partnered with local medical colleges to perform regular visits to primary health centers and additional immunisation sites. The visits provide opportunities to correct improper practices through a process of supportive supervision. After only a few months of operation, the new system made a substantial impact by improving the quality of immunisations on several fronts, e.g., through AD syringes, sharps disposal, and by ensuring that cold chain temperature charts be maintained in all areas. Moreover, dropout rates for DPT3 and measles vaccine have decreased markedly over the first three years of the project.

Increased Government Commitment: Percentage of Immunization Costs Absorbed by AP Government

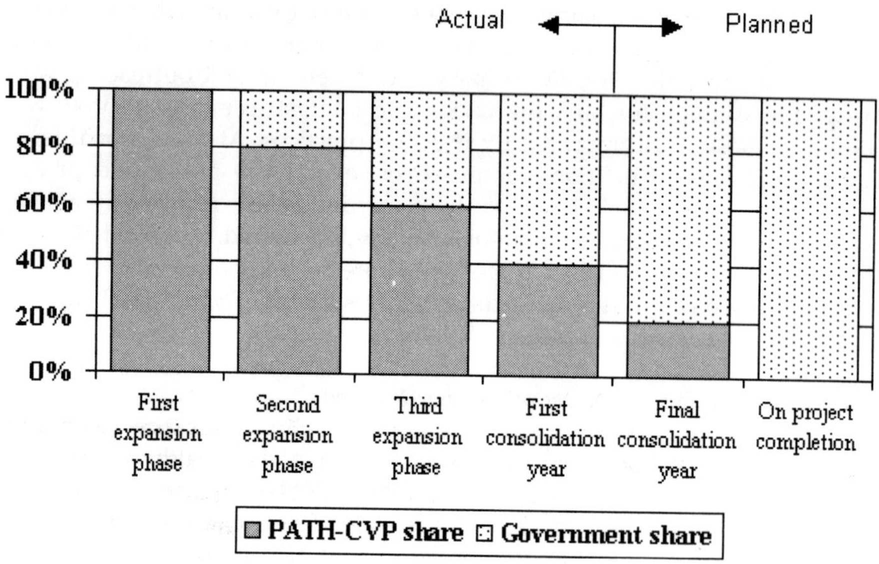

The Andhra Pradesh experience shows that commitment to measurable goals, and readiness to take on new vaccines and technologies, together with improved training and close attention to management in primary health centers, can help to substantially improve immunisation services and coverage.

WHO Review of National Immunisation Coverage 1980-02, Oct. 2003

Trends in officially reported data show an increase in coverage beginning in the early to mid 1980s reflecting the phased Geographic expansion of the EPI programme from 31 districts in 1985 to all 452 districts by 1990. In 1985 the Universal Immunisation Programme (UIP), the inclusion of immunisation in India's Technology Mission (one of 5 missions reporting directly to the Prime Minister) and the infusion of resources associated with the global Universal Childhood Immunisation (UCI) goal resulted in rapidly increasing coverage in the late 1980s. While official reports describe sustained high coverage following 1990, survey data suggests significantly lower coverage beginning in the late 1980s. Officially reported data may be over estimated due to methods for ascertaining the size of the target population. Coverage for 1990 and 1991 was estimated to have been 70% and 57% respectively based on an extensive sub-national Immunisation Coverage Survey of 1991 and results from the 1992 National Family Health Survey (NFHS). Estimates prior to 1990 were established by calibrating the data reported to UNICEF by the 1990 estimate established by an evaluation of the 1991 and 1992 surveys. The marked increase to 1990 and the subsequent decline are attributed to the extensive (but unsustained) efforts to reach UCI goals. The estimates for the periods following 1995 are based on the Coverage Evaluation Surveys (CES), MICSs, and a second NFHS (1997/98) and show a marked decline in coverage during this period. Estimates for 1993 through 1995 are interpolated between the levels established by the 1992 and 1996 surveys. The estimate for 1995-1997 are based an evaluation of the survey data. Results from previous Demograhic and Health Surveys (similar to the NFHS and MICS) suggest that coverage values based on mother's history are effected by a recall bias for the multi-antigen vaccines (i.e., OPV 1, 2, 3 and DPT 1, 2, 3) and to most likely occur in longer surveys covering a variety of indicators. It does not appear to be a problem in surveys focused on immunisation coverage such as the EPI 30 cluster surveys and the CES. To control for this bias we have adjusted the DPT3 card or history value by calculating the dropout rate from DPT1 to DPT3 based on card results and applying this multiplier to the DPT1 card or history value. This adjustment may result in an overestimate since children without a card are less likely to be immunized than children with a card. The 1996 and 1997 results of the CES seem to estimate the upper range of actual coverage. The dropout rate of 6% from

DPT1 to DPT3 in the 1998/1999 CES is unusually low (dropout from the NFHS 98/99 is 13% based on card only data). The estimate of 1997 is based on an adjustment of the NFHS (1997/98) results to account for recall bias and the CES. The estimate of 62% is supported by results from the 1997 Reproductive and Child Health Survey. The 1995 peak was established from data in the 1996 CES that described coverage in a cohort 25-36 months of age. The 1999 estimate is based on the MICS adjusted for recall bias. The recent increase is supported by the 2001 and 2002 CES surveys.

WHO/UNICEF estimates of the percent of children born in 2000-2002 protected against tetanus (PAT) by vaccination of their mothers with tetanus toxoid.

In most instances PAT reflects the number of mothers receiving two doses of tetanus toxoid during pregnancy. In some cases the mother may have received an adequate number of doses of tetanus toxoid prior to the pregnancy, protecting the child even though no doses were received during the current pregnancy. These estimates are based on data provided through the WHO/UNICEF Joint Reporting Form on Vaccine Preventable Diseases and have been supplemented by information from national household surveys conducted under the auspices of the National government and from data available in the published literature.

Vaccinations and other precautions for the travelers to India

Most travelers to India will need vaccinations for hepatitis A, typhoid fever, and polio, as well as medications for malaria prophylaxis and travelers' diarrhea. Other immunisations may be necessary depending upon the circumstances of the trip and the medical history of the traveler, as discussed below. Insect repellents are recommended, in conjunction with other measures to prevent mosquito bites. All travelers should visit either a travel health clinic or their personal physician 4-8 weeks before departure for necessary advice about medication and vaccination, etc.

Medications

Travelers' diarrhea is the most common travel-related ailment. The cornerstone of prevention is food and water precautions, as outlined below. All travelers should bring along an antibiotic and an antidiarrheal drug to be started promptly if significant diarrhea occurs, defined as three or more loose stools in an 8-hour period or five or more loose stools in a 24-hour period, especially if associated with nausea, vomiting, cramps, fever or blood in the stool. A quinolone antibiotic is usually prescribed: either ciprofloxacin 500 mg twice daily or levofloxacin (Levaquin) 500 mg once daily for a total of three days. Quinolones are generally well tolerated, but occasionally cause sun sensitivity and should not be given to children, pregnant women, or anyone with a history of quinolone allergy. Alternative regimens include a three-day course of trimethoprim-sulfamethoxazole one double-strength tablet twice daily or azithromycin (Zithromax) 500 mg once daily. Trimethoprim-sulfamethoxazole should not be given to pregnant women or those with a history of sulfa allergy. Azithromycin should be avoided in those allergic to erythromycin or related antibiotics. An antidiarrheal drug such as diphenoxylate (Lomotil) or loperamide (Imodium) should be taken as needed to slow the frequency of stools, but not enough to stop the bowel movements completely. However, Diphenoxylate (Lomotil) and loperamide (Imodium) should not be given to children under age two. Most cases of travelers' diarrhea are mild and do not require either antibiotics or antidiarrheal drugs. Adequate fluid intake is essential. If diarrhea is severe or bloody, or if fever occurs with shaking chills, or if abdominal pain becomes marked, or if diarrhea persists for more than 72 hours, medical attention should be sought. Though effective, antibiotics are not recommended prophylactically (i.e. to prevent diarrhea before it occurs) because of the risk of adverse effects, though this approach may be warranted in special situations, such as immuno-compromised travelers.

Malaria

Prophylaxis is recommended year-round throughout the country (including the cities of Delhi and Bombay), except at altitudes higher than 2000 m (6561 ft) in the states of Himachal Pradesh, Jammu, Kashmir, and Sikkim. Most malaria cases are reported from forested areas in the states of

Madhya Pradesh, Maharashtra, Orissa, Gujarat, Rajasthan, Bihar, and Karnataka. Either mefloquine (Lariam), atovaquone/proguanil (Malarone), or doxycycline may be given. Mefloquine is taken once weekly in a dosage of 250 mg, starting one-to-two weeks before arrival and continuing through the trip and for four weeks after departure. Mefloquine may cause mild neuro-psychiatric symptoms, including nausea, vomiting, dizziness, insomnia, and nightmares. Rarely, severe reactions occur, including depression, anxiety, psychosis, hallucinations, and seizures. Mefloquine should not be given to anyone with a history of seizures, psychiatric illness, cardiac conduction disorders, or allergy to quinine or quinidine. Those taking mefloquine (Lariam) should read the Lariam Medication Guide. Atovaquone/proguanil (Malarone) is a recently approved combination pill taken once daily with food starting two days before arrival and continuing through the trip and for seven days after departure. Side effects, which are typically mild, may include abdominal pain, nausea, vomiting, headache, diarrhea, or dizziness. Serious adverse reactions are rare. Doxycycline is effective, but may cause an exaggerated sunburn reaction, which limits its usefulness in the tropics.

Long-term travelers who may not have access to medical care should bring along medications for emergency self-treatment should they develop symptoms suggestive of malaria, such as fever, chills, headaches, and muscle aches, and cannot obtain medical care within 24 hours. Symptoms of malaria sometimes do not occur for months or even years after exposure.

Immunisations

The following are the recommended vaccinations for India:

Hepatitis A vaccine is recommended for all travelers over age two. It should be given at least two weeks (preferably four weeks or more) before departure. A booster should be given 6-12 months later to confer long-term immunity. Two vaccines are currently available in the United States: VAQTA (Merck and Co., Inc.) and Havrix (GlaxoSmithKline). Both are well tolerated. Side effects, which are generally mild, may include soreness at the injection site, headache, and malaise. Travelers who are less than two years old, are pregnant, or have less than two weeks before departure should receive a single intramuscular dose of gammaglobulin instead of vaccine.

Typhoid vaccine is recommended for all travelers. It is generally given in an oral form (Vivotif Berna) consisting of four capsules taken on alternate days until completed. The capsules should be kept refrigerated and taken with cool liquid. Side effects are uncommon and may include abdominal discomfort, nausea, rash or hives. The alternative is an injectable polysaccharide vaccine (Typhim Vi; Aventis Pasteur Inc.), given as a single dose. Adverse reactions, which are uncommon, may include discomfort at the injection site, fever and headache. The oral vaccine is approved for travelers at least six years old, whereas the injectable vaccine is approved for those over age two. There are no data concerning the safety of typhoid vaccine during pregnancy. The injectable vaccine (Typhim Vi) is probably preferable to the oral vaccine in pregnant and immunocompromised travelers.

Polio immunisation is recommended. In 1998, more than 75% of the polio cases reported in the world occurred in India, most from the states of Bihar and Uttar Pradesh. Any adult who received the recommended childhood immunisations but never received a booster as an adult should be given a single dose of inactivated polio vaccine. Better still is the use of polio vaccine as drops. All children should be up-to-date in their polio immunisations and any adult who never completed the initial series of immunisations should do so before departure. Side effects are uncommon and may include pain at the injection site. Since inactivated polio vaccine includes trace amounts of streptomycin, neomycin and polymyxin B, individuals allergic to these antibiotics should not receive the vaccine.

Japanese encephalitis vaccine is recommended for long-term (1 month) travelers to rural areas or travelers who may engage in extensive unprotected outdoor activities in rural areas, especially in the evening, during shorter trips. The most recent outbreak of Japanese encephalitis began in Andhra Pradesh state in September, 1999, and continued late into the year. Historically, outbreaks have occurred in Andhra Pradesh every two to three years. (An outbreak of encephalitis was reported from Andhra Pradesh in June-July 2003, suspected to be due to Japanese encephalitis, but this has not yet been confirmed.) Outbreaks have also been reported from West Bengal, Bihar, Karnataka, Tamil Nadu, Assam, Uttar Pradesh, Manipur and Goa. Urban cases have been reported (e.g. Lucknow). In India, the only states not reporting Japanese encephalitis are Arunachai, Dadra, Daman, Diu, Gujarat, Himachai, Jammu, Kashmir, Lakshadweep, Meghalaya, Nagar Haveli, Orissa, Punjab, Rajasthan, and Sikkim. The vaccine (JE-VAX; Aventis Pasteur Inc.) is given as a series of three injections on days 0, 7 and 30. Mild side effects including fever, headache, muscle aches, malaise and soreness at the injection site occur in about 20% of those vaccinated. Serious allergic reactions including urticaria, angioedema, respiratory distress and anaphylaxis occur in approximately 0.6% of vaccines and may occur as long as one week after vaccination. Any person who receives the vaccine should be observed in the doctor's office for at least 30 minutes following the injection and should complete the full series at least 10 days before departure. There are no data concerning the safety of Japanese encephalitis vaccine during pregnancy.

Influenza Vaccine

(Recommendations of the IAP Committee on Immunisation)

Influenza virus is an orthomyxovirus. There are three antigenic types—A, B, and C, with several subtypes of each based on two surface antigens—hemagglutinin and neuraminidase. Influenza virus, especially type A, is characterized by frequent mutations—antigenic drifts and antigenic shifts. It is of the utmost importance, therefore, that the vaccine should incorporate the current strain prevalent during that time.

Current inactivated influenza vaccines are produced from virus grown in embryonated hen's eggs, and are of three types: whole virus, split-product, subunit surface-antigen formulations. Whole-virus vaccines are associated with increased adverse reactions, especially in children, and are currently not used. Most influenza vaccines are split-product vaccines, produced from detergent treated, highly purified influenza virus, or surface-antigen vaccines containing purified hemagglutinin and neuraminidase.

Vaccines are usually trivalent, containing 15 mg each of two influenza A subtypes (H1N1 and H3N2) and one influenza B strain. The present vaccine contains 15 mg of hemagglutinin of each of the three WHO recommended strains (Northern Hemisphere) for the season 2004-05.

1. A/New Caledonia/20/99 (H1N1)—like strain [variant A/New Caledonia/20/99 (IVR-116)].
2. A/Fujian/411/2002 (H3N2)—like strain [variant A/Wyoming/3/2003 (X-147)].
3. B/Shanghai/361/2002—like strain [variant B/Jingsu/10/2003].

Vaccines elicit a relatively strain-specific humoral response, have reduced efficacy against antigenically drifted viruses and are ineffective against unrelated strains. The influenza vaccine is therefore unique as the precise composition has to be changed periodically in anticipation of the prevalent influenza strain expected to circulate in a given year. The vaccine is effective for only a short period, usually 6 months to 1 year and a new vaccine is brought every year. The WHO reviews vaccine composition biannually and updates antigenic content depending on prevalent circulating subtypes based on the data obtained from its chain of reference laboratories from world. over to provide antigenically well-matched vaccines.

Influenza vaccine is highly immunogenic and is associated with minimal side effects. This vaccine is currently recommended for use only in high-risk children and adolescents, e.g. individuals with chronic pulmonary and cardiac disease, sickle cell disease, immunodeficiency, HIV infection, systemic lupus erythematosus, diabetes mellitus and those on long-term aspirin therapy. Influenza vaccine is also recommended to be given for severe cases of asthma who need oral corticosteroids frequently. Two doses at an interval of one month are given to children less than 9 years of age.

Hepatitis B vaccine is recommended for travelers who will have intimate contact with local residents or potentially need blood transfusions or injections while abroad, especially if visiting for more than six months. It is also recommended for all health care personnel. Two vaccines are currently licensed in the United States: Recombivax HB (Merck and Co., Inc.) and Engerix-B (GlaxoSmithKline). A full series consists of three intramuscular doses given at 0, 1 and 6 months. Engerix-B is also approved for administration at 0, 1, 2, and 12 months, which may be appropriate for travelers departing in less than 6 months. Side effects are generally mild and may include discomfort at the injection site and low-grade fever. Severe allergic reactions (anaphylaxis) occur rarely.

Rabies vaccine is recommended only for those at high risk for animal bites, such as veterinarians and animal handlers, and for long-term travelers who may have contact with animals and may not have access to medical care. Dog bites account for most cases of rabies in India. Bites from cats, tigers, camels, and the Indian civet may also transmit rabies. A complete pre-exposure series consists of three doses of vaccine injected into the deltoid muscle on days 0, 7, and 21 or 28. Side effects may include pain at the injection site, headache, nausea, abdominal pain, muscle aches, dizziness, or allergic reactions.

Several lots of IMOVAX Rabies Vaccine (Aventis Pasteur) were recently recalled because they had been found to contain live rabies virus that had not been fully inactivated. All those who received rabies vaccine between September 2003 and April 2004 should contact their physician to determine if they received vaccine from one of the recalled lots and, if so, whether further evaluation is necessary. Any animal bite or scratch should be thoroughly cleaned with large amounts of soap and water and local health authorities should be contacted immediately for possible post-exposure treatment, whether or not the person has been immunized against rabies.The post-exposure doses are given on day 0, 3, 7, 14, 28.

All travelers should be up-to-date on routine immunisations, including Tetanus-diphtheria vaccine (recommended for all travelers who have not received a tetanus-diphtheria immunisation within the last 10 years; diphtheria reported among children in north India September 1999).

Measles vaccine is recommended for any traveler, born after 1956 who does not have either a history of two documented measles immunisations or a blood test showing immunity. Many adults who had only one vaccination show immunity when tested and do not need the second vaccination. Measles vaccine should not be given to pregnant or severely immuno-compromised individuals.

Varicella (chickenpox) vaccine is recommended for any international traveler over one year of age who does not have either a history of documented chickenpox or a blood test showing immunity. Many people who believe they never had chickenpox, show immunity when tested and do not need the vaccine. Varicella vaccine should not be given to pregnant or immuno-compromised individuals.

The Varicella Vaccine (Chicken Pox)

Recommendations of the IAP Committee on Immunisation

Chicken pox is usually a self limiting and generally benign disease affecting mostly children and young adults. Complications of varicella may be more commonly seen in immuno-compromised individuals, adults and pregnant women. Takahashi *et al.* developed a live attenuated vaccine from the Oka strain in Japan in the early seventies. The vaccine has been in clinical use in Japan since 1989 and in the United States since 1995. The vaccine can be administered to any healthy individual above the age of 12 months who has not had varicella previously.

Varicella vaccines in use today are all derived from the original Oka strain but the virus contents may vary from one manufacturer to another. The recommended dose is 0.5 ml and the minimum infectious virus content should be 1000 Plaque Forming Units. The vaccine is administered subcutaneously.

It is a highly effective vaccine and protective immunity, humoral as well as cellular, develops in 95-99% individuals. The immunity appears to be long lasting.

The IAP COI opines that varicella vaccine is not recommended for universal immunisation in India at present. One has to emphasize the generally benign nature of and rarity of complications with varicella infection in young children. It may be offered to children from high socio-economic strata of society after explaining the pros and cons to the parents on a one-to-one "named child" basis. It may be prescribed to adolescents who have not had varicella in past (or are known to be varicella IgG negative) especially if they are leaving home for studies in a residential school/college.

It is indicated in children with chronic lung/heart disease, humoral immunodeficiencies, HIV infection (but with CD4 counts above 15% of the age related norms), leukemia (but in remission and oft chemotherapy for atleast 3-6 months) and those on long-term salicylates/high dose long-term oral steroids. Varicella vaccine is also recommended in household contacts of immunocompromised children. It may also be considered in children attending creches and daycare centers.

Varicella vaccine is also indicated in susceptible adolescents and adults if they are inmates of or working in the institutional set-up, e.g. school teachers, day care center workers, military personnel and health care professionals.

The vaccine is stored at 2-8°C and can be administered subcutaneously or intramuscularly. It should be protected from light and needs to be used within 30 minutes of its reconstitution. When used for post-exposure prophylaxis it should be administered within 72 hours of varicella exposure. It should be noted, however, that the efficacy of the vaccine in preventing varicella under such circumstances is not very clear.

Varicella Zoster Immunoglobulin

Varicella zoster immunoglobulin (VZIG) is used for passive post-exposure prophylaxis in immunodeficient individuals who have been exposed to varicella or herpes zoster and are unlikely to have detectable antibody levels. It should be given to the neonate if the mother develops varicella 5 days before to 2 days after delivery. It has to be given by intramuscular injection and the dose is 125 units/10 kg body weight.

Cholera vaccine is not generally recommended, even though outbreaks occur, because most travelers are at low risk for infection. The only cholera vaccine approved for use in the United States has low efficacy and a high incidence of adverse reactions, and is no longer being manufactured or sold. Two oral vaccines have recently been developed but are not yet approved. These vaccines, where available, may be considered for certain high-risk individuals, such as relief workers or health professionals.

Yellow fever vaccine is required for all travelers arriving from a yellow-fever-infected country in Africa or the Americas, or arriving from or transiting through the following countries: Africa: Angola, Benin, Burkina Faso, Burundi, Cameroon, Central African Republic, Chad, Congo, Cote d'Ivoire, Democratic Republic of the Congo, Equatorial Guinea, Ethiopia, Gabon, The Gambia, Ghana, Guinea, Guinea-Bissau, Kenya, Liberia, Mali, Niger, Nigeria, Rwanda, Sao Tome and Principe, Senegal, Sierra Leone, Somalia, Sudan, Tanzania, Togo, Uganda, and Zambia. Americas: Bolivia, Brazil, Colombia, Ecuador, French Guiana, Guyana, Panama, Peru, Suriname, and Venezuela. Caribbean: Trinidad and Tobago. Any person (except infants up to the age of 6 months) arriving without a certificate within 6 days of departure from or transit through an infected area will be isolated for up to 6 days.

Yellow fever vaccine (YF-VAX; Aventis Pasteur Inc.) must be administered at an approved yellow fever vaccination center, which will give each vaccine a fully validated International Certificate of Vaccination. Yellow fever vaccine should not in general be given to those who are younger than nine months of age, pregnant, immuno-compromised, or allergic to eggs. Yellow fever vaccine is not recommended or required for travelers arriving directly from North America, Europe, Australia, or other Asian countries.

Recent outbreaks

An outbreak of dengue fever was reported from Delhi and surrounding areas in June 2003, resulting in 2185 confirmed cases and four deaths as of November 9. A previous outbreak occurred in Delhi from August to November 1996. Dengue fever is a flu-like illness, which is sometimes complicated by hemorrhage or shock. Aedes mosquitoes, which bite primarily in the daytime, transmit the infection and favor densely populated areas, though they also inhabit rural environments. No vaccine is available at this time. Insect protection measures are strongly advised.

Cases of typhoid fever, which show increased resistance to quinolones or third-generation cephalosporins, the antibiotics often used to treat these infections, have recently been reported among travelers to India and Nepal.

An outbreak of encephalitis was reported from Andhra Pradesh in June-July 2003, resulting in 279 cases and 154 deaths as of July 24. Preliminary evidence suggested that the outbreak was caused by Japanese encephalitis, though other tests indicated a different virus. An outbreak of pneumonic plague (plague involving the lungs) was reported in February 2002 from Hat Koti village, Shimla district, Himachal Pradesh state. As of February 19, a total of 16 cases had been identified, including four deaths. The outbreak appears to be limited to the residents of this village. The risk to travelers appears to be extremely low. The World Health Organisation recommends no special restrictions on travel or trade to or from India. A previous outbreak of pneumonic plague occurred in 1994. Eight states were involved, including Maharashtra (including Bombay), Gujarat (including the city of Surat), Karnataka, Uttar Pradesh, Madhya Pradesh, Haryana, Rajasthan, and West Bengal, as well as the federal district of New Delhi.

A malaria outbreak was reported from the northeastern state of Assam in the summer of 2002, involving more than 40,000 people. The outbreak appeared to be related to heavy rains, which amplified the mosquito population. A malaria outbreak was also reported from Assam in May-June 2001.

A cholera outbreak related to flooding was reported from Orissa State in July-August 2001, resulting in 34,000 cases and 33 deaths as of mid-August.

Visceral leishmaniasis is on the rise in India and has reached epidemic proportions in Bihar State. According to the World Health Organisation, more than 200,000 residents of Bihar became infected in 1994.

Leptospirosis occurs in India. An outbreak was reported from Gujarat State in September 2003, affecting Surat, Navasari, and Valsad districts. A previous outbreak involved Surat and Valsad districts in 1997. In India, the animal reservoir for the disease includes rats, cattle, rodents, bandicoots, pigs, dogs, and cats.

Buffalopox was reported in five children from two villages in Beed district, Maharashtra State in March 1998, at the same time that the illness was occurring locally in cattle. Fever, enlarged lymph nodes and pox lesions on the hands characterize the illness in humans. Three cases of the disease were also reported from Maharashtra State between 1992 and 1994.

Other infections

Vibrio parahemolyticus (rapidly increasing since 1996)
Hepatitis E (transmitted by contaminated food or water)
Cutaneous leishmaniasis (Rajasthan State)
Brucellosis (outbreak reported from Calcutta in August 2000).

Kyasanur Forest disease (transmitted by ticks who've fed on infected monkeys; most cases reported from forested areas in Karnataka State during dry spells; outbreaks reported from Chikmagalur, Shimoga, Uttara Kannada, and Dakshina Kannada districts in April-June 2003 and from the Western Ghats region in April-May 2000.

Anthrax (recent outbreaks in south India; reported in villagers who have direct contact with infected animals or animal products):

Typhus
Tick-borne relapsing fever (northern India)
Louse-borne relapsing fever
Scrub typhus
Tick-borne spotted fever
Leptospirosis
Lymphatic filariasis
West Nile fever (transmitted by mosquitoes)
Chikungunya fever (transmitted by mosquitoes)
Cysticercosis
Echinococcosis
Giant intestinal fluke (fasciolopsiasis)
Lung fluke (paragonimiasis)

HIV (human immunodeficiency virus) infection is reported, but travelers are not at risk unless they have unprotected sexual contacts or receive injections or blood transfusions.

Food and water precautions

Do not drink tap water unless it has been boiled, filtered, or chemically disinfected. Do not drink un-bottled beverages or drinks with ice. Do not eat fruits or vegetables unless they have been peeled or cooked. Avoid cooked foods that are no longer piping hot. Cooked foods that have been left at room temperature are particularly hazardous. Avoid un-pasteurized milk and any products that might have been made from un-pasteurized milk, such as ice cream. Avoid food and beverages obtained from street vendors. Do not eat raw or undercooked meat or fish. Some types of fish may contain poisonous bio-toxins even when cooked. Barracuda in particular should never be eaten. Other fish that may contain toxins include red snapper, grouper, amberjack, and sea bass.

Insect and tick protection

Wear long sleeves, long pants, hats and shoes. For rural and forested areas, boots are preferable, with pants tucked in, to prevent tick bites. Apply insect repellents containing 25-35% DEET (N,N-diethyl-3-methylbenzamide) to clothing and exposed skin (but not to the eyes, mouth, or open wounds). For children between 2 and 12 years of age, use preparations containing no more than 10% DEET and apply sparingly. Do not use DEET-containing compounds on children less than two years of age. Preparations containing a higher concentration of DEET carry an increased risk of neurologic toxicity, especially in children. For additional protection, apply permethrin-containing compounds to clothing, shoes, and bed nets. Permethrin-treated clothing appears to have little toxicity. Don't sleep with the window open unless there is a screen. If sleeping outdoors or in an accommodation that allows entry of mosquitoes, use a bed net, preferably impregnated with insect repellent, with edges tucked in under the mattress. The mesh size should be less than 1.5 mm. If the sleeping area is not otherwise protected, use a mosquito coil, which fills the room with insecticide through the night. In rural or forested areas, perform a thorough tick check at the end of each day with the assistance of a friend or a full-length mirror. Ticks should be removed with tweezers, grasping the tick by the head. Many tick-borne illnesses can be prevented by prompt tick removal.

Take appropriate measures to prevent motion sickness and jet lag, discussed elsewhere. On long flights, be sure to walk around the cabin, contract your leg muscles periodically, and drink plenty of fluids to prevent blood clots in the legs. For those at high risk for blood clots, consider wearing compression stockings. Avoid contact with stray dogs and other animals. If an animal bites or scratches you, clean the wound with large amounts of soap and water and contact local health authorities immediately. Wear sun block regularly when needed. Use condoms for all sexual encounters. Ride only in motor vehicles with seat belts. Do not ride on motorcycles.

Protection against Terrorist incidents and other Violence

Over the years, there have been occasional terrorist bombing incidents in various parts of India, predominantly in Jammu and Kashmir. These bomb blasts have occurred in public places as well as on public transportation such as trains and buses. In late 2002 and in 2003, there were several bomb blasts in Mumbai (Bombay), including on public transportation, at a public market and at the Gateway of India. In December 2000, terrorists attacked Delhi's Red Fort, a major tourist attraction, leaving three Indians dead, and in December 2001, terrorists attacked the Indian Parliament. Nine policemen, one Parliament staff member and five terrorists died in the incident. In September 2002, terrorists attacked the Swaminarayan temple complex in Gandhinagar, the capital of Gujarat state. Over 30 people were killed and 70 injured. Foreign visitors have been injured in some of these attacks. It is recommended that Foreign visitors avoid travel to the entire state of Jammu and Kashmir. A number of terrorist groups operate in Jammu and Kashmir, and military movements continue along the Line of Control separating Indian and Pakistani-controlled Kashmir. Since 1989, more than 60,000 people have been killed in the Kashmir conflict, including more than 1,000 civilians in 2002 alone. The state's summer capital of Srinagar is particularly susceptible to terrorist attacks. In March 2003, unidentified gunmen killed 24 Hindu Pandits, including 11 women and 2 children, in the southern Kashmiri town of Shopian. In October 2001, a bomb exploded at the Jammu and Kashmir State Assembly complex, killing 38 people and injuring over 100 others. The few tourists who go to these areas are quite visible and vulnerable and definitely at risk. In 1999, the terrorist organisation Harakat Ul Mujahideen issued a ban on tourists, visiting Kashmir. In 1995, the terrorist organisation Al Faran kidnapped seven Western tourists, who were trekking in Kashmir valley. One of the hostages was brutally murdered, another escaped, and the other five have never been found.

Sporadic incidents of violence by ethnic insurgent groups, including the bombing of buses and trains, are also reported from parts of Assam, Manipur, Nagaland, Tripura, and Meghalaya. While U.S. citizens have not been specifically targeted, visitors are cautioned not to travel outside major cities at night. Security laws are in force, and the central government has deployed security personnel to several Northeast states. Foreign citizens, traveling to or residing in rural areas of East Central and Southern India should be aware of the left-wing extremist groups called "Naxalites" and exercise appropriate caution. Urban demonstrations pose risks to travelers' personal safety and can disrupt transportation systems and city services. During the Dassera festival season and the Diwali festival of lights, American travelers to Calcutta and Eastern India should exercise additional caution. These holidays are often accompanied by large and sometimes unruly crowds, especially in the immediate vicinity of the Pandals. Such concentrations heighten the risk of petty theft, accidental injury, and crowd disturbances. Transportation, even for emergency purposes, is more difficult during the holiday season, and travelers may become disoriented amidst large, flowing crowds.

Crime

Petty crime, especially theft of personal property, is common. Pickpockets can be very adept, and women have reported having their purse-straps cut or the bottom of their purses slit without their knowledge. Theft of U.S. passports is quite common, particularly in major tourist areas. Some Westerners, including U.S. citizens, have been the victims of robberies, rapes, or other violent attacks. The common thread for most attacks has been that the victims were alone.

Traffic safety and road conditions (reproduced from the U.S. State Dept. Consular Information Sheet)

Safety of public transportation: Poor
Urban road condition/maintenance: Poor
Rural road condition/maintenance: Poor
Availability of roadside assistance: Poor to non-existent

Travel by road is dangerous. Trains are somewhat safer than buses, but train accidents still occur more frequently than in developed countries. Frequent use of one's horn to announce presence is both customary and wise. It is very important to keep in mind that if a driver hits a pedestrian or a cow, the vehicle and its occupants are at risk of being attacked by passersby. Such attacks put the vehicle's occupants at significant risk of injury or death, or at least incineration of the vehicle.

Immunisation in adolescents and adults

Immunisation in adolescents is as important as it is in infants. Even the youth from elite class in cities like Chandigarh are not aware about preventive aspects of health care in adolescent age group. When one thinks about the health care in this age group one considers only about behavioural, psychological and sexual problems of teenagers. The immunisation needs of teenagers have remained ignored. A rubella infection can strike a pregnant youth and severely affect her unborn child and an attack of mumps can lead to orchitis, causing infertility in males. Immunisations against hepatitis B, measles, mumps, rubella (German measles), tetanus (lockjaw), diphtheria and chickenpox are available for all adolescents. In addition, vaccinations against hepatitis A, influenza (flu), pneumococcal, and meningococcal disease are needed by some adolescents. However vaccination among youth has not caught the fancy of all those concerned. Even in US the adherence rate to recommended immunisations is 24% for adolescents, compared with 60% for children. In endemic zones like India, typhoid vaccines should also be given.

Should all adolescents be immunized?

Yes. All adolescents require measles, mumps, rubella, tetanus and diphtheria immunisations. All adolescents with diabetes or chronic heart, lung, liver or kidney disorders need protection against influenza and pneumococcal disease, and should consult their doctors regarding their need for these injections. Chickenpox vaccine is recommended for those not previously vaccinated and who have no history of the disease. Hepatitis B vaccine is indicated for all adolescents aged 8-18 who have not been vaccinated. Hepatitis A vaccine is recommended for adolescents traveling to or working in countries where the disease is common, and for those living in communities with outbreaks of the disease, and those living in areas that have hepatitis A. It is also recommended for adolescents who have chronic liver disease or clotting-factor disorders, use illegal injection drugs, or are male and have sex with other males.

How often adolescent need to be immunized?

Hepatitis B vaccine is generally administered in 3 doses. Adolescents not previously vaccinated with 2 doses of MMR vaccine require these. Immunisation against tetanus and diphtheria (Td vaccine) should be supplemented with a booster shot at 11-12 years of age and every 10 years thereafter. One dose of chickenpox vaccine is recommended for adolescents 11-12 years of age, or 2 doses for those 13 or older, if there is no proof of prior chickenpox disease or immunisation. The flu shot should be administered yearly to adolescents who have any medical condition that places them at high risk for complications associated with influenza, such as diabetes, asthma, or chronic heart, lung, or other diseases. Immunisation against pneumococcal disease is recommended for adolescents with certain chronic diseases who are at increased risk for this disease or its complications, and a booster dose is recommended 5 years after the initial dose for this group. Hepatitis A vaccine is administered in 2 doses. Human papillomavirus (HPV) vaccine is also advised in youngsters.

HPV Vaccine; Gardasil

This vaccine prevents cancer cervix in girls, who are sexually active. The vaccine is now available in India; offers hope for future to our female young adults. In June 2006, the FDA of America licensed a vaccine for HPV, which is targeted to preadolescent and adolescent girls, and to women aged 9- 26. HPV vaccine has tremendous potential for reducing the prevalence of both cervical disease, including cancer, and genital warts. Cervical cancer is the second leading cause of cancer death among women worldwide—and the vaccine can significantly reduce HPV-related morbidity and mortality. Full immunisation against HPV requires 3 doses of vaccine—administered in the deltoid muscle at 0, 2, and 6 months.

Should adults also consider immunisation?

Some adults think immunisation is just for kids and adolescents, or are unaware that adult vaccines exist. Each year, lakhs of people are hospitalised because of influenza. Influenza vaccination is readily available and must be repeated each year. Anyone 50 or older, or having chronic illness or immunosuppression, has a greater risk for severe complications. Vaccine against pneumococcal infection is also necessary, every 5 years, in the same age group. Booster doses of Tetanus and diphtheria are needed at 10-year intervals throughout a person's life. Hepatitis B is a sexually transmitted disease that we must immunize against. Anyone 50 and all women of childbearing age need to be safeguarded against measles, mumps, rubella (MMR). Adults have far greater risk of complications from Chickenpox; must be vaccinated against.

Remember, vaccination is the most cost effective mode of health care.

Questions and Answers

Q. What is vaccination or immunisation?

A. Vaccination or immunisation is terms used interchangeably. Both the terms mean process of giving vaccines or 'shots' to children or adults so that they develop immunity or resistance against that particular disease.

Q. How does a vaccine work?

A. Normally in many diseases the disease-forming germ enters the body, produces the disease and subsequently the body mounts immune response or fighting power against the germ and lastly one recovers from the disease. Here immunity against disease is produced after one has suffered from the disease. A vaccine is nothing else but whole or part of the disease germ, which has been processed or modified in such a way than it has lost its capacity to produce disease but it can still induce immunity or fighting power by body when administered in the body. Hence by vaccination one develops immunity without suffering from the disease.

Q. What are the types of vaccine?

A. One can look at the types of vaccines from different angles. Different vaccines work against different diseases like there are separate vaccines for poliomyelitis, measles, diphtheria, tetanus, etc. Vaccines can be oral vaccines like oral polio vaccine or oral typhoid vaccine or it can be injectable vaccine like DPT vaccine or hepatitis B vaccine. Vaccines can be single vaccine like the measles vaccine or combination of more than one vaccine like the MMR vaccine (which acts against meals, mumps and rubella) or the DPT vaccine (which acts against diphtheria, pertussis and tetanus). Injectable vaccines can be given subcutaneously, i.e. below the skin like the measles vaccine or given intramuscularly, i.e. in the muscle like DPT vaccine. Lastly vaccines are usually given prophylactically, i.e. before the exposure to the disease germs like most of the vaccines, e.g. polio vaccine, DPT, vaccine, etc. Some vaccines work when given even after the exposure to the disease germ like the rabies vaccine, which is given after the dog bite. Hence one can look at the various vaccines from different angles.

Q. Which vaccines are usually given to a baby?

A. The vaccines recommended routinely to a baby differ from authority to authority. We will mainly discuss the schedule recommended by Government of India and that recommended by Indian Academy of Pediatrics, i.e. the professional body of pediatricians of India.

Government of India schedule

The minimum vaccines that an Indian child should receive are the vaccines recommended by Government of India under the Expanded programme of Immunisation (EPI). It includes 3 doses of tetanus toxoid given to the mother during the pregnancy to protect both the mother and the newborn from tetanus. After birth the baby receives vaccines against six killer vaccine preventable diseases including BCG (against tuberculosis) oral polio vaccine (against poliomyelitis), DPT vaccine (against Diphtheria, Pertussis, Tetanus) and measles vaccine (against measles).

The time schedule of giving these vaccines is shown in the table. Individual vaccines are discussed somewhere else.

EPI schedules as recommended by Government of India.

Birth - 15 days	- BCG + OPV (ZERO DOSE)
6 weeks - 8 weeks	- OPV1 + DPT1
10 weeks - 12 weeks	- OPV2 + DPT2
14 weeks - 16 weeks	- OPV3 + DPT3
9 months (completed)	- Measles vaccine
15 months - 18 months	- 1st booster of OPV/DPT
4 years - 6 years	- DT vaccine
10 years	- Tetanus Toxoid
16 years	- Tetanus Toxoid

Vaccination schedule recommended by Indian Academy of Pediatrics (IAP)

IAP fully endorses and supports the EPI schedules as recommended by Government of India and agrees that EPI schedule is the minimum a child should receive. But IAP recommends some additional vaccines and some additional doses of EPI vaccines. Additional doses of EPI Vaccine: IAP recommends 2 additional doses of oral polio vaccine, one as the fifth dose during primary vaccination along with measles at 9 months of age and one at the age of 4-6 years during the 2nd booster dose. It also recommends DTP and not DT at 4-6 years of age as 2nd booster dose.

- Additional vaccines as routine: IAP recommends 2 more vaccines as a must for all children. It recommends 3 doses of Hepatitis B vaccines as 0-1-6 months schedules starting as early as possible after birth. 0-1-6 schedule means first dose followed by 2nd dose one month after 1st dose and 3rd dose 6 months from the 1st dose (5months after the 2nd dose). To match with EPI schedule, it recommends first dose at birth along with zero dose of OPV and BCG. The second dose could be given at 6 weeks of age along with the OPV1and DPT1 and the third dose could be postponed till 9 months of age along with measles vaccine. This will entail giving simultaneous vaccines and cut down the number of visits the parents have to make. The second vaccine recommended as a must is MMR vaccine to be given at 15 months – 18 months of age. It could be given along with the first booster of OPV and DPT to reduce an additional visit.

IAP Time Schedule of routine vaccination

Birth—15 days	BCG + OPV (zero dose)
Hepatitis B 1st Dose	
6 weeks-8 weeks	OPV1 + DPT1
Hepatitis B 2nd dose	
10 weeks-12 weeks	OPV2 + DPT2
14 weeks-16 weeks	OPV3 + DPT3
6-9 months	Hepatitis B 3rd dose
9 months (completed)	Measles vaccine
15-18 months	1st Booster dose of OPV + DPT
MMR vaccine	
4-6 years	2nd booster dose of OPV + DPT
10 years	Tetanus toxoid
16 years	Tetanus toxoid

Q. Are there some more vaccines given by doctors?

A. In addition to the extended schedule as recommended by IAP, there are some more vaccines, which may be required to be given. Such vaccines can be divided into two groups. 1st group of vaccines includes those, which protect against disease, which lead to lot of morbidity and mortality. These include typhoid vaccine and Hib vaccine. These are costly vaccines. But for the cost, they are recommended as routine vaccines for all children. Hib vaccine is given as 3 primary doses at 4 weeks interval starting at 6 weeks of age along with OPV and DPT followed by a booster at 15-18 months of age again along with the 1st booster dose of OPV/DPT and MMR given together or separately as discussed under Hib vaccines later. The currently available typhoid vaccines given are after 2 years of age and repeated every 3-5 years there after.

The second group of vaccines includes those optional vaccines, which protect against common childhood diseases like hepatitis A and chicken pox, which lead to more suffering but very less chance of death. These diseases are usually mild and self-limiting in children and hence option of routine vaccination of children is left to parents. They are severe in adults and adolescents with more chances of complication and hence are routinely recommended in that age group. These vaccines are very costly at present. This makes their use optional as per wishes of parents. A chickenpox vaccine is given routinely to all children only in USA at present. It is given at the age of 15 months. Hepatitis A is given as 2 doses in 0-6 to 12 schedule starting after 2 years of age. The first dose is followed up by 2nd dose after 6 to 12 months of first dose. Hence if all these vaccines are given to a child the schedule will be as shown below.

Time schedule of all vaccines including optional vaccines

Birth—15 days	- BCG + OPV (zero dose) Hepatitis B 1st dose
6-8 weeks	- OPV1 + DPT1 + Hepatitis B 2nd dose + Hib 1st dose (DPT + Hib can be given as a combined vaccine)
10-12 weeks	- OPV2 + DPT2 + Hib 2nd dose
14-16 weeks	- OPV3 + DPT3 + Hib 3rd dose (DPT + Hib can be given as combined vaccines)
6-9 months	- Hepatitis B 3rd dose
9 months complete	- Measles vaccines
15-18 months	- MMR vaccine - 1st booster of OPV + DPT - Booster of Hib vaccine - Varicella vaccine
2 years complete	- Typhoid vaccine and repeat every 3-5 years - Hepatitis A vaccine followed by 2nd dose at 6-12 months following 1st dose
4-6 years	- 2nd booster of OPV + DPT
10 years	- Tetanus Toxoid
16 years	- Tetanus Toxoid

Q. What if the vaccine is not given at the recommended age and is delayed?

A. The decision to give or not to give a vaccine when patient comes late depends on the natural history of the particular disease *vis-a-vis* the age of the child. BCG, OPV and DPT should be given till 5 years of age. If patient is older than 5 years only DT should be given. In a child older than 6 months, prior Mantoux test is necessary before giving BCG. If measles is delayed, it can be given as measles till 12 months or as MMR there after. If MMR is delayed, it can be given at any age till adolescence. After that one can give mumps and rubella vaccine. Hepatitis B can be given till any age including adulthood, though the response is blunted after the age of 40 years. Hib vaccine if delayed can be given till 5 years of age. For a child above 12-15 months, only one dose of Hib vaccine is enough. Typhoid vaccine can be given till adulthood. Similarly Hepatitis A and chickenpox vaccine can be given till any age provided patient has not suffered from the respective disease.

Q. What if the subsequent dose is delayed?

A. For OPV and DPT, if patient comes late for the 2nd and 3rd primary doses or the booster doses it is not necessary to restart the schedule. Instead just complete the remaining doses including 1st booster 1 year after the last primary dose and 2nd booster at 3 – 4 years after the 1st booster dose. For Hepatitis B and Hepatitis A (3 dose schedule), a maximum gap of 6 months between the 1st and the 2nd dose and a maximum gap of 1 year between the 2nd and 3rd dose is allowed, beyond which it may be prudent to restart the schedule. What is more important is to realize that the child remains unprotected or only partially protected till he completes the desired schedule. Hence it is important to complete the schedule as fast as possible to give early and complete protection and to prevent breakthrough infections.

Q. Can a vaccine be given when a child is sick?

A. Minor illness like mild cough, cold, loose stools, vomiting or even mild fever is not a contraindication for vaccination. However if a child is suffering from severe diseases, high fever, severe loose stools, pneumonia or any other illness needing investigation or admission to a hospital, vaccination should be postponed till full recovery. OPV dose can be given during diarrhea but should not be counted and an extra dose in the schedule should be given.

Q. What precautions should one take before vaccination?

A. Foremost is to complete the schedule in time. Do tell the doctor about any adverse effects seen to previous immunisation. Understand properly the implications of giving or not giving the vaccine under optional category. One can feed the child including breast feeds before and after any vaccination. There is no need to starve the child before vaccination. Maintain properly the vaccination card and take it along during each vaccination for the doctor to see record.

Q. What precautions should be taken after vaccination?

A. Keep firm pressure for few minutes at the injection site with a spirit swab. Do not massage or rub at the injection site. Wait in the consulting room for another 30 minutes should any reaction develop following vaccination. Note down carefully when to come back for next vaccination. Inform the doctor immediately if the child develops any reaction or abnormal behavior or habits following vaccination in the next few days.

Q. What are the common side effects of vaccination?

A. Most of the vaccines are very safe. Patient can get pain, redness, swelling at the injection site. It is less common with subcutaneous injections. Rarely a nodule may form which remains for few weeks especially following DPT. Patient can develop mild to moderate fever, which usually responds to paracetamol. Never give aspirin for pain or fever following vaccination especially after varicella vaccine. Rarely child can develop fussiness, irritability, anorexia, vomiting, diarrhea, excessive crying, etc. especially after DTP injection. Lastly there could develop severe reaction like convulsion, encephalopathy, depressed, responsiveness, hypotonia, altered consciousness, anaphylaxis, shock, hyper pyrexia (fever>1050C) cyanosis, etc. which must be reported immediately to the doctor.

Not all the vaccines lead to reactions. Not all the children develop reaction nor does it develop with each dose of vaccine. Equally important is the fact that development of some reaction like fever or pain is not a prerequisite of good action of vaccine.

Q. What are contraindications to vaccination?

A. Patients with severe reactions to previous immunisation should not receive same vaccine again. Patients with progressive neurological disorders should not receive DPT but instead be given DT injections. Patients will severe egg allergies should not be given measles or MMR vaccine. Patients with immune compromised state like symptomatic HIV or AIDS should by and large not receive live vaccines especially if a killed vaccine substitute is available. Of course there are some exceptions to this rule and for details refer to individual vaccines.

Q. Where should one go for vaccines?

A. The vaccines covered under EPI schedule, i.e. BCG, OPV, DPT and measles vaccines are at present given free of charge by health authorities. Private practitioners give all the new vaccines too but at a cost. It is an individual choice as to where to go for vaccination. Make sure that wherever you go for vaccination has all the facilities to maintain cold chain and proper storage facilities.

Q. What is cold chain? How are the vaccines stored?

A. Cold chain means keeping the vaccines at the recommended

temperature, usually 2-80C, all throughout from the time of manufacturing till it is given to the patients. It involves proper storage and transport facilities using walk in coolers, refrigerated vans, and refrigerators at clinic and vaccine carriers. At the site of manufacturing the vaccines are stored in big refrigeration or cold storage rooms. From there it is transported to countries, various states of countries and various cities by air or road transport with cold storage facilities. It is then supplied to the clinics in vaccine carriers. In clinic they are stored in refrigerators and taken out for use in vaccine carriers. Thus a chain of cold storage is maintained till last. In the clinic, vaccines are stored in a refrigerator. This refrigerator should not be used for storing anything else. The stock of BCG, OPV, measles, MMR and varicella vaccine is kept in refrigerator compartment or the chiller compartment. Vaccines that can not be frozen like DTP, DT, Tetanus Toxoid, Typhoid vaccine, Hib vaccine, Hepatitis B vaccine, Hepatitis A vaccine, Rabies vaccine are kept in the first and second racks. Even the diluents should be stored in the refrigerator and is kept in lower racks. No vaccine should be kept in door compartment as the temperature can reach as high as 150C once the door is opened. Instead water bottles should be stored in the door and in the extra space in refrigerator so that should electric power fail the temperature inside is maintained at 2 – 80C for long time. Do not open the refrigerator again and again. If possible use ice lined refrigerator, which can keep the temperatures at 2-80C for 10 hrs in case of power failure. Ideally a dial thermometer is fixed so that one can read the temperature inside the refrigerator from outside without opening the refrigerator from time to time. In case of power failure do not open the refrigerator. The temperature will be maintained between 2-80C for a few hours longer in an ice-lined refrigerator. If the temperature goes beyond 80C say after 1-4 hours of power failure, one will need to keep the vaccines in the vaccine carrier with the ice stuffed from all the side. While keeping vaccines in a carrier always put enough ice below and above the vaccines and keep the vaccines in plastic bag to avoid getting frozen by direct contact with ice. The temperature is maintained at 2-80C till some ice remains in the carrier. Hence make sure to replace ice from time to time usually 6-8 hours.

Q. Can you give more than one vaccine at a time?

A. More and more vaccines are recommended and available for children. Many of them overlap the age of recommendation, e.g. OPV, DTP, Hib and Hepatitis B, all 4 will be required to be given at 6-8 weeks. Unless given on same day the schedule of all these vaccines will not get completed in time. Hence one can and one needs to give these vaccines simultaneously. One can either use combination vaccine, e.g. DPT + Hib vaccine in same syringe is available or give them on same day using different syringes and at separate sites, e.g. DPT and Hepatitis B. As time goes, more and more combination vaccines will be available to reduce the number of pricks.

Q. What should be minimum gap between 2 vaccines?

A. As discussed before, any number of vaccines can be given on same day at separate sites but if not given on same day there should be gap of 4 weeks between two vaccines in general. One should not give one vaccine today, second 7 day and 3rd vaccine after another 7 days. Extra doses of OPV like in pulse immunisation or ring immunisation is notable exemption to this rule. Some vaccines like rabies vaccine have schedule where 5 doses are given in 1 month's time. Again rabies vaccine or tetanus toxoid when indicated, should be started as soon as possible, irrespective of vaccines received in recent past

Q. Does one need consent for vaccination?

A. It depends on the rule of the country and type of vaccine. In India, EPI vaccines are given by health authorities only on informed oral consent. For the other vaccines informed oral consent with documentation in the vaccination card is what should be minimally done. Patient should be informed about pros and cons of giving and not giving vaccines in the language that patient can follow. Hence so far written consent is not recommended by any authorities.

The new 2006 Recommended Childhood and Adolescent Immunisation Schedule may mean some new shots for your kids, especially your toddlers and teens.

According to the CDC and AAP, changes in the immunisation schedule since the last release include:

- The importance of the hepatitis B vaccine (HepB) birth dose has been emphasized.
- Instead of the plain tetanus booster (Td), all children at age 11 to 12 years should now get the newer Tdap vaccine, which also includes an acellular pertussis booster, to help decrease the incidence of whooping cough in teenagers. Older teens who haven't had a tetanus shot yet should get a Tdap shot too, either Boostrix or Adacel.
- Meningococcal conjugate vaccine (MCV4) or Menactra, approved by FDA on January 14, 2005, should be administered to all children at age 11-12 years as well as to unvaccinated adolescents at high school entry (age 15 years) to prevent them from getting sepsis and meningitis. It is also recommended for all college freshmen living in dormitories.
- The hepatitis A vaccine (HepA), as two doses 6 months apart, is now recommended for all toddlers between the ages of 12 and 23 months. This used to be given at age 2 and over and then only to high risk children.

References

Alberts ME, "When and where will it **stop**", *Iowa Med* 1986 Sep; 76(9):424. [When!]

Alexander, NJ, *et al.*, "**Contraceptive** Vaccine Development", *Reprod Fertil Development,* 1994, 6(3):273-280. [Why would they make a contraceptive vaccine? Who would use such a disasterous concoction? Vaccines prevent .... children!]

Allen, JM, "**Over-the-counter** Sale of Drugs and Vaccines, *J AM Vet Med Assoc,* Feb 1, 1995, 206(3):286. [I'll take two DPTs, one MMR, and one polio for the road; Oh and how about some Viagra, Prozac and Ritalin .]

Ambs, E *et al.*, "Tuberculous **Abcess** of the Upper Arm With Regional **Lymphadenitis** as a Consequence of **Injection inTwo Siblings**", *Med Klin,* July 7, 1967, 62:1050-1054. [It happened twice, what a coincidence! Must be genetic!]

Any Missed Organs?

Arnold, H, "Our Vaccination Service is **Sick**", *Oeff Egsundheitswes,* Feb 1974, 36:133-134. [Agree!]

Baker, J *et al.*, "**Accidental Vaccinia**: Primary Inoculation of a Scrotum", *Clin Pediatr* (Phila), Apr 1972, 11:244-245. [Ooops, the needle slipped.]

Barrie, H, "Campaign of **Terror**", *AM J Disorder Child,* Sept 1983, 137(9):922-923. [Qui tu - Vaccination - Et Brutus?]

Bonard, EC, "Is Vaccination Still **Necessary**?", *Rev Med Suisse Romande,* Oct 1987, 107(10):781-782. [Good question? Who are they asking?]

Bonifacio, A *et al.*, "**Traffic Accidents** as an expression of "Iatrogenic damage", *Minerva Med,* Feb 24, 1971, 62:735-740. [But officer I was just vaccinated!]

Borsche, A, "What are the **Hazards** of Vaccinations in Childhood?" *ZFA,* May 10, 1976, 52(13):666-674. [Hazards are Plenty!]

Breiman RF, Zanca JA, "Of **floors and ceilings**—defining, assuring, and communicating vaccine safety", *Am J Public Health* 1997 Dec; 87(12):1919-1920. [What is in between floors and ceilings?]

Brotherton J, Wang H, Schaffer A, *et al.* Vaccine preventable diseases and vaccination coverage in Australia, 2003 to 2005. *Communicable Diseases Intelligence* 2007;31(Suppl):viii-S152.

Budal, J, "**Hazards** of **Prophylactic** Vaccination," *Orv Hetil,* Sept 10, 1972, 113:2237-2240. [or "**Prophylactic**" Hazards!]

Buddle, BM *et al.*, "**Contagious Ecthyma** Virus-Vaccination **Failures**", *Am J Vet Research,* Feb 1984, 45(2):263-266.

Castan, P *et al.*, "**Coma** Revealing an acute Leukosis in a child, 15 days after an Oral Anti-poliomyelitis Vaccination," *Acta Neurol Bekg,* May 1965, 65:349-367. [Coma from vaccines!]

Cho, CT, *et al.*, "**Panencephalitis** Following Measles Vaccination", *JAMA,* May 28, 1973, 224:1299. [The measles vaccination is given to prevent pancephalitis; panencephalitis is a demyelination disease, too.]

Cichutek, K, Nucleic Acid Immunisations", *Vaccine,* Dec 1994, 12(16):1520-1525 (23 ref). [Gene therapy could make auto-immune diseases increase.]

Conteras Poza L, *et al.*, "An **Unusual Accident** During Smallpox Vaccination: Intramuscular Injection of the **Lymph Vaccine**", *Rev Sanid hig Publica* (Madr) Oct 1971, 45:1017-1022. [I thought that vaccines were **supposed** to be given IM.]

Converse, J L, *et al.*, "Control of Tissue Reactions in monkeys vaccinated with Viable **Coccidioides immitis** by prevaccination with killed **Coccidioides immitis**", *J Bact,* Sept 1965, 90:783-788.

Damert, C *et al.*, "**Hygenical** and Bacteriological Inspection of the Execution of Vaccination," Z *Gesamite Hyg,* Jul 1974, 20(7):439-442. [Hygiene means clean ... vaccine hygiene = oxymoron!]

Daugaard, J, "**Adverse Effects** of Vaccination. The **Liability** of Physicians and The objective Liability," *Nord Med,* Jun 1972, 87:183-184. [Who is liable .... no one!]

Davis, LE, "Communicating **Hydrocephalus** in New born Hamsters and Cats Following Vaccinia Virus infection", *J Neurosurg,* Jun 1981, 54(6):767-772. [Hydrocephalus is similar to brain swelling or "water on the brain" and vaccinia virus is used in making vaccines.]

DeRenzi, S, *et al.,* "**Damage** Caused by Vaccine Therapy and Serotherapy", *Clin Ter,* Sept 30, 1966, 38:497-500. [**Damage** Caused by Vaccines!]

Donaldson, AI, *et al.,* "**Transmission** of Foot-and-mouth Disease by **Vaccinated** Cattle Following **Natural** Challenge", *Research Vet Sci,* Jan 1989, 46(1):9-14. [Does that mean that the vaccines di work, or that the cattle put their foot in their mouth? How do they decide what is a natural challenge after a cow is vaccinated with the same virus?]

Editorial, "Are We Vaccinating without **Reason**?", *Lakartidningen,* Nov 27, 1974, 71(48):4915. [Could be! What is reasonable to a three-year old?]

Edwards, K, "Danger of **Sunburn** Following Vaccination", *Papua New Guinea Med J,* Dec 1977, 20(4):203. [Are vaccines phototoxic?]

Elliman, D, "Vaccination and **Professional Confusion**", *Br Med J,* Sept 15, 1990, 301(675):551. [Not just any confusion, but **Professional Confusion**.]

Espmark, A, "The Composition of Vaccines With Reference to **Potentially Injurious Allergens**", *Lakartidningen,* Nov 3, 1965, 62:3662-3667. [Vaccines are **Potentially Injurious Allergens**!]

Favez, G, "Tuberculous **Superinfection** Following a Smallpox Re-Vaccination", *Praxis,* July 21, 1960; 49:698-699. [Super means large/big/great!]

Forrester, HL, *et al.,* "**Inefficacy** of Pneumococcal vaccine in a High Risk Population," Am J Med, Sept 1987, 83(3): 425-430. [Ineffectiveness! We are all high risk ... at risk of getting a vaccine!]

Frerichs, GN *et al.,* "Estimation of Residual Free **Formaldehyde** in Biological Products", *J Biol Stand* 1980; 8(2):139-144. [Take your choice to be embalmed now or later ... oh I forgot to tell you ... you don't have a choice ... roll up your sleeve.] [Formaldehyde is a carcinogen., but that does not matter after you are dead. It just saves them a step.]

Freter, R *et al.,* "Oral Immunisation And Production of **Coproantibody** in Human Volunteers", J Immunol, Dec 1963, 91:724-729. [Guess what copro- means .... Feces.]

Garlick, P *et al.,* "Stimulation of Protein **Synthesis** and **Breakdown** By Vaccination", *Br Med J,* Jul 26, 1980, 281(6235):263-265. [Does not sound like normal protein synthesis.]

Gunderman, JR, "**Guillain-Barre Syndrome.** Occurrence Following Combined Mumps-Rubella Vaccine", *Am J Disorder Child,* Jun 1973, 125:834-835. [GBS is paralysis!]

Haas, R, *et al.,* "Studies on the Occurrence of **Viremia** Following Oral Poliomyelitis Vaccination with Sabin Type I Strain LSC2ab", *Deutsch Med Wschr,* Mar 4, 1968, 91:385-389. [Vaccines contains viruses!]

Hale, MS *et al.,* "**Carpal Tunnel Syndrome** Associated With Rubella Immunisation", *Am J Phys Med,* Aug 1973, 52:189-194. [Did I mention **Carpal Tunnel Syndrome**?]

Hanissian, AS *et al.,* "**Vasculitis** and **Myositis** Secondary to Rubella Vaccination", *Arch Neurol,* Mar 1973, 28:202-204. [Did I mention vasculitis and myositis?]

Harte, PG *et al.,* "**Failure** of Malaria Vaccine in **Mice** Born to Immune **Mothers**", *Clin Exp Immunol,* Sept 1982 49(3):509-516. [Of Mice and Mothers!]

Heart:

Heed, JR, "Human Immunisation With Rabies Vaccine in **Suckling Mice Brain,**" *Salud Publica,* May-Jun 1974, 16(3): 469-480. [Have you had your suckling mice brains today?]

Hillary, IB, *et al.*, "Persistence of antibody 10 years after Vaccination with Wistar **RA 27/3** Strain of Live Attenuated Rubella Vaccine", *Br Med J*, Jun 28, 1980, 280(6231):1580-1581. [RA 27/3 is made from aborted fetus; means it was first used in 1970.]

Johnson, RH, *et al.*, "**Nosocomial** Vaccinia Infection", *West J Med*, Oct 1976, 125(4):266-270. [Nosocomial means a disease **acquired** in a doctor's office or hospital.]

Knudsen, Rc, *et al.*, "Difference in the Protective Immunity of the **tongue and feet** [foot and mouth] of Guinea Pigs Vaccinated with **Foot-and-Mouth** [foot and mouth] Disease Virus Type A12 Following **intradermolingual and Footpad** [foot and mouth]Challenge", *Vet Microbiol*, May 1982, 7(2):97-107. [Some body put their foot in their mouth!]

Krudusz, J, "**Effect** of Vaccinotherapy on the **Sedimentation Rate** and On the **Hematocrit**", *Klin Oczna*, 1967, 37:191-195. [ESR is indication of health!]

Larbre, F *et al.*, "**Fatal Acute Myocarditis** After Smallpox Vaccination", *Pediatrie*, Apr-May 1966, 21:345-350.

Levaditi, JC *et al.*, "Local **Tolerance** of Vaccines Adsorbed on Immuno-Stimulating Substances", *Sem Hop Ther*, Feb 1975, 51(2):117-118. [Tolerance and sensitisation, not immunity and immunisation.]

Levenbuk, IS, *et al.*, "A Morphological Study of the **Harmlessness** of Live Dysentery Vaccines From Streptomycin Dependent Mutants of Sh. Flexnert", *ZH Mikrobiol Epidemiol Immunobiol*, Feb 1972, 49:18-22. [Listed under **Vaccinations Adverse Reactions**.]

Levine, MM, "Non-target Effects of Live Vaccines: Myth, Reality and **Demagoguery**," *Development Biol Stand*, 1995, 84:33-38.Vaccine Myths- for sure; Demagogue - false gods!]

Lewis, J, "**Iatrogenic** Malaria," *New Zeal Med J*, Feb 1970, 71:88-89. [Malaria caused by the doctor!]

Mason, MM *et al.*, "**Toxicology** and **Carcinogenesis** of Various Chemicals Used in the Preparation of Vaccines", *np*, Jun 1971, 4:185-204.[Vaccines are not "toxic" or "cancer" causing?]

Mather, C, "Cotton Mather Anguishes Over the Consequences of His Son's **Inoculation** Against Smallpox", *Pediatrics*, May 1974; 53:756. [Is it for or against?]

Michiels, J, "**Harmful Effects** of Common Drugs on the Vital Apparatus. Agents of Immunity." *Bull Sociologist Beige Ophtalmol*, 1972, 160:467-483. [Listed under Vaccinations.]

Miller, Ta, "The Possibilities for Application of the **Canine Hookworm** Vaccine Technology to the Prevention and **Control of Hookworm** Infection and Disease in **Man**", **In:** Nuclear Techniques in Helminthology Research, Vienna, International Atomic Energy Agency, 1973. [That could be great to control human heart worms, too. We could also switch from going to medical doctors to vets.]

Millichap JG, *et al.*, "Etiology and treatment of **infantile spasms**: current concepts, including the role of DPT immunisation," *Acta Paediatr Jpn* 1987 Feb; 29(1):54-60. [Did I mention Infantile Spasms?]

Motelunas, LI *et al.*, "The Potential Epidemiological **Hazard** of Parental Transmission of Epidemic **Hepatitis** as the Result of Vaccination," *Zh Mikrobiol*, Nov 1965, 42:105-108. [Hazard Plus!]

NA, "AIDS Vaccines: Is **Optimism Justified**? *Fortschr Med*, Jul 20, 1989, 107(21):13. [Sounds a bit pessimistic!]

[Many researchers feel that it is literally impossible to make an AIDS vaccine, but they are still testing the experimental ones on real people ... human "guinea pigs."]

NA, "Protection for AIDS Vaccine **Suits**", *NJMed*, May 1989, 86(5):338. [Protection from lawsuits that is. Why would there be any lawsuits if the vaccine was safe and effective?]

NA, "**Risk Language** Preferred By Mothers in Considering a Hypothetical New Vaccine For Their Children", 1991, *np*, [It is all in how you say it. Vaccines prevent disease and may cause death sometimes ... or vaccines may prevent disease and cause DEATH!]

Na, "Sibling **Accidentally Vaccinates** other Following Inoculation", *Can Med Assoc J*, Aug 4, 1973, 109:237. [I hate it when they let siblings play with needles.]

Na, "The Hen's Egg versus the Horse's **Brain**: ..." 1988, np, [Horse sense in making vaccines!]

NA, "Vaccination, **For** and **Against**", 1964, *Belg T Geneesk*, 20:125-130. [Is it for or against?]

NA, "Vaccines Made From **House-Dust Mites**", *Drug Ther Bull*, Apr 23, 1976, 14(9):35-36. [Sic!]

Nelson, ST, "John Hutchinson On Vaccination **Syphilis** (Hutchinson, J)", *Arch Derm*, (Chic), May 1969, 99:529-535. [Vaccinations and STDs!]

Nosov, SD, *et al.*, "**Systematisation** of Reactions Developing After Prophylactic Vaccination", *Pediatria*, Feb 1972, 51:10-15. [If reactions can be **systematized,** they can be **predicted**.]

Opitz, B *et al.*, "Prevention of **Iatrogenic Infections** Following Vaccination", *Dtsch Gesundheltsw*, Jun 15, 1972, 27:1131-1136. [Disease caused by the doctor!]

Pathel, JC, *et al.*, "**Tetanus** Following Vaccination Against Small-pox", *J Pediatr*, Jul 1960; 27:251-263. [Now you need a tetanus vaccination!]

Perez Diaz R, *et al.*, "[Post-vaccinal **Pericarditis**. Report of 2 Cases]", *Rev Cuba Med*, 1:49-54, Jul-Aug 1962.

Pop, A, "Production of Laboratory **Animals** for the Production of Serums and Vaccines," *Arch Roum Path Exp Mocrobiol*, 1967, 23:423-430. [Animal research for vaccine production!]

Prakken, JR, "**Syphilisation**", *Nederl T Geneesk*, Jun 13, 1970, 114:1019-1023. [Syphilis!]

Provost, A *et al.*, "Inopportune Cattle **Mucosal Diseases** Associated With Rinderpest Vaccine", Bull Epizoot Afr, Dec 1972, 20:265-267. [Those ... inopportune infections.]

Raff, MJ, "Progressive Vaccinia (**Vaccinia Gangrenosum**)", *J Ky Med Assoc*, Feb 1973, 71:92-95.

Redey, B, "**Self-Experiments** with the Ingestion of Various Bacteria", *Acta Microbiol Acad Sci Hung*, 1974, 21(1-2):45-62. [Beyond the call of duty for some scientists.]

Remsey, "**Iatrogenic** [Doctor -caused] Disease Caused by Vaccination", *Orv Hetil*, Sept 1971, 112:2245.

Rubin, R H, *et al.*, "**Adverse Reactions** to **Duck Embryo** Rabies Vaccine. Range and Incidence," *Ann Intern Med*, May 1973, 78:643-649. [Adversion to duck embryos, yuck!]

Sahadevan, MG *et al.*, "Post-vaccinal **Myelitis**", *J Indian Med Ass*, Feb 16, 1966, 46:205-206. [Did I mention myelitis?]

Simon, J *et al.*, "A new Model of **Multiple Sclerosis**. Experimental Vaccinia Infection in the Monkey", *Forschr Med*, Nov 6, 1980, 98(41):1607-1611. [Links of vaccines to MS.]

Spier, RE, "**Democratic** Governments and Vaccines", *Vaccine*, Nov 1994, 12(15):1363. [Good, let's take a **vote** on vaccinations - after every one is **educated** to their real adverse effects!]

Spless, H, "**Sterility** of Vaccination Guns", *Dtsch Med Wochenschr*, Jun 27, 1975, 100(26):1445-1446. [Make sure the gun is sterile, because what is inside it isn't.]

Starke, G, *et al.*, "Requirements for the Control of a **Dog Kidney Cell-adapted** Live Mumps Virus Vaccine", *J Biol Stand*, Apr 1974, 2(2):143-150. [DKC = Dog Kidney Cells]

Stewart, AM, *et al.*, "**Aetiology** of Childhood Leukaemia", *Lancet*, 16 Oct, 1965, 2:789-790.

Stickl, H, "Discussion on the **Most Favorable Age** For Primary Smallpox Vaccination of Children", *Monatsschr Kinderheilkd*, Sept 1970, 118:541-544. [Answer - none!]

Stickl, H, "Estimation of **Vaccination Damage**", *Med Welt*, Oct 14, 1972, 23:1495-1497. [Safety?]

Stickl, H, "**No Negligence** in Preventive Vaccinations", Fortschr Med, July 20, 1989, 107(21):14-15. [No negligence because they are supposed to do that ... have adverse reactions ... that is .]

Stickl, H, *et al.*, "**Purulent [pus] meningitides** Following Smallpox Vaccination. On the Problem of Post- Vaccinal Decrease of Resistance", *Deutsch Med Wschr*, Jul 22, 1966, 91:1307-1310. [Vaccines are the injection of viruses cultured from pus ...]

Stroder, J, "**Incorrect Therapy** in Children", *Folia Clin Int* (Barc), Feb 1966, 16:82-90. [Agreed.]

Sun, M, "Compensation for **Victims** of Vaccines", *np*, Feb 27, 1981, 211(4485):906-908. [They call them victims, not patients.]

Tesovic, G *et al.*, "**Aseptic Meningitis** after Measles, Mumps and Rubella Vaccine", *Lancet*, Jun 12, 1993, 341(8859):1541. [AM has same symptoms as poliomyelitis!]

Thoman M, "The **Toxic Shot** Syndrome", *Vet Hum Toxicol*, Apr 1986, 28(2):163-166. [Animals are not exempt from vaccination damage either!]

Webster, AC, "The Adverse Effect of **Environment** on the Response to Distemper Vaccination", *Aust Vet J*, Oct 1975, 51(10): 488-490. ["The terrain is everything" ... Pasteur's famous last words.]

Wehrle PF, "**Injury** associated with the use of vaccines," *Clin Ther* 1985;7(3):282-284. [Dah!]

Weissmann, G, "In Quest of Fleck: Science From the **Holocaust**", *Hosp Pract*, Oct 1980, 15(10):48-49.52, 54-55 passim. [Which Holocaust are they speaking of?]

What About AIDS Vaccines?

Williams, Go, "Vaccines in Older Patients: Combating the Risk of **Mortality**", *Geriatrics*, Nov 1980, 35(11):55-57, 63-64. [Does not sound good for the elderly ... it is your time to go ... I mean go be vaccinated!]

APPENDIX

INTRODUCTION OF COMBINED PENTAVALENT (DTP-HEP B- HIB) V,ACCINE INTO THE EPI

EPIDEMIOLOGICAL UNIT
Department of Health Services
Ministry of Health Care and Nutrition
231, de Saram Place, Colombo 01000, Sri Lanka
EPI/81/VII/2007 22nd October 2007

A decision has been taken to introduce Hib (Haemophilus Influenzae B) vaccine into the EPI programme in Sri Lanka from year 2008. This decision is based on the recommendation by the National Advisory Committee on Communicable Diseases. The Hib vaccine will be in the form of a combined pentavalent (DTP-Hep B-Hib) vaccine, which would include DTP and Hep B and therefore would replace both DTP and Hepatitis B in the present schedule.

Background

The bacterium, *Haemophilus influenzae type B* (Hib), is an important cause of infections in infants and young children; severe disease in adults due to Hib is uncommon. Where it has been studied carefully, Hib is the leading cause of acute bacterial meningitis in infants and children less than five years old, accounting for one-third to one-half of all cases of bacterial meningitis in this age group. Bacterial meningitis is fatal unless treated immediately with antibiotics. Even with proper treatment 3-25% of affected children may die. Permanent disability with sequelae that include deafness, learning disabilities, and difficulties in movement is not uncommon among those who survive the infection.

Studies have also shown that Hib accounts for up to one-quarter of the severe pneumonia cases in young children. WHO estimates that without vaccination 400,000 children die each year of Hib disease. The disease burden study on 'Haemophilus Influenzae B' carried out in 2004 has indicated that it is an emerging public health issue in Sri Lanka. The study has revealed that Hib meningitis incidence under 5 years population in the Colombo district is 20.1 per 100,000, and it estimated all Hib disease incidence to be 124.5 cases per 100,000 under 5 years. This rate is the highest incidence reported in the south Asian region.

Hib Vaccine

Safe and effective vaccines against Hib infections exist. These vaccines have been routinely used to vaccinate infants in many countries for over 10 years. The experience with these vaccines has shown that they are very safe and highly effective in preventing severe Hib disease, including meningitis and pneumonia. Studies have shown that vaccination reduces the risk of invasive Hib disease in young children by >90%, and in some cases, has even led to protection of un-immunized populations by 'herd immunity'. WHO has recommended that Hib conjugate vaccine be included in routine infant immunisation programmes in all countries where the resources permit its use and the burden of disease is established. Hib conjugate vaccines are available in several different formulations. They can be obtained as a liquid or freeze-dried powder (lyophilised), in single or multi-dose vials, and as monovalent vaccines (Hib

conjugate vaccine only) or in combination with other routine vaccines (e.g., DTP, DTP-Hepatitis B). Pentavalent (DTP-Hep B-Hib) vaccines are available in both liquid and freeze-dried forms. However in the freeze-dried form combined DTP-Hep B is available in liquid form and Hib component as freeze-dried and therefore the latter should be reconstituted (mixed) before use. It has been decided to use liquid form Pentavalent (DTP-Hep B-Hib)vaccine in the national EPI programme considering the convenience of using liquid form of Pentavalent (DTP-Hep B-Hib)vaccine at busy immunisation clinics,. At present, only single dose liquid form Pentavalent (DTP-Hep B-Hib) vaccine is available.

Donor support for introduction of Pentavalent (DTP-Hep B-Hib) vaccine

With the support of the GAVI Alliance combined pentavalent (DTP-Hep B-Hib) vaccine will be introduced into the national EPI programme in 2008 in all districts of the country. During Phase I GAVI support (2003-2007), all countries were supported to introduce new vaccines as a donation. Hence Sri Lanka received Hep B vaccine for 5 years as a donation. However, in Phase II GAVI support is based on co-finance policy, where both the recipient country and GAVI share the vaccine cost.

Initially the contribution from the country will be minimal. Subsequently it will be increased and by 2015 each country will have to bear the total expenditure.

Since the Government is committed to share a significant amount of the cost in introduction of Pentavalent (DTP-Hep B-Hib) vaccine, it is important to give due consideration to the accountability. Therefore, the Ministry of Health will take necessary measurers to ensure accountability at national, district (RDHS) and divisional (MOH) levels.

Schedule

The Pentavalent (DTP-Hep B-Hib) vaccine will be introduced into the **current** EPI schedule at completion of 2, 4 and 6 months of age. First three doses of OPV also will also be given with the Pentavalent (DTP-Hep B-Hib) vaccine at the same time as done in the past with DTP and Hep B vaccines at the completion of 2, 4 and 6 months of age.

Please note that no pentavalent fourth dose will be given at the age of 18 months but the fourth dose of DTP given at this age will be continued. If any dose of Pentavalent (DTP-Hep B-Hib) vaccine is missed or delayed, it should be given at the next earliest available opportunity for immunisation. The immunisation **regime** should not be restarted if a dose is missed.

Eligible children for Pentavalent (DTP-Hep B-Hib) vaccine

All children presenting to immunisation clinics for DPT1 and Hepatitis B 1 on or after the 1st January 2008 will be eligible to receive the Pentavalent (DTP-Hep B –Hib) vaccine. Children who have received their first or/and second dose(s) of DPT and Hepatitis B before the 1st January 2008 will not be eligible for Pentavalent (DTP-Hep B-Hib) vaccine as their subsequent DTP and Hep B vaccination.

Dosage

The standard dose for infants and children is 0.5 ml.

Route and site of administration of the Pentavalent (DTP-Hep B-Hib) vaccine

Pentavalent (DTP-Hep B-Hib) vaccine should be given as an INTRAMUSCULAR (IM) injection to the anterolateral aspect of the thigh in infants. Pentavalent (DTP-Hep B-Hib) vaccine SHOULD NOT be given in the buttock or administered intradermally because this route of administration does not produce an adequate antibody response. In addition there may be a risk of injury to the sciatic nerve, if it is given in the buttock. Unlike the present practice of administering two injectable vaccines (DPT and Hep.B) in the same clinic session, where it is advised that the two injections are administered in different sites/thighs, in Pentavalent (DTP-Hep B-Hib) there is no special concern of which side/site to be used. However, it is advisable to use the left thigh/deltoid muscle to maintain an uniform practice.

Contra-indications

There are very few reasons to withhold or postpone administration of Pentavalent (DTP-Hep B-Hib) vaccine. It should be avoided only for children with:

- A history of a severe allergic reaction (e.g. generalised urticaria, difficulty in breathing, swelling of mouth and throat, shock) to a previous dose of Pentavalent DTP-Hep B-Hib vaccine or with known hypersensitivity to any vaccine component
- A history of an encephalopathy of unknown aetiology after a previous immunisation with a vaccine containing pertussis. In these circumstances, the vaccination course should be continued with DT and Hepatitis B,which are available in all government immunisation clinics. Since the monovalent Hib vaccine is not available in the government clinics, these children may not be able to receive the Hib vaccine in the routine immunisation clinics.

- A severe acute illness with temperature above 38.5°C. As with other vaccines, vaccination should be postponed in children suffering from acute febrile illness
- A progressive neurological disease.

The following are NOT contra indications;

- Minor illnesses such as respiratory tract infection or diarrhoea with temperature below 38.5°C
- Allergy or asthma
- Family history of convulsions
- Treatment with antibiotics
- Treatment with topical corticosteroids or systemic use of corticosteroids at low dosage (<0.5 mg/kg of prednisone or equivalent) in case of skin diseases like dermatitis, eczema, or other localised skin disorders
- Infection with HIV
- Breast feeding
- History of seizures (Convulsions, fits)
- Chronic illnesses such as those of heart, lung, kidney or liver
- Stable neurological conditions, e.g. cerebral palsy, Down syndrome
- Pre-maturity or low birth weight
- History of jaundice at birth.

Precautions for Use

Precautions should be taken to avoid undesirable reactions before administering the vaccine. These precautions include review of the child's medical history, particularly regarding hypersensitivity reactions to previous administration of any type of vaccine and the child's history of recent health problems.

Administration of any subsequent dose of Pentavalent (DTP-Hep B-Hib) should be carefully considered if, in connection with the administration of vaccine, one or more of the following effects have been observed: 40°C temperature within 48 hours following vaccination (not due to other identifiable causes); collapse or shock (hypotonic hyporesponsive episodes) within 48 hours following vaccination; persistent crying lasting more than 3 hours during the 48 hours following vaccination; convulsions, with or without fever, within 3 days following vaccination. Pentavalent (DTP-Hep B-Hib) vaccine should be administered with caution to subjects with thrombocytopenia or a bleeding disorder since bleeding may occur following an intramuscular administration of the vaccine to these subjects.

Storage temperature and shelf-life

Penta valent (DTP-Hep B-Hib) vaccine should be stored and transported between 2C. 8C. IT SHOULD NOT BE FROZEN. Hence this vaccine should **NEVER** be stored in the freezer compartment and should preferably be kept in the middle shelf of the main compartment of the refrigerator in all places storing the vaccine including MOH offices. While transporting the vaccine vials should **NOT** be kept in contact with ice in vaccine carriers/flasks and during clinic sessions Penta valent (DTP-Hep B-Hib) vials should **NOT** be kept in contact with ice.

Injection Safety

At present only auto- disable (AD) syringes are used in the national EPI in the country. Therefore, administration of Pentavalent (DTP-Hep B-Hib) vaccine will be carried out using AD syringes. AD syringes and safety boxes for the national EPI will be provided by the Medical Supplies Division in coordination with the Epidemiology Unit and the RDHS, MOH and head of medical institutions will be responsible to ensure the availability and use of injection safety items at all immunisation clinics in their respective areas. Further it is emphasized that appropriate and safe disposal of sharps waste should be ensured in all aspects of the programme

Role of MOH in introduction of Pentavalent (DTP-Hep B-Hib) vaccine into EPI

- Training of MOH staff on Introduction of Pentavalent (DTP-Hep B-Hib) vaccination
- Creating public awareness regarding new additions to EPI by organizing public education programmes
- Timely request of adequate vaccine stocks for the area, supervision of storage and transport of vaccines and maintenance of cold chain
- Timely request of adequate stocks of AD syringes for the area, identifying mechanisms for disposal of AD syringes and sharps waste for the area and monitoring the implementation and sustenance of the activity.
- Monitoring and supervision of immunisation coverage, vaccine wastage and reporting of AEFI at MOH level with regard to Pentavalent (DTP-Hep B-Hib) vaccine quarterly, according to the quarterly EPI Return for the area and taking corrective measures when required.
- Monitoring of dropouts from immunisation with regard to Pentavalent (DTP-Hep B-Hib) vaccination.
- Monitoring of record keeping at clinic level and MOH level.
- Monitoring timeliness of EPI returns sent from MOH Office to RDHS/RE.
- MOH is responsible for vaccine management accountability: More than 1% vaccine wastage should not be allowed since single dose liquid pentavalent vaccine is used. Each vial of vaccine is accountable and any significant wastage should be

clearly documented and should be reported to both Epidemiology Unit and RDHS. Any losses due to unacceptable reasons will be recovered from the responsible officer.

Role of Public Health Nursing Sister in introduction of Pentavalent vaccine into EPI

- Training of PHMM on Pentavalent (DTP-Hep B-Hib) vaccination.
- Education of public regarding the new addition to the EPI.
- Monitoring and supervision of maintenance of cold chain and proper storage of vaccine stocks.
- Supervision of organisation of immunisation clinics to facilitate administration of Pentavalent (DTP-Hep B-Hib) vaccine.
- Supervision of disposal of sharps waste in the area with regard to AD syringes and other injection material.
- Monitoring of immunisation coverage, vaccine wastage, AEFI and dropout from immunisation with regard to Pentavalent (DTP-Hep B-Hib) vaccination at Clinic/PHM level and MOH level.
- Monitoring and supervision of record keeping at clinic level and MOH level.
- Accurate, timely compilation of EPI data at MOH level.

Role of Supervisory Public Health Midwife in introduction of Pentavalent vaccine into EPI

- Training of PHMM on Pentavalent (DTP-Hep B-Hib) vaccination.
- Education of public regarding the new addition to the EPI.
- Monitoring and supervision of maintenance of cold chain and proper storage of vaccine stocks.
- Supervision of organisation of immunisation clinics to facilitate administration of Pentavalent (DTP-Hep B-Hib) vaccine.
- Supervision of disposal of sharps waste in the area with regard to AD syringes and other injection material.
- Monitoring of immunisation coverage, vaccine wastage, AEFI and dropout from immunisation with regard to Pentavalent (DTP-Hep B-Hib) vaccination at Clinic/PHM level and MOH level.
- Monitoring and supervision of record keeping at clinic level and MOH level.
- Accurate, timely compilation of EPI data at MOH level.

Role of Public Health Midwife in introduction of Pentavalent vaccine into EPI

- Education of the public on the new addition to the EPI.
- Maintenance of cold chain during transport of vaccines and during clinic sessions. Enforcing vigilance and providing personal attention to prevent dropouts from immunisation and to detect AEFI with regard to Pentavalent DTP-Hep B-Hib vaccine.
- Safety assurance of the sharps waste disposal activity in the immunisation clinics.
- Maintenance of accurate records regarding all immunisation at clinic level especially on Pentavalent (DTP-Hep B-Hib) vaccination: Birth and Immunisation Register, Clinic Immunisation Register, Clinic AEFI Register, Part A/B of CHDR, Clinic Summary, Quarterly MCH Clinic Return.

Role of Regional Epidemiologist/MO-MCH in introduction of Pentavalent vaccine into EPI

- Conduction of district training programme for MOH and hospital staff at district level and active participation, co-ordination and supervision of training programmes at MOH level.
- Close monitoring of vaccine storage and maintenance of cold chain at Regional Drug Stores and at MOH level.
- Close supervision of vaccine and AD syringes supply in the region.
- Overall supervision of mechanisms developed in the region for disposal of AD syringes and sharp waste.
- Close monitoring and supervision of immunisation coverage and vaccine wastage quarterly and reporting of AEFI monthly with regard to Pentavalent (DTP-Hep B-Hib) vaccine.

Role of Heads of Health Institutions in introduction of Pentavalent vaccine into EPI

- Timely requisition of adequate vaccine stocks and AD syringes for the immunisation clinic.
- Close monitoring of vaccine storage and maintenance of cold chain at the institutional level.
- Close supervision of vaccine and AD syringe supply to the clinic.
- Overall monitoring of immunisation coverage, vaccine wastage and AEFI with regard to Pentavalent (DTP-Hep B-Hib) vaccination at hospital level.

- Overall monitoring and supervision of record keeping at hospital level.
- Officer Incharge of the EPI clinics is responsible for vaccine management accountability: More than 1% vaccine wastage should not be allowed since single dose liquid pentavalent vaccine is used. Each vial of vaccine is accountable and any significant wastage should be clearly documented and should be reported to both Epidemiology Unit/RDHS. Any losses due to unacceptable reasons will be recovered from the responsible officer.

Role of Officer In-charge/Regional Medical Supply Division (RMSD) in introduction of Pentavalent vaccine into EPI

- Timely request of adequate vaccine stocks and AD syringes for the district.
- Timely distribution of vaccines and AD syringe to MOH and medical institutions.
- Maintenance of cold chain for vaccine during storage at RMSD and transport.
- Preparation of the correct monthly stock return for the district.
- OIC RMSD is totally responsible for vaccine management accountability at the RMSD. More than 1% vaccine wastage should not be allowed since single dose liquid pentavalent DTP-Hep B-Hib vaccine is stored. Each vial of vaccine is accountable and any significant wastage should be clearly documented, to be reported to both Epidemiology Unit and RDHS. OIC RMSD will be held responsible for any losses due to unaccepted reasons.

Training of Health Staff

Introduction of Pentavalent (DTP–Hep B-Hib) vaccine into the routine immunisation programme, EPI, requires training and educating of field health staff to provide the knowledge and skills to sustain a successful programme. This training should include the use of AD syringes and methods adopted for safe disposal of used AD syringes and other sharp waste. Following have been identified as important issues that should be clearly and completely addressed during all training sessions.

- Hib diseases.
- Hib Vaccine (contraindications, vaccine administration, storage).
- Use of Injection safety items (AD syringes, safety boxes).
- Vaccine logistics (vaccine wastage, accountability, maintaining adequate stocks).
- Record Keeping: maintenance of records and registers, completeness, accuracy and timeliness of returns.

- Vaccine Safety: Adverse Events Following Immunisation Training programmes at the national level will be conducted for Regional Epidemiologists and MO.

(MCH) who will be the trainers for their respective health staff. They will be responsible for training MOOH and hospital staff who conduct EPI clinics in their respective districts/medical institutions. MOOH will be responsible for training their own staff and this activity should be assisted and monitored by RE and MO/MCH of the district.

This guideline on introduction of Pentavalent DTP-Hep B_Hib vaccine into the EPI may be used as the training material and this will be available in all 3 official languages. Further, electronic version of training material will be developed by the Epidemiology Unit and will be given to each district. It is the responsibility of REE and MOO (MCH) to share this with all MOOH and Hospitals staff during the district level training. This document contains the background of the programme, implementation strategies, information on Haemophillus Influenza B infection, details of the vaccine and AD syringes.

Records and Returns

With a new addition to the present immunisation schedule it is important to monitor the programme very closely. This should be done with records and returns presently in use in the EPI.

Child Health Development Record (CHDR)

Three doses of Pentavalent (DTP-Hep B-Hib) immunisation should be recorded in the 3 empty rows provided under corresponding rows for Hepatitis B vaccines. The name of the vaccine ('Pentavalent') and does should be clearly written in the first column followed by the date, and batch number. AEFI from previous dose should be entered in the corresponding space provided in the same row. It is mandatory to fill the same in formation in both A and B parts of the CHDR.

Clinic Immunisation Register

All immunisations carried out in the clinic should be entered in this register. The 3 columns provided for 'Other' vaccines should be used to enter 03 doses of Pentavalent (DTP-Hep B-Hib) vaccine.

Clinic Summary

As there are no columns are available in this register for other vaccines, the columns allocated for the Pre School DPT 1, DPT2 and DPT 3 should be used for entering 3 doses of Pentavalent vaccine. Pre School fourth dose of DPT should be entered in the 4th column. Similarly, 3 columns allocated for the preschool OPV 1, OPV2, and OPV3 should be used for entering Hep B1, Hep B2 and Hep B3 vaccine and two preschool OPV doses (4th and 5th) should be entered in the 4th and 5th columns of the Preschool polio spaces. This procedure will be followed until such time that the new formats are printed with relevant changes. Even though originally the pre school DPT (1, 2 and 3) and OPV (1, 2 and 3) columns were allocated for the entering of delayed DPT and OPV immunisations, this information is not readily available form the source document (clinic immunisation register). Hence these spaces are often kept redundant and using these columns for Pentavalent vaccines will not effect the Medical Information System. It is important to record this clearly because only a group of infants would receive Pentavalent vaccine in an immunisation clinic while many others will receive DTP and Hep B separately.

Clinic AEFI Register

A register should be maintained at each clinic to record all adverse events reported following immunisations. The name of the child, the type of adverse event and the vaccine following which the adverse event appeared, should all be entered in the register against the date of the clinic in which it is reported.

Quarterly MCH Clinic Return

At the end of every month, entries in the clinic summary should be added up (totaled) and immunisations performed during the whole month should be recorded in this return monthly. This return should be sent to the MOH office by each PHM at the end of each quarter before the 5th of the following month.

As in the case of the clinic summery the corresponding spaces (rows) available for the entering preschool DPT 1 to DPT3 will be used for entering 3 doses of Pentavalent (DTP-Hep B-Hib) immunisation. It is important to note that in this return the spaces are horizontally aligned in contrast to the vertically aligned columns in the clinic return.

1st dose (Penta 1), 2nd dose (Penta 2), 3rd dose (Penta 3)
Triple (DPT) preschoolers, 4th dose (DPT 4)

Monthly AEFI Return

All adverse events reported from the area following immunisations should be summarized into this return by MOH and copies of the return should be sent to RE and the Epidemiological Unit. Adverse events from Pentavalent (DTP-Hep B-Hib) vaccine should be entered in the column "Other" and it should be named so.

Monthly Stock Return of Vaccines and ORS

The number of Pentavalent (DTP-Hep B-Hib) doses required for the institution for the month should be requisitioned under the column "Other" in the monthly return and it should be named so.

Vaccine Movement Register

This register should be maintained at the MOH office and used for each immunisation clinic session held in the area. The number of doses of immunisations used at the clinic and the number of immunisations performed at the clinic should be entered under each clinic session in this register. An extra column should be added to enter Pentavalent (DTP-Hep B-Hib) immunisation for the purpose. This register is vital in compiling vaccine wastages.

Quarterly EPI Return (EPID/EPI/2/98)

Entries in all Quarterly MCH Clinic Returns received at the MOH office and data on immunisation activities carried out in schools, estates and, hospitals in the area should be summarized on to this return. The number of Pentavalent (DTP-Hep B-Hib) immunisations for the quarter should be entered under the heading 1-4 year DPT 1st to 3rd dose of the return. This arrangement is similar to that of Quarterly MCH clinic return.

Triple vaccine (DPT)

1-4 year
1st dose (Penta 1)
2nd dose (Penta 2)
3rd dose (Penta 3)
4th dose (DPT 4)

Calculation of Pentavalent (DTP-Hep B-Hib) coverage should be done as for other EPI antigens.

$$\text{Coverage} = \frac{\text{Total number of Pentavalent immunisations from Health Unit, Hospitals and, Estates of the area for the quarter}}{\text{Estimated number of infants for the quarter}} \times 100$$

Vaccine wastage for Pentavalent (DTP-Hep B-Hib) vaccine should be entered in page 3 of the quarterly EPI Return in the table provided. It should be entered on the row marked as 'other'. Name of the antigen—'Pentavalent' should be clearly written on the first column (A) of the row. Calculation of Pentavalent (DTP-Hep B-Hib) vaccine wastage should be done similar to other EPI antigens.

Monitoring and Evaluation

Close monitoring and evaluation of the introduction of Pentavalent (DTP-Hep B-Hib) vaccine into the national immunisation programme from its initiation is important for sustenance of the programme. Presently used EPI indicators:, i.e. vaccine coverage, vaccine wastage and rate of AEFI will be used for this purpose. Monitoring of Pentavalent (DTP-Hep B-Hib) immunisation coverage, vaccine wastage and adverse events reported following Pentavalent (DTP-Hep B-Hib) immunisation should be done at MOH level by MOH and PHNS and at district level by RE and MO/MCH.

Epidemiological Unit will be responsible for monitoring at national level as for other EPI antigens. Monitoring of Pentavalent (DTP-Hep B-Hib) Immunisation Coverage Monitoring of Pentavalent (DTP-Hep B-Hib) vaccine coverage will be incorporated into the routine immunisation monitoring mechanism, the Quarterly EPI Return as soon as the vaccine is introduced. Special inputs to improve coverage have to be provided by responsible monitoring authorities for areas with poor coverage of Pentavalent (DTP-Hep B-Hib) immunisation. It is also very important that data are recorded in the return accurately and clearly. MOH should be responsible for sending a timely, Wastage = 100 – usage:

$$\text{Usage}^{*} = \frac{\text{Number of DTP-Hep. B-Hib immunisations performed during the quarter}}{\text{Number of DTP-Hep. B-Hib doses used in all clinics during the quarter}} \times 100$$

At national level, analysis of Pentavalent (DTP-Hep B-Hib) immunisation coverage will be dealt with separately to monitor the progress of the activity in its early years. A completely immunized child for Triple, Hepatitis B and Hib will be defined as a child immunized with all 3 doses within his/her first year and this indicator will be important to assess the progress of the programme.

Monitoring of Pentavalent (DTP-Hep B-Hib) Vaccine Wastage

Since DTP-Hep B-Hib single dose liquid pentavalent vaccine is more expensive than other EPI vaccines, it is important to monitor the wastage and to implement strategies to minimize it, at all levels concerned. Also since the Government of Sri Lanka is committed to co-finance the Pentavalent (DTP-Hep B-Hib) Immunisation Programme from the beginning of introduction, minimizing vaccine wastage is crucial.

The routine immunisation monitoring tool of EPI, the Quarterly EPI Return will be used to monitor the wastage of Pentavalent (DTP-Hep B-Hib) vaccine. It is therefore important that reliable and accurate data is provided through the Quarterly EPI Return. Assessment of causes for vaccine wastage at each MOH level is important as these vary widely between different settings. Strategies for reducing wastage could then be designed accordingly.

Possible causes for high vaccine wastage

- Breakdown of cold chain or inadequacy of cold chain maintenance system,

- Freezing of vaccines, and
- Poor monitoring of proper vaccine movement between MOH office and immunisation clinics.

Strategies that could be designed

- Careful planning in vaccine indentation and distribution,
- Strict maintenance of cold chain,
- Careful planning of immunisation clinic locations,
- Monitoring of proper vaccine movement at MOH level,
- Maintenance of accurate records and utilisation of these to minimize inadequacies of vaccine stocks at MOH level, and
- Improvement of safe vaccine storage.

Minimizing Vaccine Wastage at Outreach Immunisation Clinics

MOH should identify an officer at each individual outreach immunisation clinic to be responsible for proper vaccine movement at individual clinic level.

Vaccine Movement Register should be rigidly maintained to monitor the flow of vaccines in each outreach immunisation clinic.

Only correct amounts of vaccine stocks should be sent to the outreach clinics based on the expected and estimated number of children to be vaccinated.

Note: Pentavalent DTP-Hep B-Hib vaccine should not be provided to the private sector immunisation services.

Monitoring of Immunisation Safety

Pentavalent (DTP- Hep B-Hib) vaccine is safe. A list of possible minor adverse events that could occur following immunisation of this vaccine has been mentioned above.

All adverse events associated with Pentavalent (DTP-Hep B-Hib) vaccine that are reported by mothers and public should be reported by field health workers using the Monthly AEFI Return. All field health officers should specifically inquire about AEFI following the previous immunisation from mothers at the next immunisation session. Please bring the contents of these guidelines to the notice of all officers concerned in your Province/ District/Institution/Unit.

A note about some vaccines in Commonwealth countries

All children aged six to 14 years are now eligible for free meningococcal conjugate C vaccine through school-based programmes only in Australia. Children aged one to five years, and those 15 to 19 years not attending school, are still eligible to be vaccinated in GP or local government settings. School-based programmes will be provided by local government immunisation services targeting children from Prep to Year 9 in school. Local governments will visit all schools in Victoria. The school based meningococcal C programme will vary between local government services however all primary and secondary schools should be visited by mid 2004.

Recording and reporting of meningococcal C vaccine

As with Phase 1, please continue to send meningococcal C vaccine notifications for children under seven years to the Australian Childhood Immunisation Register (ACIR). Vaccine administered to children seven to 19 years is reported to the Department of Human Services (DHS) Immunisation Program. If you record vaccines on a computerised database, please continue to do so and a follow up of extracting that data will be provided at a later stage. For immunisation providers who do not have computerised recording systems, please continue to fax through data on vaccine administered for the seven to 19 year age group.

Statistics from the Australian Childhood Immunisation Register as at 31 May 2003 shows Victoria has immunised 41.50% of children aged between one and five. In Australia overall, 33.7% have been immunised. This is a great effort by Victorian immunisation providers to achieve this result. Perhaps there are children under seven years who have received meningococcal conjugate C vaccine and it has not been reported to ACIR. The Health Insurance Commission will pay $6 per meningococcal conjugate C vaccine 'catch-up' dose administered and reported to ACIR for children less than six years of age.

Meningococcal C vaccine is now part of the 12-month-old immunisation schedule along with MMR and Comvax vaccine. It is important that all vaccines due at 12 months of age should be strongly encouraged to be given by all immunisation providers for disease protection. This means three separate vaccines in three separate limbs. As of January 2004, the ACIR will not pay the 12 month immunisation encounters unless all appropriate vaccines have been administered. IMMUNISATION PROGRAM NEWSLETTER Issue 6 August 2003A.

Childhood Pneumococcal Vaccine

It has become increasingly important for immunisation providers to be well informed about the 7-valent conjugate pneumococcal vaccine. This vaccine is currently selectively funded for Aboriginal and Torres Strait Islander infants and children with certain medical conditions. This limited funding may have inadvertently given doctors and nurses the impression that this vaccine is not important for all babies and infants. This safe and effective vaccine is recommended for all infants <2 years by ATAGI (the Australian Technical Advisory Group on Immunisations) and by the Royal Children's Hospital Immunisation Service. The three doses of conjugate pneumococcal vaccine are recommended to be given at the same time as the routine 2, 4, and 6 month immunisations. The earlier this immunisation is given the better because the age peak it affects is very young. As a public health measure introducing this vaccine as a single dose at 18 months will not prevent a large number of the cases and is not a good option. Catch-up doses are recommended for infants who have missed out on the early three dose primary course. From 7-17 months, 2 doses are required, approximately 2 months apart. Toddlers 18 months and older are given a single dose. Catch-up doses can be given at the same visit as the routine 12-month or the 18-month immunisations.

Children between 2 and 5 years of age are also at risk of pneumococcal disease, however, the incidence of pneumococcal disease declines in this age group. The age cut-off point is therefore a little arbitrary, however, it is appropriate to offer children 2-5 years of age a single catch-up dose, though this practice is not universal. It should be noted that this accepted dosage regimen differs from the product information that states 3 doses are required for the 6-12 month age group and a booster dose is at 1 year for babies given the 2, 4, 6, month primary course.

A booster dose is not currently considered to be necessary following the 3 dose primary schedule.

Pneumococcal bacteria cause meningitis, septicaemia, pneumonia and otitis media and other conditions. The 7 strains, included in the vaccine, cause about 90% of invasive pneumococcal disease in the non-indigenous population of Australia. Pneumococcal meningitis is currently the commonest cause of meningitis in children under 5 years of age. Though this vaccine is expensive, and therefore at times awkward to discuss, we can not deny families being informed about its availability and importance.

7-valent conjugate pneumococcal vaccine

Age	*Number of doses*
2-6 months	3
7-17 months	2
18 months-5 years	1

Optimal interval ≥ 2 months

Questions about the 7-valent conjugate pneumococcal vaccine can be answered by the Royal Children's Hospital on 9345, 6599 or the Immunisation Program DHS on 9637 4180.

Written by Dr Jenny Royle, Royal Children's Hospital, Melbourne.

Are they due their routine preschool vaccines?

If **yes**, the Immunisation Service at the Royal Children's Hospital would like your help with a new study. The study compares a new preschool low dose vaccine (Boostrix™), with the vaccine currently given to children at 4-5 years of age, to see whether the new vaccine reduces the frequency/severity of local reactions.

Hepatitis B Vaccine for Year 7 Students

All students in Year 7 are offered free hepatitis B vaccine through a school-based programme. These students receive a two-dose course of adult hepatitis B vaccine (HBVax II by CSL). Following the initial dose of Adult HBVax II hepatitis B vaccine 1ml IM, the second dose is given four to six months later.

This vaccine regime is approved for use in children aged 11 to 15 only. If a student is absent from school on immunisation day, it is important this regime is followed to ensure continuity and the unnecessary requirement of receiving three vaccines. Two doses of Adult HBVax II in this age group have been proven to be safe and effective and provide long lasting protection against hepatitis B.

ADT Vaccine Schedule

Adult diphtheria and tetanus (ADT or dT) vaccine is recommended for use in people eight years and over. ADT vaccine is used for 'catch-up' vaccination in people who have no documentation of previous diphtheria and tetanus containing vaccines. A primary course of ADT consists of three doses one to two months apart and then two boosters are given at ten yearly intervals. It is routinely offered to all year 10 secondary school students or adolescents aged 15 to 17 who are not attending school. ADT is also routinely scheduled at age 50 if a dose has not been administered in the previous 10 years. (*Source:* 7th Edition Immunisation Handbook and Draft 8th Edition Immunisation Handbook).

Tetanus Prone Wounds

In the event of a tetanus-prone wound a booster dose of tetanus containing vaccine should be given if more than five years have elapsed since the last dose. If there is any doubt about the adequacy of prior tetanus immunisation, tetanus immune globulin should be given as well as a tetanus toxoid containing vaccine.

Use a combination vaccine of Td or DTPa (for children who have not reached their 8th birthday) in preference to tetanus-toxoid alone in order to boost community protection against diphtheria *(Source: Draft 8th Edition Immunisation Handbook).*

Pertussis Cases

Seven children under 12 months of age with pertussis have been notified to the Communicable Diseases Section of DHS since the start of July. The youngest infants were 23 days old, 35 days old and 60 days old (all too young to be immunised), a four month old infant (first dose of Infanrix given and not yet due for second dose), ten-month-old twins (fully vaccinated) and a 20 month old child (unvaccinated). One infant had a mother with a cough and there was no case of illness with cough reported in any of the other close contacts.

The product information for Infanrix vaccine states its efficacy for the pertussis component is about 84%. Because of this efficacy level, in communities where there is high immunisation coverage above 90% it is likely that some vaccine preventable diseases will occur in vaccinated people. Maintenance of cold chain for vaccines is also important to ensure vaccines administered are effective.

A pertussis containing vaccine (Boostrix) is licensed as a booster for people aged 10 years and over but it is not currently recommended as a routine vaccination.

On an individual basis, any adult expressing an interest in receiving this vaccine should be encouraged to do so provided there are no contra-indications.

Maternal antibody does not give adequate protection against pertussis, so babies can be infected before they are old enough to be vaccinated. In recent years among highly immunised communities, many cases of pertussis have been recognised in adults and adolescents due to waning immunity. *Source*: Draft 8th Edition Immunisation Handbook.

Reporting Immunisations Promptly

Delays in reporting immunisation encounters to the ACIR impact not only the ACIR reporting and coverage rates, but can also affect parents claiming family assistance payments, delay payments to providers and cause Immunisation History forms to be completed unnecessarily. Twenty per cent of immunisations are reported to the ACIR within five days of the service date. Sixty–two per cent of immunisations have been sent to the ACIR within two weeks of the service date. Seventy–five percent of services have been notified, however, 25 per cent remain unreported three weeks after the service date. Ninety per cent of services have been notified within six weeks after the service date.

Reporting delays can impact

- *Family payments and Immunisation History*
  (IMMU-13) forms.

Two family assistance payments are linked to the immunisation status of a child; the Child Care Benefit and the Maternity Immunisation Allowance. Parents can authorise the Family Assistance Office to check the immunisation status of a child, as recorded on the ACIR, when applying for these benefits. Delays in reporting immunisation services to the ACIR often result in families receiving letters from the Family Assistance Office informing them that their child is not up-to-date with their immunisation. Unless the parent can confirm that their child is up-to-date or has an approved exemption, their payment could be cancelled. When this happens parents often ask immunisation providers to complete an Immunisation History (IMMU-13) form. This places a time burden on both the parent and provider that could have been prevented if the immunisation service had been reported promptly to the ACIR.

- *Immunisation history statements*

When immunisation services are not notified promptly to the ACIR, a child up-to-date with immunisation will be shown as due or overdue on immunisation history statements sent to parents by the ACIR. This can result in parents making unnecessary enquiries with their provider about their child's incomplete immunisation history.

- *GPII Outcomes payments*

The immunisation status of children is currently assessed for the GPII Outcomes payment using strict age appropriate immunisation rules and does not allow for children following a catch-up schedule. From July 2003, GPII will adopt the ACIR's due and overdue rules to determine immunisation status. These new arrangements will provide a more consistent approach in determining immunisation status and will cater for children following a catch-up schedule.

The new assessment process will use the immunisation status recorded on the ACIR for each child at the time the GPII Outcomes calculation is made. It will be important, therefore, that immunisation services are promptly registered on the ACIR.

- *ACIR reports*

When immunisation services are not reported promptly to the ACIR a child who is up-to-date with their immunisation will be shown as due or overdue on the ACIR reports used by providers. This can result in immunisation providers unnecessarily trying to follow-up children reported as overdue.

- *ACIR coverage*

Immunisation coverage rates are calculated every three months. A child may be up-to-date with immunisation but will not be assessed as such when these details are not recorded on the ACIR in time to be included in the assessment. This can result in immunisation providers unnecessarily trying to follow-up children reported as overdue.

Immunisation 'Catch up' Scenario

'Catch-up' immunisation is a regular occurrence that can either be very simple or be quite complicated depending on the records presented. If the child is under 7 years and has received previous vaccines in Australia, then the ACIR can be contacted if a parent does not have documentation or holds incomplete documentation of an immunisation history. To assist in planning 'catch-up' immunisation, a table has been provided with a scenario to give an example of planning a 'catch-up' programme. The following information is from the *Draft 8th Edition Immunisation Handbook.*

- Plan the 'catch-up' on the basis of documented evidence of previous vaccination.

- As a child gets older the recommended vaccines change or they might need to be omitted from the schedule. For example, DTPa containing vaccines are used up to the eighth birthday and thereafter dT (ADT) or dTpa (Boostrix if a primary course of DTP was administered) can be used.
- For incomplete or overdue vaccinations, build on previous documented doses. Never start the schedule again, regardless of the interval (unless there are no written vaccination records).
- If more than one vaccine is overdue, it is appropriate to give all the vaccines at one visit (in separate syringes and separate sites).
- The intervals between doses can be reduced when implementing a 'catch-up' immunisation programme but the optimal intervals recommended in the ASVS should be used once the child or adult is back to the recommended vaccine and dose number for their age.
- Or use the Immunisation 'catch-up' calculator on the web as follows:
  www.health.sa.gov.au/immunisationcalculator

A child aged two years attends your clinic. The mother states the child is behind in immunisations. The yellow book has a record of the 2 month and 4 month immunisations completed but no record of a sixth month or 12 month immunisation being given. After contacting ACIR on 1800 653 809, it is confirmed that both these vaccine schedules are missing.

USFDA says

The Rotarix vaccine is a liquid and given in a two-dose series to infants from 6 to 24 weeks of age. Rotavirus causes an estimated 2.7 million cases of gastroenteritis in U.S. children each year—and about 55,000 to 70,000 of those children require hospitalisation. Between 20 and 60 deaths are attributed to the infection. Without vaccination, nearly every child in the United States would likely be infected at least once with rotavirus by age 5, the FDA said in its late-Thursday announcement.

4

Overview of Blindness and Ophthalmic Services

A. BLINDNESS

Blindness is an enormous burden to the society, and the cost from lost productivity and labour and from rehabilitation of blind is immense and is growing. Efforts to prevent blindness will not only reduce human suffering but also enormously help save national economy.

1. Problem

A major portion of the blindness in the developing countries is due to infections, trauma, poor nutrition, uncorrected refractive errors and glaucoma, which is easily preventable. Cataract surgery is so safe that cataract blindness is easily curable. Corneal opacities are often a sequlae of infection, trauma, nutritional deficiencies, dystrophies and degenerations. Corneal grafting can restore eye-sight to large number of these patients. As much as 80% of the blindness is either preventable or curable in most of the developing nations including India. Systematic preventive and curative community-based plan is required to reduce the blindness rate of the targeted 0.5% at national level by the year 2000. Vertical blindness prevention viz., trachoma or xerophthalmic control need to be broadened to include or co-ordinate with activities relevant to the prevention and cure of other blinding problems. Emphasis should be on developing activities at the primary, village level as these will benefit the greatest number. However, secondary and tertiary facilities should also be developed to provide continued training and management of complicated cases and to gradually raise the level of competence of the ophthalmic services.

2. Visual Impairment

About 28 million are blind in the world of which as many as 9 million are in India. Blindness is usually measured in terms of ability of the patient to count at 3 metres. Although, priority is accorded to these most affected, there are many more with different levels of visual impairment (Table 4.1).

TABLE 4.1

Categories of Visual Impairment

Category	*Visual acuity with best correction*
1	>6/18—<6/60
2	>6/60—3/60
3	>3/60—< 1/60
4	>1/60—light perception
5	No light perception

Cataract and blindness due to corneal disorders constitute the major (upto 80%) causes of blindness in almost all developing countries including India. In India, the major causes of blindness include cataract (56%), infections (20%), smallpox (3%), injuries (1.2%), malnutrition (2%), glaucoma (0.5%) and others (18%).

3. Levels of Eye Care

3.1 Primary Eye Care

Primary eye care implies the first provision of promotive, preventive and curative measures for eye health both to the individual and community. It should form a part of primary health care. Primary eye care needs to be sustained and supported by an adequate referral system requiring regular short-term training courses for primary health workers. Clinical activities include recognition and treatment of conjunctivitis and lid infection, ophthalmia neonatorum, trachoma, allergic conjunctivitis, trauma, superficial foreign bodies, nutritional deficiencies by the primary health care worker; recognition and referral after early treatment for conditions like corneal ulcers, lacerations of eyeball, lid lacerations, entropion, bums and quick referral for cataract, visual loss or pain in the eye. Promotive and preventive activities should include health education in personal and environmental hygiene, nutrition, sanitation and protection of eye. Primary care workers should be actively involved in community care efforts, viz., prevention of xerophthalmia and follow up of eye in mobile clinics.

3.2 Secondary Eye Care

Eye care facilities available at the secondary level should provide for the definitive management of common blinding conditions such as cataract, entropion, trauma, glaucoma and corneal and intraocular infection. Such services are usually available at district level. This level of eye care should be integrated into general medical infrastructure.

3.3 Tertiary Eye Care

Facilities to provide diagnostic and curative services for conditions such as corneal grafting, retinal detachment, etc. are more efficiency provided in national centres. It is important that the staff of tertiary eye centres are involved in the training of health personnel in eye care. The tertiary eye care centres should provided technical leadership in various aspects of public health ophthalmology including research related to delivery of eye care.

3.4 Mobile Eye Services

Mobile ophthalmic terms help fulfil the function of delivering primary and secondary eye care in areas where such services are looking. These services are of a temporary nature and must eventually.

4. Planning Strategy in India: A Mode

4.1. Eye Health Education

Strategy to control visual impairment includes eye health education forms a vital component of measures for the prevention and cure of avoidable blindness. Important areas of influence should be identified and the behavioural changes desired to be achieved defined with particular reference to:

(a) nutrition,
(b) personal hygiene and sanitation,
(c) early detection of visual defects,
(d) occupational hazards to eye-sight and other injuries,
(e) glaucoma and other blindness diseases,
(f) eye surgery and protection from quack surgeons, and
(g) appeals for voluntary eye donation.

There is a great need to make the people aware that blindness in most cases is preventable and in others curable by medical or surgical intervention. The strategy of communication to be employed shall be both interpersonal communication and through mass media. The curriculum and content of the material and software should be carefully drawn out and pretested by the experts and should be periodically evaluated. All such materials should be produced in national language and in regional languages.

4.2 Intensification and Utilisation of Available Resources

Although the available resources do not match the growing requirements, there is enough scope for utilisation of all available resources to the maximum. This can be done by enlisting support of voluntary and private sector, and identifying the available resources within the service network. The strategy to meet this need and prepare the needed manpower as early as possible is outlined below:

(i) Involve all available ophthalmic surgeons in the Government and private sector.
(ii) Encourage their involvement through suitable incentives and material support.
(iii) Introduce a short-term course in ophthalmology.
(iv) Increase the seats in post-graduate course in ophthalmology.
(v) Increase the number of schools for preparation of ophthalmic assistants.
(vi) Encourage participation of the voluntary sector in training programme.

4.3 Expansion of Infrastructure

The existing infrastructure is unable to cater to the full needs of the eye care particularly at the peripheral level. It is necessary to create a nucleus of primary eye care at the Primary Health Centre level with extension of services by the Community Health Guides. All existing PHCs should, therefore, be equipped with basic ophthalmic equipment. In-service training to Medical Officer, PHC and outreach staff should be arranged gradually. Simultaneously, the secondary tier of service should be built up at taluka and district levels. The sight-saving medicines should be supplied to all PHCs in the country.

(i) The existing School Health Programme should be further strengthened and periodic check up of eyes of the students, including testing of vision must be ensured in co-ordination with the PHCs, existing Mobile Units and the proposed District Mobile Units.
(ii) Screening of glaucoma be done at the PHCs and through the eye camps. If detected and treated early, glaucoma can be controlled and blindness due to it can be avoided. In addition, Mobile Units should also undertake the mass-screening programme for detection of glaucoma during the eye camps being organised by them.

4.4 Eye Donation Movement

Sight can be restored to many corneal blind by corneal graft. Efforts in this direction need to be intensified to popularise the movement. Simultaneously information for collection of donor material and its proper preservation needs to be developed. District hospitals should be considered as a Unit for a purpose of collection of donor material with its outreach upto the PHC level.

4.5 Free/Subsidised Spectacles to the Poor

People who seek cataract operation in eye camps usually belong to the poorer sections of the society. Often most of them cannot afford to buy spectacles which are essential after the operations. These individuals should be provided with spectacles, free of cost, or at subsidised rates. Similarly, during the screening of school children for visual defects, a number of school children may be found to need glasses. Some of them belong to families below poverty line. A provision should be made for supply of free spectacles for such needy children. The funds for implementation of this scheme can be explored from the Ministry of Rural Reconstruction under their anti-poverty Programme.

4.6 Programme Evaluation and Monitoring

Implementation of the programme based on the above strategy needs to be concurrently monitored to get the feedback for timely modifications. In addition, a public health programme of this magnitude requires periodic surveys to understand the epidemiological phenomena and to achieve reduction in the prevalence of blindness. A centre that can undertake this task may be established at Central level with its outreach in every district of the country.

4.7 Research and Development

Problems like cataract, trachoma and many other eye diseases need further basic and applied research efforts. Emphasis in this direction should be given to clinical drug trial, surgical procedures, camp methodology and operational research in eye care delivery.

4.8 Rehabilitation

One of the problems associated with blindness is that of rehabilitating the blind in his own socio-economic setting and giving him an opportunity to be useful to the society. The ophthalmic personnel have a vital role to play in providing psychological support to the blind or those who are likely to become blind. Some of the aspects which need to be argumented are:

(i) Psychological preparation of the victim to accept the reality.
(ii) Providing low vision aids.
(iii) Elementary principles of mobility and the art of daily living.
(iv) Providing information about available rehabilitative services.

4.9 Legislation

Widespread quackery, difficulty in getting the door material and the profession and trade of optician are some of the vital areas which need legislative control. Some of these aspects are covered by legislation but need to be implemented more vigorously while others need fresh legislative measures.

5 Planning for Eye Care

Planning process should be comprehensive, feasible and compatible with future upgradation of technology. Components of planned eye care should include:

(a) Identification of manpower and facilities already available.
(b) Implementation of primary eye care.
(c) Strengthening of secondary and tertiary health services.
(d) As a temporary measure, utilisation of mobile units (when applicable) and organisation of other outreach activities related to prevention of blindness.
(e) Plans to deal with technical aspects of managing the blinding disorders in the country.
(f) Training and continuing education of personnel in activities related to prevention of blindness:
  (i) Primary health care workers,
  (ii) Specialised ophthalmic auxiliary staff,
  (iii) General physicians, and
  (iv) Ophthalmologists, including sub-specialities.
(g) Supervision, motivation and evaluation of personnel at all levels, including provision of appropriate career structures.
(h) Promotion of community participation and health education.
(i) Provision of logistic support:
  (i) Salary and necessary expenses for personnel,
  (ii) Equipment, supplies and transport, and
  (iii) Use of local industries and appropriate technology, e.g., low-cost spectacles and diagnostic equipment.
(j) Mobilisation of financial and other resource inputs:
  (i) National inputs from government and private funds or donations,
  (ii) Governmental oganisations,
  (iii) Non-Governmental agencies, and
  (iv) Inter-governmental agencies.
(k) Evaluation of implementation:
  (i) Measurements of programme activities in terms of time cost and performance,
  (ii) Effect on blindness rates and on the prevalence of specific disorders, and
  (iii) Assessment of other useful indicators, such as development of eye health services, community participation and changes in social and economic factors related to visual disability and its prevention.

5.1 Ophthalmic Surgeons

It is estimated that there are about 6000 ophthalmic Surgeons in India. They are mostly in big cities. Every year 250 to 300 ophthalmologists are being trained in various medical colleges. At present, there is one ophthalmologist for every 2.7 lakh of population. In most of the advanced countries, the present ratio is one ophthalmic surgeon for 20,000 population. The population of India is expected to reach 900 millions by the year 2000 A.D. Even on the basis of one ophthalmologist for every 50,000 we shall need at least 18,000 eye specialists.

There is a proposal to establish one Primary Health Centre for every 30,000 population by the year 2000 A.D. The existing Primary Health Centres will be upgraded to 30 beded General Hospitals or Community Health Centres which shall have an ophthalmic surgeon. 6,000 ophthalmologists will be needed to fill up these community health centres. Another 12,000 ophthalmologists will be required for district hospitals, medical colleges, State Institutes, the Apex institution and the private sectors.

5.2 Ophthalmic Assistance

There is a need to provide an Ophthalmic Assistant in each Primary Health Centre for primary eye care, testing of vision, prescription of glasses, assisting Mobile Units in conducting eye camps, and screening referrals for district hospitals. Such an ophthalmic assistant is also required for district and sub-divisional hospital. It is estimated that in all about 6,000 ophthalmic assistants would be required.

5.3 Orthoptists

Orthoptists are technicians trained for investigations for giving exercises and treatment of squint and allied conditions. In India, at present, there are only? or 6 schools for training of orthoptists, which produce about 560 candidates after two years training. With the development of services at the intermediate and tertiary sections the need for orthoptists would be increased manifold. To meet this need, it is recommended that 30 more centres for training of orthoptists be identified and established. Each institute may take 10 candidates for 2 year course.

5.4 Optical Technician

Optical technician is a person who is trained in the manufacturing of glasses. With the increase in demand for spectacles, the need for such technicians is likely to be increased. There are very few schools in optometry which turn out such technicians.

5.5 Opticians

Opticians are technicians trained to grind and make spectacles prescribed by the opthalmologistic optometrist. There is hardly any institutional facility for training these workers. It is recommended that institutional training for opticians be worked out and established in different parts of the country.

5.6 Community Health Volunteer

The medical officer incharge of the PHC and the Ophthalmic Assistant attached to the PHC should periodically organise training and orientation sessions for CHV and MPWS. They should be trained in giving advice for common eye ailments, preventions and education for eye care. Similar orientation may also be arranged for MCHS and workers engaged in integrated child development.

(a) Practicing Ophthalmologist

Efforts should be made to involve and motivate the practicing ophthalmologists to adopt their neighbourhood community for eye camp and eye care by providing suitable and appropriate incentives to them. They may hold eye camps with the help of voluntary organisations or with the Government Mobile Units. They may be encouraged to establish eye clinics and perform more surgical work.

(b) Private Medical Practitioners

There voluntary participation in the community in eye care education, medical management of emergencies and screening of referrals, should be appreciated and encouraged. They must be given orientation for ophthalmic care work.

5.7 Ophthalmic Drugs

Drugs like corticosteroids need to be categorised under scheduled drugs so that they are available only on prescription. To sight saving, anti-viral, anti-fungals and anti-glucoma drugs should be included in the list of drugs to be made available at PHC level. The combination of corticosteroids with other drugs like sulphas/antibiotics and atropine should be banned.

There should be colour coding of bottle and cartons of drugs like the miotics, mydriatics, antibiotics, corticosteroids and others. The testing of drugs and clinical trials should be strengthened in the national and regional institutes in collaboration with the Indian Council of Medical Research and Drugs Controller of India. The Central Drug Research Institute, Lucknow, may also collaborate in this.

5.8 Ophthalmic Glasses (Spectacles): Contact Lenses

Mass-scale production of ophthalmic lenses and protective glasses should be encouraged through Government or Public Sector. There is a need for the production of inexpensive but safe ophthalmic glasses for use as spectacles, protective glasses, etc. The cost should be reduced by setting up mass production units of standard size lenses and frames.

Till such times they are manufactured in sufficient number in the country import of those items should be allowed, and exempted from customs duty. The material for contact lenses (soft and hard) should be produced in the country.

Intra-ocular implants should be put in scheduled category as in USA in order to avoid their injudicious use. Its usage should also be evaluated and restricted to a few identified centres till its results are evaluated and found satisfactory.

5.9 Surgical Instruments

There is a scarcity of special quality of steel required for the manufacture of sharp surgical instruments for ophthalmic use, particularly the micro-surgical instruments.

For standardisation and further development in the instruments and equipment, a well-equipped workshop should be established with a certification cell on the quality and reliability of the manufactured equipment. ISI specifications for all the essential instruments should be developed.

6. Planning of Eye Camp

All organisations conducting eye camps should follow guidelines laid out for organisational procedures and operative interventions and maintain scientific approach.

(a) The criteria for selection of camp site should take into consideration the following but not necessarily all
   (i) Where no surgical and special and specialist ophthalmic services are available.
   (ii) Where no such camp has been organised for the last six months.
   (iii) Where local community (voluntary organisation, social workers, etc.) and Government Agencies (B.o.o., P.H.C., Medical Officers, Law and Order Officer, etc.) have opted for co-operation. This may be assessed during a pre-camp visit.
   (iv) Proper accommodation at the camp site, i.e. a pucca building from PHC/School/Dharamshala with 2-3 rooms should be available to house operation theatre, etc.
   (v) Camp side should be clean. It should be sprayed with insecticides.
   (vi) Where adequate arrangement for the stay of mobile team is available. There should be good water supply and provision for drainage.
   (vii) It is preferred if electric supply is available at the camp site. It is preferable to have portable electric generators.

(b) Staff of a Mobile Camp
   (i) In a mobile camp, one ophthalmic surgeon must be accompanied by 1 operation theatre assistant and 4 para-medical personnel.
   (ii) It is preferable to have two eye surgeons in one camp.
   (iii) Where the facilities are available especially medical colleges, institutes, participation of more surgeons and para-medical

personnel should be encouraged to provide better facilities to the patients.

(c) Local ophthalmic surgeon and doctors should be involved in the management and conduction of the camp irrespective of it being Government sector or voluntary sector camp.

(d) A local eye camp committee should be made for:
   (a) Publicity,
   (b) arrangements of accommodation and food for the patients,
   (c) funds collection,
   (d) to provide volunteers and social workers, and
   (e) to look after arrangements for the team organising the camp.

(e) The transport system developed or provided should be appropriate to the environment and operational need.
   (a) (i) The civic amenities should be provided proportional to the inpatients strength.
      (ii) For one hundred patients 4 Safai Karamchari (two male and two female) should be deputed round the clock.
      (iii) If pucca lavatories are not available, arrangements must be made for trench lavatories.
      (iv) Lavatories for males and females should be separate.
      (v) Abundance supply of dean water should be available at the site. Electric supply in all wards, lavatories and passages be provided.
      (vi) The place be properly sprayed by insecticides to get rid of fly and mosquito menace.
   (b) *Minimum Standards for Mobile Camp Ward*
      (i) The wards are to be provided for male and females patients.
      (ii) Clean sheet be provided for each bedding.
      (iii) Overcrowding should be avoided, 25 sq. feet should be area per patient allotted.
      (iv) Each ward be kept under the charge of one worker who will look after them and other house-keeping staff to help catering and to provide other comforts to the patients.
   (c) *Minimum Standard for Operation Theatre*
      (i) The O.T. should be located in a pucca room of minimum 12' x 15' for running at least 2 operation tables. There should be a separate annexe for sterilisation of instruments and storage.
      (ii) The room should be made free of any cobwebs, hangings, white-wash scrappings, etc., the floor should be pucca cemented or brick flooring.
      (iii) It should preferably have electric fittings.
   (d) *Sterilisation of Operation Theatre*
      Fumigation or carbolisation of the operation theatre should be done.

(e) *Operating Instruments*

(i) These should be of good quality, stainless steel instruments and several sets of instruments should be available for proper sterilisation.

(ii) Quality control of the surgical instruments should be ensured at the time of the purchase.

(iii) The instruments should be put in sets and should be of adequate number so that no borrowing from one set to the other is there. There should be minimum of seven sets for cataract surgery for two surgeons.

(iv) The sterilisation should be best in quality for blunt as well as for sharp instruments. It is ideal to use small autoclaves for this purpose as boiling is not a satisfactory method.

(f) *Life-Saving Emergency Measurers*

Camp equipment should also be equipped with life-saving drugs, suction apparatus and oxygen cylinder and oxygen regulating apparatus.

(g) *Case Selection*

(i) One-eyed patients must be given a special care and should be done by senior surgeon.

(ii) Operations of both eyes at a time should be avoided.

(iii) The following cases should not be operated at the camp:

- Very tense and psychic patients.
- Children if general anaesthesia facilities are not available.
- Cases of poor surgical risk (severe diabetes, severe hypertension and with cardiac problem).
- Cases with definite history of urinary problems.

(h) *Minimum Standards for the Pre-Operative Care*

On admission for surgery the patient is examined for:

(i) Blood pressure,

(ii) Urine analysis,

(iii) Intra-ocular pressure, and

(iv) Lacrimal sac patency test.

The eye to be operated is marked (on the forehead) with mercurochrome. The local drops of antibiotics are instilled in conjunctival/sac 6-8 times before surgery and the patient is given pre-operative instructions.

(i) *Premedication and Anaesthesia for Surgery*

(i) Premedication should be given. Surgeons may choose the premedication of his choice.

(ii) Standard methods of anaesthesia should be used (facial block and retrobulbar).

(j) *Standardisation of Operation Techniques*

(i) Standard scientific techniques should be adopted which give best results in the hands of the camp eye surgeon who should be qualified with adequate experience.

(ii) Corneao-scleral sutures must be given.

(iii) Sub-sonunctival injection of antibiotics must be given at the end of the surgery.

(k) *Post-Operative Care*

(i) At least one eye surgeon should stay in the camp till each patient is discharged.

(ii) Post-operative Dressing, one eye bandaging is preferred and use of cartella shield is desirable.

(iii) First dressing should be after 24 hours and subsequent dressings be done by competent ophthalmic surgeon.

(iv) Medication

- Local antibiotics drops and ointments instillation daily.
- Systemic antibiotic or chemotherapeutic agent is ordinarily not necessary as a routine but should be given wherever otherwise indicated.
- Local cortico-steroid usage should depend on local eye reaction.
- Cough and constipation should be taken care for.

(l) *Mobility*

- The patients are made mobile after 24 hours. This warrants application of more suture at the time of surgery.

(m) *Discharge*

- The patients are advised about do's and don'ts and post-operative instructions printed on discharge slips, antibiotic/steroid and ointment atropine is prescribed depending on the need of the individual patient.
- Temporary glasses can be dispensed for better mobility of these patients.
- The follow-up date should be announced at the time of discharge of patients.

(n) *Post-Eye Camp Follow-up*

One ophthalmic surgeon with the help of Ophthalmic Assistants must conduct follow up examination after 2-3 weeks of the closing of the camps for examination, suture removal and supply of aphakic glasses.

7. Planning Approach to Specific Blinding Conditions

7.1. Xerophthalmia

Primary Level

Where xerophthalmia is known to be a major public health problem, thought should be given to instituting emergency and generalised prophylaxis by periodically administering large doses of vitamin A to the population at risk. The vitamin should be administered by village or urban primary health care workers and under five clinics as part of their regular routine. In addition to routine distribution, the primary health care worker should examine every child for xerophthalmia (inquiring about the presence of night blindness and seeking evidence of Bitot's spots and corneal ulceration).

Because vitamin A deficiency clusters in families and neighbourhoods, families of affected children, their neighbours and, if at all possible, the rest of the village should be made aware of the potential seriousness of the problem and the care with which it can be prevented. They should be provided with specific instructions about which locally available food to use to feed their children and how best to prepare them.

Secondary Level

Where village-level workers are not available, primary xerophthalmia control is provided by static centres (clinics, hospitals, etc.). For the most part, these only reach children presenting of their own accord. Since vitamin A deficiency clusters in communities, a modest outreach programme can be a cost-effective means of dealing with the problem. Staff of centres can visit the neighbourhoods in which the xerophthalmia cases arises, administer a massive vitamin A dose to all pre-school-age children and provide nutritional education to their families. Among cultures that readily recognize night blindness, teachers can instruct school children to report the condition when present among younger siblings. Staff of centres should respond to a positive report in exactly the same way as to a self-referred case.

Static centres often have better-trained staff, more plentiful medical supplies, and inpatient facilities. They are, therefore, better able to handle cases of corneal ulceration and necrosis (and the severe illness commonly accompanying them) than are village-level workers. Their personnel may also be able to supervise primary health care workers and provide them with refresher course feedback and encouragement.

Tertiary Level

There is little need for sophisticated, tertiary-level care in the treatment of blinding malnutrition. Prompt vitamin A therapy will usually preserve useful vision whenever that is still possible. Those blinded by xerophthalmia rarely benefit from corneal transplantation..

7.2. Cataract

Primary Level

The initial intervention usually takes place at the primary level where locally available health care personnel such as the village health worker or volunteer can be trained to screen for visual acuity and identify those patients whose acuities are equal to or less than a predetermined level, usually 3/60 or 6/60. Further examinations to detect cataract can be carried out at the primary level or can be referred directly to the secondary level.

Secondary Level

The usual secondary level of care in most developing countries is the local hospital, which is staffed by a general medical practitioner and medical auxiliaries who have been well-trained to assist the general practitioner. Occasionally an Ophthalmologist may be available, or at least a surgeon or General Medical Officer who has received training in cataract surgery. Cataract surgery should be available at the secondary level, where it can be performed in local hospital! satellite eye hospitals or mobile eye camps.

Tertiary Level

Tertiary facilities are primarily towards taking care of more complicated cases such as congenital cataracts requiring general anaesthesia, cataracts, accompanied by other diseases of the eye such as glaucoma or iritis, or cataracts associated with systemic diseases such as diabetes that may complicate the pre- and post-operative care of the patient. In addition, the tertiary hospital may serve as a base for the development of satellite hospitals and mobile eye units.

7.3 Trauma

Primary Level

The treatment and management of ocular injuries is an important part of primary eye care in both rural and urban settings. Basic supplies of drugs, instruments and dressing materials should be provided to manage eye injuries at primary health care level. It is of particular importance that antibiotic ointment be made available in rural areas.

The primary health care worker may remove conjunctival foreign bodies, but deeply embedded corneal foreign bodies are best dealt with by personnel with special training. If referral to the secondary or tertiary levels is not practicable because of distance, etc. It may be desirable to train primary health care workers in the removal of corneal foreign bodies, and to provide instruments, topical anaesthetics, antibiotic eye ointment and dressing material.

The industry should have a provision for first aid and proper referral facilities for specialised care. Plants with potential risk of serious chemical hazards should evolve and maintain an emergency care service, emphasizing preventive aspects, giving periodic dummy demonstrations, and providing for quick irrigation and flushing of injurious toxic substances from the eye.

Secondary and Tertiary Levels

In addition to these emergency measures, some cases will need further treatment in the district hospital and more specialised treatment in special centres. Information regarding the eye casualty service should be readily available and liaison with the hospital authorities should be maintained.

7.4. Glaucoma

Primary Level

All primary health care workers should be able to recognize that an acute red eye, with reduced vision or pain or corneal clouding or dilated pupil, requires immediate referral.

There is little the primary health care worker can do to identify patients with early open-angle glaucoma. He should recognize the need, however, to refer any patient with decreased acuity, particularly when unilateral and any patient with relatively fixed, dilated or asymmetric pupils.

Secondary Level

Personnel at the secondary level should be capable of differentiating the various causes of red eye and providing appropriate medical therapy. Whenever possible, they should have available both pilocarpine and oral hyperosmotic agents, such as glycerol, to treat angle closure. Depending upon their degree of training in ophthalmic disease, secondary-level personnel may perform peripheral iridectomies. Otherwise these operations should be performed at the tertiary level.

For chronic open-angle glaucoma, the challenge at the secondary level is case-detection. Cases should then be referred to the tertiary level for evaluation and filtering surgery if needed. Following successful surgery, the patient should return to the secondary-level worker for periodic evaluation, and referral if the pressure should again begin to rise.

Tertiary Level

Depending upon the quality and relative availability of secondary and tertiary services, tertiary personnel may be required to perform peripheral iridectomies. Because of their superior training and facilities, they are best equipped for carrying out filtering surgery and managing its early post-operative complications.

7.5 Trachoma and Infections

Primary Level

The actual application of antibiotics to the eye is often carried out by local health aides with little, formal training in health work.

In the long-run, most of the antibiotic treatment must be carried out by the affected people themselves. To do this, they need to have an understanding of the disease and of the measures that can be taken for treatment. Provision of water, reduction of household crowding, identification and control of breeding sites of eye-seeking flies and improvement of personal hygiene should be actively encouraged and assisted, in order to reduce the transmission of eye infections.

Secondary Level

Simple eyelid surgery in the community itself is essential to block the chronic route to blindness from trachoma. This surgery can be provided by either health centres or mobile teams. Experience has shown that selected and appropriately trained medical auxiliaries can provide most of the lid surgery needed.

Once the backlog of trichiasis and entropion has been dealt-with there will be a continuing need for surgery on a lesser scale because cases of potentially blinding lid distortions will continue to arise long after infective stages of trachoma have been controlled in the community. In severely affected communities periodic surveillance with provision of lid surgery will therefore be required for many years.

B. A MODEL OF OPHTHALMIC OUTPATIENT SERVICES

The Royal College of Ophthalmologists

The Ophthalmic Outpatient Department (OPD) handles a significant proportion of all Ophthalmology workload and activity. An increasing amount of Ophthalmology treatments such as laser photocoagulation, chalazion treatment, botulinum treatment and intra-vitreal injections are now undertaken in OPD. As diseases of the ageing eye (cataract, glaucoma, AMD) are the most prevalent diseases in developed societies the majority of adult patients attending ophthalmic OPDs are over 65 years of age. Similarly, the majority of people with sight problems are aged over 60. These large number of older people attending ophthalmology OPDs are added to by large numbers of diabetic individuals with or at risk of eye disease. Importantly Ophthalmology OPDs also deal with significant numbers of children. Furthermore OPD activity in ophthalmology is proportionately greater than in other surgical specialties. It is recognised from NHS Hospital Episode Statistics returns that Ophthalmology clinics account for 10% of all hospital outpatient visits. At present a significant proportion of both ophthalmic primary care and management of long-term care for ophthalmic chronic conditions takes place in the Hospital Eye

Service in OPD. All of these factors make the Ophthalmic OPD a hub of activity and underpin the importance of quality OPD architecture, layout and patient flows. Some of these factors may change due to staff working practices; such as the development of the extended role of optometrists in the community and the GP with a Specialist Interest (GPwSI) in ophthalmology. Novel Integrated Clinical Assessment and Treatment Services (ICATS) may change the traditional 'divide' that separates primary and secondary care and are being developed in ophthalmology. In some areas NHS Commissioners are aiming to move aspects of ophthalmic care into the community. The standards for appropriate OPD care and facilities are the same regardless of whether care is delivered in the Hospital Eye Service, in independent sector treatment centers or in the community. This document seeks to refresh the College's commitment to the maintenance of proper professional standards in the ophthalmology OPD and to see the quality of care improve. The Health Care Commission provides generic or core standards with which all providers of health care in England must comply, and which are regularly inspected. For up-to-date information and to examine reports of inspections and 'health checks' of ophthalmology providers visit the Health Care Commission's website www.health care commission.org.uk The College has provided a discussion paper on Ophthalmic Primary Care.

Eye Clinic set-up

Many departments have open plan eye clinic areas with multiple workspaces. This allows an ideal environment for both teaching and clinical supervision whilst maintaining a reasonable degree of privacy. With the evolving requirement to reduce health care associated infections and the Department of Health aim to ensure MRSA screening for all admitted/day care patients, facilities for undressing for ophthalmology patients for swabs may be needed in the ophthalmology OPD if 'swabbing centres' are not provided centrally at hospitals. This matter is under review at the time of writing. Raised expectations of confidentiality and some 'noisy' paediatric refractions would favour some separate examination rooms. It should be possible to vary the lighting level in the clinic room, preferably via a dimmer switch near the slit lamp or by remote control. Window blinds are needed to ensure darkened examination rooms and air conditioning should be present throughout the department. All rooms should include an illuminated Snellen visual acuity test chart although there should be provision in the eye clinic for logMAR charts and contrast sensitivity testing. For adult clinics the 6 metre distance between patient and chart can be reduced to 3 metres by using a mirror. Scaled down vision charts for 3 metres direct are also available. Increasingly logMAR charts are needed for low vision use and in age-related macular degeneration patients as well as in children. Each clinic room or workstation must be equipped with a slit lamp, tonometer, indirect ophthalmoscope as well as a reclining chair or examination couch. A portable slit lamp and tonometer should be available for occasional use. There must be adequate hand washing facilities and alcohol gel dispensers to allow clinical staff to decontaminate their hands between each patient contact. Guidance on instrument decontamination from the College relevant to ophthalmology should be followed. Ease of access to the Eye OPD for visually impaired and wheelchair patients is critical. Often Eye Clinics are best located on ground floor levels. Directions to OPD should be very well signposted bearing in mind the need of low vision users. Navigational aids, sometimes tactile, embedded into walls or floors are in use for low vision users in some hospitals. If ground floor provision is not possible adequate elevator access is vital. Rooms must be large enough to allow visually impaired and wheelchair patients to be transferred—use safe manual handling techniques—to the slit lamp or examination couch. Cantilever mounted slit lamps can be used to examine patients in wheelchairs as an alternative. However, such cantilever mounts need to be adaptable to a range of patient and wheelchair sizes to be effective. Many eye units use a modular system incorporating the slit lamp along with other diagnostic equipment combined with an electrically adjustable chair, suitable for most patients. The clinician's chair must also be adjustable and provide good lumbar support. Equipment for obtaining microbiology and virology specimens from the ocular surface should be available. Equipment needed for undertaking examination of lacrimal drainage apparatus should be readily available as should any surgical equipment as needed if minor eyelid procedures, such as treatment of chalazion are undertaken in the OPD. Specific guidance on disease specific equipment requirements for assessment or treatment of specific eye conditions or interventions undertaken on an outpatient or daycare basis will be found in the relevant College publications, such as Cataract Surgery Guidelines, AMD or Diabetic Retinopathy Guidelines. These are available on the College website and regularly updated. Additionally guidance on Emergency Eye Services, which are often undertaken in the Ophthalmology OPD should be read in conjunction with this document. Many ophthalmology OPDs may undertake some teaching of medical and or optometric students who often 'sit in' during clinic sessions. Where such teaching is undertaken video screen display of slit lamp images is helpful. As part of the electronic patient record programme, it is important to have easily available high speed access to internet resources such as: NICE guidelines, Royal College websites as well as clinical information sources and databases. All clinic rooms should thus have access to the hospital's network and internet access. Such computers must have adequate quality flat screens for viewing of patient images captured from retinal angiograms or diabetic retinal screening and OCT and other digital examinations, including radiology images. College guidance on ophthalmic imaging equipment requirements and on informatics has been provided but must be considered in the context of continuing rapid developments of such technology. Access to the hospital's radiology imaging network is desirable in all cases and is mandatory if digital imaging is only performed, as is increasingly the case in modern radiology departments. Visual field testing should be undertaken in a room with appropriate lighting conditions and laser rooms should conform to regulations governing the safe use of class 4 lasers. There must be emergency resuscitation equipment available if fluorescein angiography is carried out. In the orthoptic department, clinic rooms should be at least 6m in length and appropriately equipped for the examination and assessment of children. There should be a separate waiting area for children and parents/guardians. Where possible children should be seen and treated in dedicated paediatric clinics. The College has provided advice on services for children. Optometric examination rooms should have appropriate facilities for visual acuity testing and refraction and there should be a slit lamp and keratometer available for contact lens fitting. Clinic waiting areas should be well lit and ventilated, preferably with air conditioning and be clearly signposted, bearing in mind that there will be many patients and carers present, some of whom may themselves be visually impaired. Separate 'sub-waiting' areas are usually provided for patients who have had their visual acuities measured and are waiting to see the clinician or who are waiting for drops to dilate their pupils. Provision should be made for patients in wheelchairs. Ideally there should be a separate waiting area for young children and families. Toilets (including facilities for the disabled) and facilities for refreshments should be available and clearly signposted. Public telephones and direct taxi lines should be available.

Location

Ophthalmologists should seek to be involved at the earliest stages of any planning and design of buildings used for clinical activities. There are examples of excellent layouts of dedicated facilities that can be drawn upon by those planning such projects. Ideally, the layout of both the ophthalmology OPD, ophthalmology day unit or ward area and ophthalmology theatre should lend itself to high volume day case surgery and to eye volume OPD throughput. For instance, the day unit should be in close proximity to theatres to enable patients to walk to and from theatre for cataract surgery as suggested in *'Action on Cataract'* and recently refreshed in *'Focus on Cataractix'*. Similarly if the OPD area is close to the theatre or treatment area patients can be progressed directly to treatment where this is appropriate, such as might be the case for intravitreal injections for AMD patients. Self-contained Ophthalmology units which are discrete within a hospital's design often demonstrate better patient flow. This has been the principle underlying the architecture of treatment centres, either NHS or independent sector.

Workload and staffing

While NHS care is becoming increasingly consultant led and based, ophthalmology however remains heavily reliant upon Staff and Associate

(SAS) grade doctors and especially so in OPD. Allied clinical professionals (nurses, nurse specialists, optometrists, orthoptists, photographers and medical technicians) play an increasing role in OPD settings in areas such as cataract assessment management and glaucoma monitoring. The College has been active in outlining the skills required for allied health care practitioners in such settings. There are many new challenges, in addition to the challenges of the ageing of the population, to face in ophthalmic OPDs including waiting times targets, 'Choose and Book' and the advent of the electronic patient record. In a general ophthalmic clinic with full nursing support, 15 to 20 minutes should be allocated for each patient and adequate space must be left on the clinic template for emergency/urgent referrals. The clinic session should last 3-3.5 hours depending upon local circumstances and there should be adequate time to allow for dictation of clinic letters and phone calls to GPs and to other specialists. The number of patients that can be accommodated in an OPD clinic session is dependent upon the team of doctors and health professionals working in the clinic. The consultant in charge must have sufficient time to review patients seen by SAS grade doctors, trainee ophthalmologists and increasingly non-medical staff. Junior trainees require close supervision and doctors in the early years of specialty training are now unlikely to have any previous ophthalmology experience and clinic template must reflect this. Methods available to increase clinic numbers and productivity are; longer clinics, more staffing, better use of technology, service redesign and or role redesign. Specialist eye nurse practitioners/ophthalmology technicians and optometrists are playing an increasingly important role in ophthalmology clinics particularly in areas of chronic disease management, e.g. glaucoma and in the initial assessment of new patients. Better quality patient care and enhanced productivity will be achieved by completing as many examinations and investigations as is needed at one clinic visit rather than having patients re-attend to complete investigations at subsequent dates. *'Do it once and do it well'* is a concept to remember. More time per patient thus often needs to be allocated to one stop clinics. Similarly, in special or treatment clinics it will be necessary to allocate more time for each appointment so that proportionately fewer patients will be seen. Many ophthalmology departments have an Eye Clinic Liaison Officer who provides an effective link with Social Services and or local charities for the visually impaired and low visual aid provision in the hospital and or community setting. The College recommends such provision.

Patient pathway

It is helpful to use service improvement techniques to identify and reduce any bottlenecks in the patient flow in OPD. On arrival patients should be directed to a clearly signposted reception desk and then advised where to wait until they are called into the clinic rooms. The clinic nurse should be aware of any patients with special needs. Clinics work more efficiently if thought is given in advance to patient flows. For new patients a patient letter vetting process can usefully include a series of initial instructions when the patient arrives in the clinic (in addition to visual acuity testing) such as—1. Examination for afferent pupillary defect, 2. Field of vision examination, 3. Orthoptic assessment, 4. Refraction examination undertaken on arrival, 5. Instillation of mydriatic eye drops. However, it is recognised that the arrival of both 'Choose and Book' and the 18 Weeks referral to treatment time target place additional strain on the administration and smooth flows and logistics of such quality and efficient OPD care. An experienced ophthalmic sister in charge and or clinic proformas for retinal or glaucoma clinics may make a significant contribution to the smooth running of clinics to take into account such matters. For follow-up patients instructions placed in notes at the end of the previous consultation can help improve the quality and efficiency of later subsequent contact.

Information for patients

Letters advising patients of appointment detail times and location should be printed on a high quality printer with a font size of at least 14 points. The patient should be advised to bring their spectacles and a list a current medications and the letter should explain what they may expect to happen during the appointment. It should be clearly stated that as patients may require dilating eye drops this might temporarily impair their ability to drive. Patient information leaflets (of appropriate size and quality print) explaining common ophthalmic conditions and surgical procedures should be readily available as should information leaflets on patient support groups and access to social services. This information should also be available on audio cassettes or CDs for patients with severe visual impairment and where possible should also be available in languages other than English. Most NHS hospital trusts have a translation or link worker service available. The College also recommends that posters and leaflets highlighting the ocular hazards of lifestyle, such as smoking, as well as details highlighting access to NHS smoking cessation services be displayed in Ophthalmic OPD.

Governance

Staff should wear identification badges so that patients are aware of the name and professional status of individuals involved in their care. The nurse in charge of the clinic must keep patients aware of the general progress of the clinic and the likely waiting time. Displays with such information have been found helpful while taking into account the needs of low vision users. Patient safety incidents in the ophthalmology OPD, may be administrative such as missing patient records, patient mis-identification, etc. or clinical such as missed diagnosis. The College recommends that such events should be recorded on local clinical risk incident reporting forms and discussed at departmental clinical governance meetings with a view to improving quality by learning from such events.

C. CASUALTY OPHTHALMIC CLINICS

The number of patients referred to the casualty clinic is usually unpredictable. In a study, the casualty clinics initially had quiet a variation in the distribution of patient numbers (7-23 patients per clinic). This resulted in some clinics being short and others too heavily overbooked. There were large number of patients attending for review in casualty clinics, which in turn reduced the number of appointment slots available for new patients; this contributed significantly for overbooking of casualty clinics.

After implementing the recommendations the subsequent clinics were more uniform, regular (10-14 patients per clinic) and identical inpatients distribution and workload. There was significant reduction in total number of review patients in casualty clinics and hence more slots were available for new referrals. The clinic format developed on PAS comprised of alternate appointment slot of a new and review patient helped in running the casualty clinic on time (as we found that new patient needed longer consultation time whilst review patient needed shorter consultation time). The departmental triage protocol also helped the nursing staff to make appropriate decisions regarding when to accept new referrals to the casualty clinics for most of the time. Hence they concluded that a proper and organised **ophthalmic** casualty clinic can help the medical and nursing staff to provide the high standards of clinical care in the best possible and efficient way.

D. MANAGEMENT AND ADMINISTRATION OF INTEGRATED CORNEA SERVICES

Alleviating blindness remains a daunting task for the eye care agencies in India. Government and non-Government agencies are actively engaged in taking care of blindness in India. A three-tier system for providing health care in general and eye care in particular is an accepted norm. To provide comprehensive eye care to our population: primary, secondary and tertiary eye care centers all have a role to play. Cataract remains the major cause of blindness and to take care of cataract blindness emphasis has been on eye camps. However, recent surveys have identified that in addition to cataract, other causes like corneal diseases, refractive errors, glaucoma and retinal diseases contribute significantly to blindness. Tertiary eye care centres are essential to develop state of the art technology for the patient care, teaching of the residents, training of the ophthalmologists and research activities. An eye center should have facilities for modern cataract surgery (suture less surgery, phacoemulsification), cornea service, retina service, glaucoma service, and oculoplastics and community ophthalmology. Each sub-speciality should be well equipped with latest gadgets for diagnosis and treatment of ocular disorders. Trained and experienced ophthalmologists should make full use of the technology available to them. Integrated cornea service should consist of cornea clinic, contact lens clinic, refractive surgery, corneal transplant surgery and eye banking. Active support of ocular microbiologist and immunologist is of paramount help.

Cornea Clinic

Cornea clinic should provide facilities for diagnosis and treatment of various corneal disorders. Corneal service is usually a part of major ophthalmic care delivery center or it may be an independent subspeciality hospital. Corneal clinic would get patients referred from the outdoor of the hospital or directly from the primary or secondary eye care centers. Facility for complete ophthalmic examination is a must. A preliminary examination of the patients is being done either by the residents/fellows or ophthalmic assistants. Slit lamp biomicroscopy is performed on every patient. Corneal lesions are documented on color-coded diagrams in specially designed corneal disease workup sheets. All the relevant clinical microbiological, biochemical, immunological and other systemic tests are performed. Depending upon the area of special interests special disease proformas can be prepared. Major workload in a cornea clinic is of managing infective corneal diseases. These include bacterial keratitis, fungal keratitis, herpes simplex keratitis and acanthamoeba keratitis. Vernal keratoconjunctivitis, dry eye, pterygium, meibomitis, limbal tumors, Mooren's ulcer are other common corneal diseases managed in the corneal clinic. Infective keratitis resulting threatened or actual corneal perforations need cyanoacrylate tissue adhesive applications. Corneal perforations need to be co-firmed on Seidel's test. Chemical injuries require urgent in emergency management. Immediate continuous conjunctival lavage with normal saline, plain water or any other fluid, even milk decreases the contact time of the chemical implicated. This helps in limiting the severity of chemical injury and improves the prognosis.

Microbiological support is the backbone of the corneal service

Speciality trained microbiologist with special interest in ocular infections may be an asset to the cornea service. Alternatively cornea surgeon has to rely upon hospital resources like combined microbiology department of the concerned hospital. Corneal surgeon should be able to perform direct microscopic examination of KOH wet mount, gram stained and giemsa stained, corneal smears. Collaboration with local laboratory for microbiological tests including bacterial, fungal and Acanthamoeba cultures may be useful. Quality control of the laboratory is an important issue. Patient should be explained all the medicines to be used in detail. On the subsequent follow-up visit, a sheet is attached to the patient files. Data is entered into the computer and sheet is preserved as a hard copy. Computerized data is coded and time spent in preparing coded sheets saves the time during data entry and analysis.

Contact Lens Clinic

Contact lens clinic should be carefully designed and special care should be taken to prepare the interiors. Recent magazines, journals, contact lens care literature should be available in plenty. A well-trained optician may be able to take care of non-medical aspect of contact lens practice. However, the ophthalmologist himself should do the complete ophthalmic examination of these patients. Patients should be carefully selected. They need to be evaluated for dry eye, allergic conjunctivitis, blepheritis and superficial punctuate keratitis. Special care should be taken to keep the appointments on time. Inventory should contain contact lenses of various base curves and powers so that minimal time spent on trial. Once contact lens trial is complete, a pair of contact lenses is prescribed to the patient. It is important to impart training to the patient so that the patient is confident to insert and remove his contact lenses. Patient should be advised on contact lens care regimen. Patient should be counselled on wearing schedule and do's and don'ts regarding the contact lenses. Patient should be provided with a copy of written instructions. Patient wearing soft contact lenses should be explained the risk of contact lens associated keratitis and giant papillary conjunctivitis. Patients following radial keratotomy, post-keratoplasty, corneal scars, keratoconus and PRK/LASIK require expertise while prescribing contact lenses.

Conreal Transplant Surgery

Corneal transplant surgery is the most important component of cornea service. Patients requiring corneal transplants should be thoroughly evaluated. Those requiring corneal transplants are registered under different categories. Patients requiring emergency grafts for corneal perforations with or without infective keratitis should be registered under separate categories. One eyed patients, bilateral blinds and children under the age of 8 years, at risk of developing amblyopia should be given priority. The success of corneal transplant surgery largely depends upon the nature of the corneal disease. Patients suffering from corneal diseases including dystrophies, keratoconus and mascular corneal scars have higher chances of having a successful corneal transplant. Patients having deep corneal vascularisation, herpes simplex keratitis, chemical injury, dry eye or ocular surface problem will have higher chances of graft rejection. Patients having pseudophakic corneal edema have more than 90% chances of having a clear graft but around 50% chances of getting good vision. This may be due to pre-existing cystoid macular edema or age-related macular degeneration changes. Prognosis should be discussed with the patient and/or his relatives in advance.

Results of modern corneal transplant surgery have significantly improved. Quality donor tissue, better preservation, use of suction trephines, micro-surgery improvements, viscoelastics have contributed the improvement is results. Patients should be adequately counselled for allografts rejection. In addition patient should be apprised of later development or worsening of pre-existing glaucoma. Patient should also be made aware of developing post-keratoplasty astigmatism and possible need of contact lens wear after surgery. It is commonly believed that surgery is 30% and follow up in corneal transplant surgery contribute 70%. The importance of regular and long-term follow up need to be stressed.

Cornea transplant service needs a dedicated team of eye bank professionals. Facility for attending eye donation calls immediately is a must. Effective communication system consisting of mobile phones, pagers, e-mail and fax are essential components. An independent vehicle is required for attending eye donation calls, transportation of donor eyes and for publicity programmes. Several sets of pre-sterilised instruments should be kept ready in advance to attend eye donation calls. Eye bank should be equipped with slit lamp, eye bank specular microscope, laminar flow system and a good refrigerator. Sufficient supply of latest media including MK or optisol should be available for corneal preservation. Eye bank technician should be proficient in distortion free corneal excision without premature collapse of the anterior chamber. Depending upon the set-up whether in Government or Non-Government agencies eye bank need to have ties with some major hospital. Active hospital retrieval programme should be initiated to have continuous supply of donor eyes. Adequate facilities for histopathology of corneal buttons, HIV test, HbSag test for eye donors and culture of donor rims should be available. Computerized documentation of data on eye donors on age, sex, cause of death, death-enucleation interval, type of preservation and recipient details should be done. Grade of donor eyes and endothelial cell counts should also be entered. Patients follow up records and results of corneal transplants should be analyzed. Stories on successful patients should be published in press, to enhance publicity on eye donation.

To start eye bank activities afresh requires lot of patience and determination. Active and interested individuals should be identified and a core group should be formed. Initial groundwork to create awareness should be done by delivering lectures during the eye screening camps. Influential people of the area preferably local leaders should be involved and persuaded to appeal general public to pledge eye donation. Heads of the voluntary societies should be requested to include eye donation as one of activities. Information and publicity material on eye donation should be made available in plenty. Once people are aware of eye donation, eye donation center should be opened to keep up the momentum. The magnitude of the corneal blindness, need of eye donation and the existing disparity between the demand and supply of donor eyes should be projected repeatedly in the press.

A local society comprising of people from various spheres of life, corneal surgeons, eye specialists and heads of the administration should be formed and registered. The heads of the local hospitals should also be involved in the movement of eye donation. During the National Fortnight on Eye Donation publicity measures should be stepped up. Public awareness lectures and film shows should be organised in the schools and colleges. Once there are voluntary eye donation calls, the local society should make a donor eye collection center. A list of trained corneal surgeons should be prepared. Arrangements to attend voluntary eye donation calls should be made. Stepwise facilities for communication including telephones, e-mail and fax should be added. Eye donation counsellors should be recruited to enhance awareness and procurement of donor eyes. An independent means of transport, vehicle should be acquired. This will help the eye bank in both publicity and procurement of the donor eyes. With each added facility the number of eye donations and number of corneal transplant surgeries increases. The rising graph shows increasing eye donations and corneal grafts with each added facility to the Eye Bank Society, Chandigarh

Refractive Surgery

Refractive errors are the commonest ocular problem encountered in practice by the ophthalmologists. A small myopic refractive error (0 to –2 dioptres) occurs in about 30% of population and 5% have myopia in the range of –2 to –6 dioptres. The same is the prevalence of hypermetropia more than 1 dioptre in the general population. Refractive laser corneal surgery has improved the results of surgical correction of these refractive errors. There is tremendous growth of refractive surgical procedures in the United States and it is estimated that more than one million laser procedures may be performed during the year 2001. Increasing population in India is becoming aware that surgical correction of refractive errors is possible and patients seek advice on the outcome of these surgical procedures. It is true that refractive laser surgery may not be the domain of all the practicing ophthalmologists, but it is important that they are aware of the procedures performed and their likely outcomes to counsel the patients.

Photo refractive keratotomy (PRK) and Laser *in-situ* keratomileusis (LASIK). Both the procedures are based on same fundamental principles of using ultraviolet laser (wavelength 193 nm). In PRK the corneal epithelium is removed either mechanically or with laser and then laser is applied on the corneal surface to produce a predetermined change in the corneal power. In myopic correction the corneal curvature is flattened by ablation of Bowman's membrane and part of the superficial stroma. Epithelial hyperplasia and regeneration accounts for stromal haze, unpredictability and regression with this technique. Burrato first described LASIK, the procedure. An automated keratome is used to cut a lamellar flap of epithelium, Bowmans membrane and superficial stroma (160 to 180 microns thickness). Excimer laser is used to ablate the stromal bed and lamellar flap is reposited back.

Cornea service needs active facility for refractive laser corneal surgery. Use of incisional refractive keratotomy may be restricted to the correction of post-cataract or corneal transplant astigmatism. Four incision radial keratotomy still may be an option in low or moderate myope not able to afford photo refractive keratotomy (PRK) or laser assisted in site keratomileusis (LASIK). LASIK is preferred over PRK because of lower incidence of regression, less epithelial haze and procedure being less painful. Patients having myopia upto 12D, hypermetropia up to 8D and astigmatism up to 6D are good candidates for LASIK. Patient needs to be counselled adequately and should have realistic expectations. Patients aiming for performing most of the activities without glasses even if uniocular unaided visual acuity is less than 6/6 are ideal candidates. With advances in automated lamellar keratomes, the keratome-related complications are negligible. With introduction of laser for making flap, necessity of automated mechanical keratomes may be eliminated. With the advent of wave front technology being linked to ablation of the cornea, results of LASIK are going to be still better.

The main constraint of laser corneal surgery is the high cost of excimer laser and automated lamellar keratomes. Utilizing a common laser facility by a group of ophthalmologists is a useful alternative.

Quality Control

Quality is also equated with excellence and comprise of effectiveness, safety, efficiency and satisfaction to the patients. In the era of technology revolution, the cornea service providers should not be forget the patient. Ultimately, it is essential that the patient is satisfied with eye care, reasonable cost and satisfactory outcome. Stokes (1971) stressed that communication and compassion is equally important. The patient should be made aware of the fact that he or she is a part of the care and not the meek recipient.

Good medical practice requires a high level of professional knowledge, personal dedication, the ability to communicate, and—most of all—the ability to make time. It also demands difficult balance between self-confidence and self-questioning. Too much of the former leads to arrogance, and too much of the latter to indecision. Sheldon in 1982 defined a clinical audit as "A study of some part of the structure, process, and outcome of medical care carried out by those personally engaged in the activity concerned, to measure the set objectives have been attained and thus assess the quality of the care delivered." Clinical audit is helpful in two ways. The first is clinical research. The complete details of the condition, treatment outcome of every patient is available for retrieval and analysis. The second objective of undertaking the clinical audit is quality assurance.

Continued Medical Education

Cornea service should have website, to inform of the various facilities available. The requisite patient information on contact lens wear, corneal transplant surgery and eye banking should be available on the website. Patients should also be able to fill registration forms, fix appointments and some other necessary documents online. This will reduce the workload during the visit and the corneal surgeon will get more time to discuss the patient's problem. Computerized recordkeeping is more efficient and time saving. A programme consisting of data entry module, reporting module and back up module is useful to secure the patients data. Even if the facility for the computerized data recording is available one need to retain the hard copies. Effective communication system, e.g. phone, fax, e-mail should be freely accessible to the cornea service and eye bank. Cornea service should have an access to the library containing latest reference books and current journals on cornea and related subjects. In addition, access to an online database system such as meddlar, pub med or Medline is extremely useful. Academic programme of the cornea service clinical meetings, journal club review and seminars should be prepared in advance. The programme should be circulated to all the interested ophthalmologists. In addition, a small or clinical update on a specific topic should be organised every six months. A news letter containing articles, details on the services available, facilities add recently and future programmes will help in achieving the desired publicity. Ultimately, the center should be approved for fellowship training in various sub-specialities by the international bodies.

Administration and Management

Administration of a Cornea service depends upon whether it is a part of an Eye Center or a sub-speciality hospital in itself. If it is a part of the Eye Center it comes under the administration of the center otherwise as an independent hospital it has to have its own administrative set-up. An effectively organised medical staff assume its role in the supervision and evaluation of patient care. Their contribution will bring greater improvement in the quality of the care. It is important to make sure that the services of the hospital are organised, supervised and evaluated from time to time. It does require extra time and specialised knowledge to effectively administer even a moderate sized hospital.

The concept of introducing a position of a medical director has a positive influence not only on the functioning of a hospital, but also on their medical staffs and patients. The medical Director should look after the management of professional activities of the hospital. The appointment of a medical director should encourage the medical staff to play an active, more meaningful and an effectives role in the hospital organisation. There are two ways of incorporating a medical director into the hospital administration. First medical director may be a part of the administrative team and reports to the chief executive officer. Alternatively there can be a certain dichotomy of the authority and responsibility with the internal organisation of the hospital. The various services chiefs on important issues and decisions assist the medical director. A service chief is in addition in-charge of his own service area and is responsible for the administration and management of that particular area. The joint commission on accreditation committee of a hospital has stated: "A good Chief of a service must have professional competence, administrative adequacy and in addition he must have a quality. Quality besides the above compassion, will, economy, understanding, sympathy, integrity and character." In addition, the medical director may ask for inputs from the management consultants. Financial matters, income tax-related issues may be sorted out with the help of the concerned professionals.

Medical director should ensure that the medical staff adhere to the laid down ethics. The hospital authorities should also carry on some charitable activities in the rural areas where the medical facilities are not accessible. In addition in the hospital also there should be provision for the free treatment of the poor patients.

E. EXPERIENCES IN DRY EYE MANAGEMENT

Dry eye is a rising menace of modern day living in pollution and stress and is the commonest problem of eye. Most of us have suffered from dry eye at one time or the other. Environmental smoke, chemicals, dust, sun, fumes, cosmetics, infrequent blinking (looking at computers, T.V., films, long driving, etc.) fluorescent and dazzling lights, over use of contact lenses, infections and allergies, injuries and scarring, air-conditioners, heaters and fans, malnutrition and dehydration all play their role in causing dry eye. Understandably, hot weather brings more of such cases. Paradoxically, neither the tests are done routinely nor any clinical studies have been conducted to find out the incidence of this commonest problem affecting eyes-tears production, distribution or evaporation. Since tears provide oxygen, nutrition and immune response, they are essential for maintaining transparency and integrity of cornea.

When dry eye (due to lacrimal gland dysfunction) is found associated with decreased saliva and other body secretions and joint pains like rheumatoid arthritis, a label of Sjorgren syndrome is given, but typical Sjorgren is not a common condition and whereas dry eye is. When meibomian glands are affected, usually due to chronic blephaitis, the lipid layer is lost and tears appears more watery, but deficient in quality.

The third layer of tear film contributed by conjunctival glands may become deficient in quality, due to chronic conjunctivitis or toxic effects of various chemicals/medicines, etc. The ophthalmologists in the metropolitan cities like Delhi/Bombay have repeatedly warned that the people are being forced to smoke through their eyes, due to increased vehicular smoke and chemicals. This has virtually caused an epidemic of dry eyes in these areas. They have also suggested to conduct clinical studies in this field and appealed to the courts and Government to ban the vehicles polluting the air and to upgrade technology in combustion of their fuel.

Relevance of Blink Rate

Blinking is essential for inducing tear secretion and spreading the aqueous, mucin, and lipd layers of the cornea. Between blinks, the tear film thins as a result of evaporation and drainage, exposing a bare cornea if the interval is too great. In a study, among workers at 22.5°C and 40%

humidity, blink rate averaged 22+9 per minute under relaxed conditions, 10+6 per minute while the subjects were reading a book at table level, and 7-7 per minute while the subjects were viewing text on a VDT. The corresponding exposed ocular surface areas, calculated by measuring the palperbral fissure width, were 2.2+0.4 cm^2, 1.2+0.4 cm^2, and 2.3+0.5 cm^2, respectively. Not only did tear evaporation increases alongwith exposed ocular surface area, but the evaporation rate per unit area also increased, suggesting a qualitative instability of the tear film over larger surfaces.

Of course, any activity or occupation that requires particular visual concentration predisposes individuals to developing ocular fatigue and other dry-eye symptoms. Takano and associates reported that the interval between blinks for ophthalmologists under normal circumstances is 2.1 + 0.4 seconds, but increases to 3.7 + 2.6 during biomicroscopy, 4.3 + 2.2 during tonometry, and 4.8 + 2.0 while performing a fundus examination, Surgical procedures substantially increase this interval further to 10.5 + 4.2 seconds during photocoagulation and 30.5 + 27.9 seconds during cataract surgery. Importance of frequent blink to prevent eye fatigue and to have stable vision cannot be over-emphasised.

My experiences

I wish to share my experiences of managing 4 cases of chronic intractable unilateral corneal ulcers, who had visited several eye centres before coming to me. They were treated with myriads of antibiotics and other drops, ointments, *sl* conj. Injections, oral antibiotics, vitamins and so on but showed only down the hill journey, i.e. formation of widespread ulcers over the cornea with profound loss of vision and other attendant symptoms. In fact, they were totally disillusioned and disappointed with the treatment and had almost written off the affected eye. Their desire to rid them off the troublesome symptoms, brought them from one centre to the other viz. Mrs. Chauhan, a housewife from Panjab University, Sultan, a farm worker from a Haryana Village, Gurnam, a driver from Punjab Roadways and Paul, an executive from Amritsar. Could dry eye be the underlying cause, I suspected. Shirmer's test performed on the other eye showed 0-1 mm reading. The diagnosis was established. Hourly regimen of preservative free tear substitutes was started. In addition 2.1. Methylecellulose, twice a day was added.

More startling was the fact that the vision continued to improve further, as the treatment continued. The complete healing of the ulcer occurred in a 2 monthly follow-up. The opacity also appeared to had become less dense, with time with continued use of tear substitutes. The experience with the use of tear substitute was gratifying indeed.

Clinical Studies

Several studies were conducted at Dr. Kumar's eye and vision centre to unravel some mysteries of dry eye.

In a study, on those persons who complained of burning, irritation, fatigue, sensitivity to light, eye strain, grittiness, sand in the eye, lack of visual comfort, unexplained redness, itching, etc., the incidence of dry eye was found to be 50%. In another study, conducted on contact-lens users, the incidence was 50% as compared to non-user youth, mostly young females, where the incidence was just 2% (Shirmer test values 0-1 mm). In another study on 60 + aged subjects, the incidence of dry eye was 50%. Many of them did not complain of any symptoms, but were more comfortable with lubricants. The incidence of dry eye was 100% among patients suffering from Pterygium or pingeculum.

Most cases of dry eye who came to the clinic and were included in the study, had some vague complaints, but otherwise they looked normal. It is only after it was suspected to be dry eye and the tests performed, that one could assess the tendency towards dryness. It would be interesting to quote a few representative examples.

(i) Neeru (45), a house.wife, suffers from continuous irritation in her eyes as though there is some dust particle, which refuses to be washed away with repeated splashing of water on the eyes. Neeru watches T.V. for long hours and has tendency towards dry eye. Use of air-conditioner often aggravates her feelings.
(ii) Neera (22) works in a private bank and is extremely tired in her eyes after daylong work on computer. If she comes out in the sun she can hardly open her eyes. She suffers from dry eye.
(iii) Harnam (50) a driver by profession is fed up with his eyes, though he is under treatment all these months and has used all possible brands of antibiotics and steroids. On Shirmer's test, it has been found that he suffers from dry eyes. Now damage to his eyes can be prevented.

Diagnosis

One has to proceed systematically for the diagnosis of a case of dry eye.

(a) History

One has to suspect from the symptoms/history, since the patient does not complain of dryness of eye, as such in most cases. The patient comes with symptoms of foreign-body sensation, burning and photophobia. Those with acute external disease have maximum symptoms. Those with chronic disease have minimum symptoms. The term discomfort may be the summation of his symptoms.

Ask "do you get tears when you peel onions? can you cry and produce tears when you feel sad or hurt." Inpatients with KCS, symptoms are usually less pronounced on awakening and worsen as the day progresses. Patients with blepharitis are highly symptomatic on awakening, better within an hour or so, and worse again later in the day. Are symptoms worsening as the patient is ageing? Is there a seásonal component? What effect does the environment cause on his symptoms?

Ask the patient what is being done now and what has been done in the past to treat the dry eye condition. A detailed list of any topical lubricants and medication must be obtained, including drops as well as ointment. Patients should be asked whether they have had previous placement of temporary collagen plugs. If so, note whether there was improvement in symptoms and whether epiphoral occurred (and, if so, for how long). Ask if and when silicone punctual plugs were placed or whether previous permanent occlusion with laser or cautery has been performed. If punctual occlusion was done, did symptoms improve or, at least, did it allow a decrease in the use of topical lubricants?

The use of systemic medications must also be noted, as many systemic medications affect tear secretion. The use of systemic steroids and other immunosuppresives, such as hydroxychloroquine (Plaquenil), methotrexate and cyclophosphamide (cytoxan), which may be used in treating patients with Sjorgren's syndrome and other collagen vascular diseases should be noted. Patients with decreased tear secretion are at risk for ocular surface infections owing to decreased levels of tear immunoglobulins, lactofferin, and lysozyme. The use of systemic immunosuppressives puts the patient at even greater risk.

It is important to determine whether the patient has any associated systemic symptoms for diseases. Therefore, a careful review of organ systems is required. Important questions should be directed towards detecting a history of dry mouth (xerostomia) or dental and gum disease. Patients with Sjogren's syndrome and xerostomia are at increased risk of dental and gum disease owing to lack of saliva. Questions that help in determining whether the patient has significant xerostomia include the following: can you feel saliva in your mouth? Can you swallow bread or meat without additional fluids? Women should be asked whether they have experienced a noticeable decrease in vaginal secretions. Patients should be questioned about whether they have ever been told; they have Sjorgren's syndrome, systemic lupus erythematous (SLE), rheumatoid arthritis (RA) systemic sclerosis (Scleroderma), vasculitis, thyroid disease, lymphoma or AIDS.

(b) Clinical Examination

Before the eyes are examined, the facial skin is examined for evidence of acne rosacea and the malar rash of SLE. The scalp is examined for seborrhric dermatitis (dandruff). Salivary gland enlargement is seen inpatients with Sjorgren's syndrome. The thyroid gland is palpated for enlargement and nodules. Exophthalmos and decreased blinking, which occur in Graves' disease, can cause symptoms and findings of dry eye due to increased evaporation. The mouth is examined for presence or absence of saliva and for oral candidiasis, and the conditions of the teeth and gums are noted. The tongue also is examined for evidence of dryness. The hands are assessed for joint inflammation and changes indicative of RA and scleroderma. Petechial rashes and eczema should be sought on the extremities.

On a look at the eye, note the severity of dermatochalasis, the palpebral fissure width and the presence of brow wrinkling or elevation. Patients with significant dermatochalasis often maintain a chin up posture to improve their vision. Function of the eyelids, completeness of the blink, and the blink rate are assessed: Do the eyelids meet with each blink? Is ptosis present? Is there lagophthalmos with a normal blink, gentle, sleep like closure, or forced eyelid closure?

The size of the lacrimal glands is evaluated by asking the patient to look down and out while the upper eyelid is retracted.

Slit lamp examination should be done in a consistent, orderly fashion, examining the marginal tear strip, the eyelid margin and lashes, the puncta, and the plaperbral and bulbar conjuctiva, concluding with the cornea. Examination of the fornices and the conjunctiva of the everted upper eyelid should be a part of every evaluation. Normal height of marginal tear skip is approximately 0.3 mm.

The conjuctiva is examined for the presence of papillae, follicles, symblepharon, subepithelial fibrosis, concreations, injection, scarring, etc.

The cornea is examined for the presence of adherent mucin and filaments, which are seen in more severe cases of KCS. Patients with increased inflammation, incomplete eyelid closure, or poor "wiper" action of the eyelids. Inpatients with KCS, filaments form inferiorly where the incomplete blink stops. The presence of corneal irregularity, punctuate epithelial erosions or punctat epithelial keratopathy is noted. Episcleritis, scleritis, and iridocyclitis can be seen inpatients with Sjorgren's syndrome and collagen vascular disease. Finally, a baseline intracoclar pressure should be obtained in all patients. If possible, as patients may be using or may require topical or systemic corticosteroids. Specular microscopy for the health of endothelial cells should also be done.

(c) Clinical Tests

Several tests are done to measure tear secretion. The important ones are Schirmer's and Jone's Tests. The Schirmer's test often is used as the basis (often the only basis) for diagnosis of the dry eye. Originally, this test was introduced to quantify reflex tearing due to conjunctival irritation (Schirmer's 1). Jones's basal secretion test used topical anesthesia to eliminate reflex stimulation of tearing. But, because topical anesthetics cause irritation and resultant reflex tearing. Jones suggested waiting 2 minutes after topical anesthetic application before performing the test. These tests all use a filter paper strip with a folded end placed between the lower eyelid and globe. The paper should be placed either to moral *or* nasal to the cornea to avoid corneal irritation and further reflex tearing. Even with topical anesthesia, there is a rapid initial wetting phase lasting 1 to 2 minutes due to absorption of the tear reservoir and local irritation. Over the next 3 to 5 mintues, there is a slower, more linear wetting rate. The most variability occurs the first 2 minutes. Therefore, readings taken at the end of 2 or 2½ minutes will have a higher rate of wetting than those taken after

5 minutes. Doubling the reading at 2½ minutes may yield erroneously high results. These tests are indirect measures of lacrimal gland secretion, measuring fluid from the tear lake after the fluid has moved across the surface of the eye. They are also subject to the effects of temperature, humidity, and evaporation.

Controversy surrounds the issue of which is the best test to use, Schirmer's or Jones's, to determine the maximum amount of tear secretion, use a Schirmer's test without anaesthesia, whereas to determine the minimum amount of tear secretion, use Jones's, basal tear secretion test. For example, inpatients with moderate to severe KCS, where it is important to determine whether a functional lacrimal gland is present, use a Schirmer's test. In suspected mild KCS or contact lens-induced dry eye, where it is important to determine the basal level of tear production, Jones's test is more appropriate.

Measurement of Tear Stability (TBUT)

Fluorescein or Invasive Tear Breakup Time

The time elapsed from the blink to appearance of the first random dry spot after application of topical fluorescein to the ocular surface is called the tear breakup time (TBUT).

Rose Bengal Test

Of all the clinical tests available, rose Bengal staining is the most useful and must be part of every dry-eye workup.

Also Fluorescein stains areas of epithelial cells loss and may actually be a vital dye. Sterile fluorescein impregnated strips or a 2% solution can be used. A drop of fluorescein is applied to the inferior marginal tear strip, and the patient is asked to blink and roll the eyes to ensure mixing. The amount of conjunctival and corneal staining can be graded similarly to rose Bengal scoring or on a scale of 0 to 4+. As with rose Bengal dye, conjunctival staining occurs in mid to moderate KCS and corneal staining. in more severe KCS.

(d) Laboratory Tests

It will include:

(i) Physical characteristics of the Tear Film viz. Tear Film Osmolality Tear Film pH, Ferning, Tear Film evaporation,
(ii) Chemical composition of the Tear Film viz. Electrolyte composition, Protein composition, Lysozyme, Lactoferrin, and
(iii) Histological Evaluation viz. Conjunctival Impression Cytology, Lacrimal Gland Biopsy.

(e) Response to Treatment Trials

Often a treatment trial will aid in diagnosis of the dry eye. Treatment with artificial lubricants will result in one of three responses— improvement, worsening, or no change. Patients with keratitis medicamentosa due to preservatives improve with discontinuation of preservatives and non-preserved artificial lubricants. Patients with moderate to severe KCS usually improve with very frequent use of topical non-preserved lubricants, whereas patients with milder disease may worsen with frequent artificial lubricants due to washing out of their own tears. If inflammation is present, patients may require topical steroids (non-preserved, if possible) for improvement. Oral tetracycline usually results in significant improvement inpatients with rosacea blepharitis. Patients with blepharospasm respond dramatically to botulinum toxin infiltration (Botox, Allergan Pharmaceuticals, Irvine, CA).

Treatment

The definitive cure remains elusive, dry eye can often be successfully controlled with available therapies, including artificial tears, lacrimal punctual plugs, and treatment of accompanying diseases such as meibomianitis and allergic conjunctivitis.

Four approaches to dry eye treatment are:

(i) The preservation of tear evaporation.

(ii) Research on artificial tear is now focused on the mechanisms of tear stability on the ocular surface rather than simply the maintenance of a certain tear volume. Recent studies have shown that the mucin layer is more critical to maintaining tear integrity than was previous believed.

(iii) Such drugs as epidermal growth factor (EGF) and aldose reductase inhibitors (ARI) although not direct treatments for dry eye, dohelpto protect the corneal epithelium.

(iv) There is considerable interest in the immunological aspects of dry eye. Immune targeted eye drops can modify the lymphocytic activities in the conjuctivita and lacrimal gland. Indeed, cycloporine A has been reported to be effective for the treatment of canine dry eye and may also be effective for certain types of dry eye in humans.

(a) Tear Substitutes

The mainstay of therapy for dry eyes is the replacement of deficient tear production with tear substitutes. Initially normal saline was used and was found to provide immediate relief in many cases. Later artificial tear containing cellulose ethers such on methylcellulose and hydroxymethyl cellulose were added. These thick preparations did indeed last somewhat longer than normal saline, but they tended toblur vision. Further developments included the use of polyvinyl alcohol, a film forming polymer that was believed to have an attraction of the ocular surface.

A wide variety of artificial tear preparations now exist, among which are preparations containing adsorptive polymers, some viscous and others non-viscous. Further attempts to devise a beneficial artificial tear include the use of sodium hyaluroanate (Healon) solution and concentrated preparations of methylcellulose. Some years ago, sustained release artificial tear inserts (Lacriserts) became available. These 5 mg hydroxypropylcellulose rods dissolve on contact with the ocular surface and release a viscous watery coating. The effects of one of these inserts can last 6 to 12 hours after insertion. The inserts provide a thick recorneal tear film and are particularly useful in KCS with an exposure component. Drawbacks include the development of a shimmering vision, particularly 2 to 3 hours after instillation, which is noted most on attempted reading.

Their cost and the difficulty in managing them has limited their usefulness. Lacriserts are effective inpatients with severe symptoms, who cannot be managed with frequent instillation of artificial tears.

Preservatives in the artificial tears retard the growth of microbial organisms but also usually have toxic effects on the ocular surface. The frequent use of drops containing preservatives can induce a significant degree of iatrogenic surface disease. The most commonly employed preservatives are benzalkonium chloride, chlorobutanol, thimerosal and chlorhexidine, the most toxic of which is benzalkonium chloride. This cationic detergent emulsifies lipids of cell walls. Chronic use of preservatives containing solutions, particularly in an otherwise compromised ocular surface, can result in irritation, lacrimation, hyperemia, photophobia and even corneal edema. Clinically, the following conditions have been associated with the use of benzalkonium chloride containing drops: puctate keratitis, grav corneal epithelial haze, pseudomembrane formation in the conjuctiva, a decrease in corneal epithelial microvilli and possibly, a delay in corneal wound healing.

Over the past several years, a number of preservative free products have been formulated. It probably is wiser to recommend the use of preservative free artificial tears to avoid the likelihood of worsening the ocular surface condition from preservative toxicity.

The application of an ointment before retiring provides a long-lasting (e.g. Lacrilube or Dualube) means of increasing lubricity between the eyelid and the ocular surface during sleep. Approximately 1/8 inch of ointment is sufficient to provide lubrication during the night without substantially blurring vision the following morning. The use of lubdcating agents is an adjunct to the use of artificial tears throughout the day.

(b) Tear Preservation

It is possible to take measures to preserve existing scanty tear production. The most commonly used approach involves occlusion of the puncta. The decision to occlude all the puncta should not be taken lightly. A hasty decision to occlude all the puncta permanently can lead to the development of epiphora, which can be very disturbing to the patient. Nonetheless, there has been a resurgence of interest in his procedure over the last several years as a useful way of managing patients with more severe forms of KCS. A silicon plug has been developed that can be inserted into the inferior and superior puncta after punctal dilatation. For trial of the efficacy of punctual occlusion, temporary collagan plugs can be tried.

Permanent punctal occlusion usually involves the application of heat to the puncta to effect a permanent seal. This has traditionally been done throughout the extensive portion of the superior part of the canaliculus; sufficient epithelium must be destroyed so that a good scar will result, otherwise in only temporary occlusion can occur, which generally open within 1 week's time. In some cases, use of driving glasses or swimming goggles can be recommended.

Occasionally useful in managing dry eye conditions is the attempt to reverse some of the desiccation seen on the corneal surface, which can be accomplished with bandage soft contact lenses. These water filled lenses provide a moist covering and exchange some of their fluid with the epithelium, thus playing a role in rehydrating desiccated epithelium. Bandage contact lenses are particularly useful in cases of filamentary keratitis as they have been associated with the rapid dissolution of the filaments and prompt relief of severe discomfort. These lenses must be used in conjunction with preservative free artificial tear preparations as they tend to dry out quickly. The considerable risk of infection associated with bandage soft contact lens wear in dry eyes leads to recommend their use in only a very small number of patients with intractable filamentary keratitis that cannot be managed by other treatment modality.

(d) Decreasing Tear Viscosity

Some patients with KCS have particularly viscous, stingy mucus that may be associated with filaments or coarse mucus plaques on the ocular surface, which appear to be major source of irritation and discomfort. The use of solution of acetycysteine four to five times daily can help decrease the viscosity of mucus on the ocular surface. The solution itself tends to be irritating on application: a milder 10% solution is more tolerable in this regard.

(e) Surgery

In severe cases, mucus membrane grafting from buccal mucosa, which is particularly useful inpatients with severely scarred conjuctiva such as occurs after chemical burns. Another surgical procedure that had been employed was parotid duct transplantation, in which ducts leading from the parotid gland are transplanted so that they empty out to the conjunctival surface.

Inpatients with severe ocular surface disease, particularly persistent epithelial defects and non-infectious corneal ulcers, a tarsorrhaphy can be extremely useful. One theory supporting its use inpatients with KCS attributes efficacy to decreasing the exposed surface of the eye.

(f) Newer Modalities

In some cases modulation of the underlying immune response may prove more efficacious than the frequent use of artificial tears. Investigations of the use of interferon—a drop for the treatment of dry eye in Sjogren's syndrome are ongoing. Preliminary results show that concentrations as low as 20 units/ml can suppress EBV *in vitro*. Concentrations of upto 2 million units/ml, used four to five times daily, are being tested in clinical trail. Approximately half the patients reported subjective improvement.

Epidermal Growth Factor (EGF) is present in tears and may play a role in the normal maintenance and wound healing of the corneal epithelium. Because dry-eye patients have a paucity of tears, the epithelium may receive insufficient EGF. The use of EGF in dry-eye patients is now under investigation. It has been found that the corneal epithelial morphological changes in diabetic patients can be reversed by topical Aldose reductase inhibitor (ARI) 0.25% of CT112; Senju Pharmaceutical, Osaka. A promising results with artificial tears containing retinol, 500 IU/ml (Vitamin A) were obtained in some cases. Researchers had some success treating dry eye with a new artificial tear compound containing 18 peptides with the RGD sequence, combined with chondroitin sulfate. Both the RGD and chondroitin sulfate portions can mediate adhesion to the corneal epithelium. RGD peptide drops may thus serve to diminish both dryness and infection.

Recently, drops containing very high concentration methylcellulose (hydroxypropyl methylcellulose) have been introduced and used for the treatment of dry eye in Sjogren's syndrome and found decreased rose bengal as well as fluorescein staining, although patients with only mild to moderate symptoms disliked the high viscosity preparation. In a recent study in Israel L02A drop, a mixture of glycerol and hyluronate, were tried, with significant relief (Ocular Pharmacology, 1998). In another study in Florida (Ophthalmology, 1999), 21 patients with bothersome symptoms, not responding to usual tear substitutes, topical non-preserved methyl predinosolone sod. succinate 3-5 times a day, was given for 2 weeks, who showed remarkable improvement in all cases.

Special glasses that employ wet sponges inserted on side panels to increase the humidity surrounding the eyes have been devised. The side panels serve both to hold the sponges and to act as additional barriers to evaporative loss. All patients who used these special glasses reported greater comfort and showed objective improvement.

References

Bacheff, E.M., Davies, A.M. and Petros-Barrazian, A., The Risk Approach in Health Care, 1984, WHO, Geneva.

Black, D. (1981), Preface to Reviewing Practice in Medical Care. Steps to quality, Assurance, edited by G. McLachlan. Nuffield Provincial Hospitals Trust, London.

Cheung WW, Heeney L, Pound JL. An advance triage system. *A&E Nursing* 2002;**10**:10-6.

Department of Health. *Action on cataracts—Good Practice Guidance*. NHS Executive. Feb 2000 http://www.dh.gov.uk/assetRoot/04/01/45/14/04014514.pdf

'*Focus on Cataract*' NHS Institute for Improvement and Innovation. Coventry 2008 x Royal College of Ophthalmologists. *Patient safety in ophthalmology*. 2005 http://www.rcophth.ac.uk/docs/profstands/ophthalmicservices/PatientSafetyinOphthalmologyJuly2.

Guidelines for Programme for Prevention of Blindness, 1979, WHO, Geneva.

Hahault, D. and Roemer, M.I., Leadership in Primary Health Care, 1986, WHO, Geneva. National Seminar on Eye Camp Organisation, 1986, Government of India.

Ilango B, McGalliard JN, Hughes A. The role of nurse practitioners in a primary care eye clinic. *A&E Nursing* 2000;**8**:43-5.

Indian Council of Medical Research, National Conference on Evaluation of Primary Health Care Programmes (1979), New Delhi.

Jones NP, Hayward JM, Khaw PT, *et al.* Function of an ophthalmic accident and emergency department:results of a six month survey. *BMJ* 1986;**292**:188-90.

Klechowshi, N.M., Roemer, M.I. and Van Derweff, A., National Health Systems and their Reorientation Towards Health for All, 1984, WHO, Geneva.

Kleckowshi, B.M., Elling, H.R. and Smith, D.L., Health System Support for Primary Health Care, 1984, WHO, Geneva.

Klezykoweshi, B.M. and Pioulean, R. (1977), Approaches to Planning and Design of Health Care Facilities in Developing Areas, WHO, Geneva.

Mach, E.P. and Abel-Smith, B. (1983), Planning the Finances of the Health Sector, WHO, Geneva.

Management Process in Health Care (1982), S. Srinivasan (Ed.), MHoon Publishers, New Delhi.

McMahon, R. (1980), On being incharge: A Guide for Middle Level Management in Primary Health Care, WHO, Geneva.

Methods of Assessment of Avoidable Blindness, 1980, WHO, Geneva.

Pan American Health Organisation, Health Planning Problems of Concept and Method (1965).

Report of the Working Group on Control of Blindness, 1982, Government of India.

Royal College of Ophthalmologists, *Hospital Eye Services, Decontamination*. 2006 http://www.rcophth.ac.uk/docs/profstands/ophthalmic-services/DecontaminationJan006.

Royal College of Ophthalmologists, *Hospital Eye Services, Informatics*. 2006 http://www.rcophth.ac.uk/docs/profstands/ophthalmic-services/InformaticsJan2006.

Royal College of Ophthalmologists, *Hospital Eye Services, Ophthalmic Emergency Services*. 2006 <http://www.rcophth.ac.uk/docs/profstands/ophthalmic services/OphthalmicEmergencyServicesJan2006>.

Royal College of Ophthalmologists, *Hospital Eye Services, Ophthalmic Imaging*. 2006 http://www.rcophth.ac.uk/docs/profstands/ophthalmic-services/OphthalmicImagingApril2006.pdf

Royal College of Ophthalmologists, *Ophthalmic Primary Care*. 2006. http://www.rcophth.ac.uk/docs/profstands/ophthalmic-services/OphthalmicPrimaryCare2005.

Seven Commonwealth Health Ministers' Meeting (1983), Commonwealth Secretariat, London.

Sheldon, M.G. (1982), Medical Audit in General Practice. Royal College of General Practitioners, occasional paper 20, pp. 1-21.

Stokes, J.F. (1971), Aims of evaluation. In Proceedings of conference on evaluation in Medical education, edited by J.A.L. Gilbert, Bulletin Commercial Printers, Edmonton, pp. 9-17.

Strategies for Prevention of Blindness in National Programmes, 1984, WHO, Geneva.

The National Service Framework for Children, Young People and Maternity Services vii Royal College of Ophthalmologists, *Hospital Eye Services, Ophthalmic Services for Children.* 2005. http://www.rcophth.ac.uk/docs/profstands/ophthalmic-services/OphthalmicServicesforChildrenMay2005.

Timmappaya, A. (1967), Hospitals in India: History, Number of Beds, Targets Regionalisation Concepts, Hospital Administration, 4: 7.

Vernon SA. Analysis of all new cases seen in a busy regional centre **ophthalmic** casualty department during a 24 week period. *JR Soc Med* 1983;**76**:279-82.

Wong D, Brazier DJ. Primary **ophthalmic** care: why did patients choose to come to the accident and emergency department? *Trans Ophthalmol Soc UK* 1986;**105**:510-2.

5

Hepatitis Clinic in a Hospital

Jaundice is emerging as a major health problem and contributes to poor health and morbidity of the affected individuals in a large measure. The number of viruses affecting the liver is increasing by the day. Diagnosis and management of such cases requires specialised knowledge, modern laboratory equipment and setting up of exclusive hepatitis clinics/ departments of hepatology. As a part of this service, a detailed knowledge about the various viruses, on going research for preventive vaccines and the development of medicinal and non-medicinal remedies would be essential. (Also see appendix attached to this chapter for Management aspects)

Many viruses can affect the liver functions and its morphology indirectly as a result of systemic infections, only a minority of these viruses are truly hepatotropic; that is they are infectious to the liver itself producing hepatitis. Jaundice as a major classical manifestation. The term viral hepatitis is referred to this group of patients affected by several viruses, the characterisation of whom in recent years has been one of the most spectacular successes of modern classical research.

While viral hepatitis has been known to occur since ages, the first description of Hepatitis B dates back to 1885 where an outbreak occurred in Germany amongst workers of a local company who were vaccinated against small pox. That two types of hepatitis viruses exist have been known since 1930s. During the Second World War when two military outbreaks occurred; one outbreak was related to Hepatitis A virus and the other to Hepatitis B. Feco-oral route of transmission was responsible for Hepatitis A, while transmission by blood was attributed to Hepatitis B. Professor Blumberg and his associates in mid-60's discovered the Australia antigen now called Hepatitis B surface antigen. With this started the era of intensive research in the field of hepatitis.

Rizetto and his associates discovered the delta antigen in 1977, which subsequently was related to a new RNA virus; the hepatitis delta virus (HMV). Feinstone *et al.* in 1973 identified the hepatitis A virus in feces by immunoprecipitation to which serum of a patient from hepatitis A had been added.

With tests being available for HAV and HBV, there was still a group of viral hepatitis patients who lacked makers of either infection. This new variant of viral hepatitis was called "Non A, Non B hepatitis; a diagnosis made on exclusion. In 1989, Hougton and associates provided a breakthrough by identifying a clone that met the criteria for being a new viral genome and provided the key to the characteristics of hepatitis C virus (HCV). At the same time a new agent responsible for outbreaks of hepatitis in tropical and sub-tropical areas was named hepatitis E virus.

The five viruses recognized by the end of 1980s account for 85-90% of viral hepatitis. Two new viruses have seen since been proposed to fill the nosological gap. Hepatitis F virus was identified in 1994 transmitted through orofaecal route by a French group. The existence of this virus has further not been substantiated. More recently hepatitis G virus has been also identified (1996). The hepatitis viruses have a very narrow host range and man seems to be their reservoir. Although they manifest in a similar way they have completely different genomic organisation.

Hepatitis A and E are transmitted via the feco-oral route. They are prevalent in virtually all areas with sub-optimal hygiene of water supply and food production. The uptake of these viruses occurs orally, but in rare cases, may be transmitted by transfusion of blood or clotting factors. The virus is taken up by some unknown receptors on the hepatocytes and the genome is released into the cell. Replication then occurs, within the cytoplasm and the virus particles are released into blood and bile.

Hepatitis B, C and D are transmitted by the parenteral route. Their entry into the hepatocytes is via hepatocyte receptors. Replication and release into the circulation is the same as in case of Hepatitis A and E except that they are released mainly into circulation.

Clinical Presentations

All the hepatitis viruses produce hepatitis of the anicteric variety in majority of the patients. Fulminant hepatitis occurs in 1% of cases with acute hepatitis. Prognosis is poor in this group of patients, being worse in sporadic, Hepatitic E. Pregnant females are more prone to develop fulminant hepatitis in the third trimester of pregnancy. While Hepatitis A primarily affects children, most of the adults in India develop antibodies to Hepatitis A; hence are usually immune to a fresh Hepatitis A virus infection. Hepatitis A along with Hepatitis E do not lead to chronicity. Patients with Hepatitis B on other hand lead to chronicity in 90% of cases, if the infection is acquired in the perinatal period, and 5-10% if acquired in adulthood. These patients of chronic hepatitis may ultimately develop cirrhosis and hepatocellular necrosis and even carcinoma. Similarly, hepatitic C which is usually acquired at adulthood, leads to chronicity in 60-70% of patients and constitute almost 20% of patients with cirrhosis/

chronic hepatitis coming to a referral center. It also forms an important etiology in causing hepatocellular carcinoma. Hepatitis D is transmitted by parental route; and causes hepatitis in the setting of hepatitis B infection.

Diagnosis

The diagnosis of different hepatitis viruses rests on the serological markers. The viral markers commonly used are with their interpretation.

1. IgM anti-HAV ⟶ acute hepatitis A infection.
2. HBsAg ⟶ carrier/acute hepatitis B.
3. IgM anti-HBc ⟶ acute hepatitis B.
4. HBeAg ⟶ replicative phase of hepatitis B.
5. anti HCV ⟶ hepatitis C (acute/chronic hepatitis).
6. IgM anti-HEV ⟶ acute hepatitis E.

Treatment of Acute Hepatitis

I. Hepatitis A

No specific therapy is required as the disease is self-limiting. Management is mainly supportive. There is no significant benefit of either bed rest, or restriction of physical activity. Alcohol however should be avoided. Steroids should be avoided. Occasionally if cholestasis occurs such patients may benefit with ursodeoxycholie acid and cholestyramic?

Prevention of Hepatitis A

India is endemic for Hepatitis A infection. Since the disease spreads by the feco-oral route, improvement in environmental hygiene, including a clean, safe water supply, adequate disposal of waste and improvement in living conditions, common-sense hygiene measures like hand washing, universal precautions, avoiding raw tap water, uncooked food are likely to decrease the incidence of Hepatitis A. With these measures a small proportion of susceptible population now includes adults who if infected with Hepatitis A infection are likely to have a more severe course. Epidemiological data from India also shows a shift in the susceptibility of the population from children to adults

Passive Immunisation

This is done with immunogrobulins prepared from larger plasma pools containing anti-HAY with levels above 100 u/ml which are protective. It is most effective if it is given before exposure intramuscularly with a dose of 0.02 ml/kg for short exposures 0-2 mo.) or 0.06 ml/kg for longer exposures (3-5 mo.) If given within 2 weeks of exposure, it is likely to be protective in 85% cases. The earlier the immunoglobin given after exposure, the more effective it is likely to be. This prophylaxis should be given to household, sexual and institutional contacts of patients with acute hepatitis A. This prophylaxis however is not necessary for casual contacts like classmates, office and factory chowkidars.

Active Immunisation

Inactivated whole virus vaccine has been available since 1992. It has shown to have a high protective efficacy when used prophylactically. It is likely to be effective for a period of 20 years with the data available. Response to hepatitis A vaccine has been used to interrupt community wide outbreaks. There are no recommendations for universal vaccination but it is indicated in school children who are the most prone group to develop acute hepatitis A. Patients with cirrhosis liver in the west are susceptible to Hepatitis A infection which may lead to decompensation. This however is not justified in the Indian setting since these cirrhotics are already immune to HAV infection as demonstrated by anti-HAY positivity in their blood. In the Indian setting this vaccine which is given as 2 doses 6 mo. apart is indicated in young children who come from an elite class, who are likely to have a higher standard of hygiene and would be also able to afford the vaccine.

2. Treatment of Hepatitis B

The emphasis in the management of hepatitis B should again be conservative with education of the patient and protection of contacts. Supportive measures are the same as with treatment of hepatitis A. Patients should avoid unnecessary activities and excesses travel during the period of jaundice. A good nutritious diet is recommended. Patients may find fatty foods induce indigestion or early satiety. Alcohol should be avoided. Most of these patients recover especially in adults. There is little role of anti-virals.

Chronic Hepatitis B

Chronicity that occurs in 5-10% of adults who suffer from acute hepatitis and 80-90% of neonates who acquire perinatal hepatitis B infection from infected hepatitis B mothers, may result in cirrhosis and hepatocellular carcinoma. The major goal of therapy is to stop viral replication and thereby obtain remission of the liver disease and prevent long-term complications of this disorder.

Interferon has proven to be an effective means of achieving these goals, which ultimately can hasten the conversion to an HBsAg negative status, signifying cure of the disease. Interferons are primarily produced by nucleated host cells in response to viral infection. It has an antiviral effect by causing viral RNA degradation through ribonuleases and protein kinases. It also inhibits viral entry, into hepatocytes. Inferferon has immunomodulatory effect as well, mediated by an increase in expression of HLA class on the surface of hepatocytes. It is given by subscutaneous route at a dose of 5 million units every day for 4 months.

It is indicated inpatients who have raised transaminases at least 1½ times the upper limit of normal, HbeAg positive indicating replicating virus and evidence of chronic hepatitis on liver biopsy. Response occurs in 25-40% of patients after 4 months of therapy as evidenced by normalisation of trasaminases, HbeAg converting to anti-HBe and histology showing evidence of inactivity. Interferon is contraindicated inpatients with decompensated cirrhosis, neuropsychiatric illness, and patients with autoimmune diseases.

It is likely to be effective inpatients of chronic hepatitis with high aminotransferases and HBV DNA load of less than 200 pg/ml. Interferon therapy is associated with significant side effects and hence should be given by physicians who are well conversant with the drug. The drug is costly which forms a major handicap.

Inpatients with chronic hepatitis B who have a precore mutant HBV virus diagnosed by the presence of HBsAg, anti-HBe and HBV DNA, lamivudine an oral nucleotide analogue is of use. This drug given in a dose of 100 mg per day, given for a period till HBeAg seronconversion occurs, which usually takes 6-9 months. The drug needs to be given for another 3 months after the seroconversion. The drug does not have any side effects except pancreatitis in children. Mutations in the YMDD moting of DNA polymerase is also described inpatients on lamivudine therapy leading to resistance. This may be associated with a rise in transminases, but rarely decompensation inpatients with cirrhosis has been described.

This drug is also indicated inpatients with decompensated cirrhosis who are HBeAg positive which forms a contraindication for patients to be given interferon therapy. Both the therapies are effective in 40% of cases. Hence, the need for preventing Hepatitis-B infection.

Hepatitis B Vaccination

Initially plasma derived Hepatitis B vaccination consisting of HBsAg particles, that produce an antibody to it has been found to be effective in preventing individuals from Hepatitis B infection. It is prepared from pooled HBsAg particles separated from the blood of individuals infected with HBV.

Later recombinant Hepatitis B vaccine became available. Most of the countries now use this vaccine which is given in a dose of 20 ug at 0.1 and 6 months intramuscularly for adults and 10 ug for children below 10 years. It gives a seroprotection in 95% of persons. The response may be poor in obese; males, severely immunnosuppressed individuals, e.g. with renal failure, post-transplant, and HIV positive patients. This poor response is due to a defective macrophage function or a poor B cell response which may be HLA mediated. It could also be due to subcutaneous injection.

Vaccine is indicated in high risk groups like health case workers which includes doctors, nurses and laboratory technicians. In India, perinatal transmission of Hepatitis B infection forms an important group which needs to be controlled. Vaccination to newborns of HBsAg positive mothers should perhaps be the only recommendation in developing countries. A practical suggestion would be to give HBV vaccine to all infants soon after birth, which would remove the necessity to screen pregnant women for HBsAg. The best use of limited available resources should not be on screening mothers, but in procuring enough HBV vaccine for all infants.

The HBV immunisation programme should integrate with the existing expanded programme on immunisation. It has been a concern that the added HBV vaccination may jeopardize the acceptance of the existing vaccines used in the EPI. In Indonesia on the contrary the added HBV vaccination did not decrease the coverage of EPI, but increased it. It has been proven that vaccination during the first week of life is effective in preventing vertical transmission of HBV. In countries where births occur mostly in hospitals or clinics, this can be easily done. However, in areas where Illost deliveries occur in the home, how to vaccinate the neonate in the first week will pose problems that definitely require additional efforts. The World Health Organisation has played an important rôle in the implementation of immunisation programmes globally. In the coming years the price of HBV vaccines will continue to fall and with active participation of government as well as non-government organisations' control programmes should be able to expand further.

With the institution of universal HBV vaccination in Taiwan, the hepatocellular incidence per 100,000 children 6-9 years of age has decreased from 0.52 for those born before 1984 to 0.13 for those born after 1984. So the prevalence of HBV infection has effectively decreased from 10% before 1984 to less than 1% after 1990. The unvaccinated population is also protected through the elevation in the group immunity level.

3. Hepatitis C Infection

Hepatitis C virus is an important cause of chronic liver disease world-wide. HCV has 6 major genotypes and it circulates within an infected individual as a number of closely related but distinct species termed as quasispecies. Majority of patients who acquire HCV infection are asymptomatic, hence they are detected just by chance. Some of them may complain of vague ill-health, exhaustion and fatigability. Routine blood examination on them leads to detection of raised transaminases and on further investigation HCV may be positive. The route of transmission is the same as HBV, i.e. through blood transfusions and blood products. A history of blood transfusion in chronic hepatitis is obvious in only 50% of cases.

The diagnosis of Hepatitis C virus infection is based on detection of antibodies to Hepatitis C antigens based on the ELISA technique. This test is able to diagnose HCV infection after 4-8 weeks of exposure. In the early part of infection the diagnosis may be made by detecting HCV RNA in the blood. While 15-20% of patients with HCV infection recover, almost 80% of them develop chronicity. A number of factors are important in the evolution of chronic hepatitis C to cirrhosis. These include the length of time that the patient has been infected, the age at exposure, dual infection with other viruses, alcohol use and genotypes. Diagnosis of cirrhosis is made by clinical assessment of the patient, the use of imaging studies; a thoughtful laboratory evaluation and histological examination of liver tissue. See Appendix to this chapter for more on Hepatitis C.

These patients develop cirrhosis after 20-30 years of getting infection. The goal of antiviral therapy for chronic hepatitis C is to normalize the liver enzyme and become HCV RNA negative. Interferon as in Hepatitis B is the sheet anchor of therapy for eradication of the disease. A 12 months course of interferon alone can eradicate HCV RNA from serum in 15-30% of cases, whereas a combination of interferon and ribavaian achieves a sustained viral clearance in approximately 40-50% of cases.

Recent long-term studies show that HCV is not detectable in the serum or liver in more than 90% of patients who experience a 6 month virologic sustained response after a course of interferon therapy. Retreatment of patients who relapse after an initial course of therapy with combination achieves 49-55% virological sustained response. Current treatment strategies for prior non-responders to interferon therapy are not satisfactory. A favourable response is dependent on low HCV RNA level, absence of fibrosis, genoa types 2 and 3 and prolonged duration of treatment. Treatment of patients with normal transaminases do not have a satisfactory response with combination therapy.

Since, the response to treatment is unsatisfactory, it is prudent for preventing this disease by making anti-HCV testing in blood banks mandatory. Patients detected HCV positive should be treated so that the general pool of HCV infection is decreased in a community.

Unlike Hepatitis B, vaccine against Hepatitis C is not yet available. An optimal HCV vaccine should elicit protective oral and cell mediated immune responses that are capable of preventing chronic HCV infection. The major challenge in clinical development of a suitable HCV vaccine lies in demonstrating its efficacy.

4. Hepatitis D

It has a presentation similar to other viruses. It is uncommon in India, and is diagnosed by demonstrating anti-HDV in blood of patients with hepatitis. It occurs only in individuals infected with Hepatitis B. Treating and preventing HBV infection is likely to decrease the prevalance of HDV infection.

5. Hepatitis E

The manifestations are similar to other hepatotropic viruses. It is diagnosed by demonstrating IgM anti-HEY in blood. Treatment is the same as other viruses. No vaccine is yet available for preventing Hepatitis E infection.

References

Dienstag JL, McHutchison JG. American Gastroenterological Association technical review on the management of hepatitis C. Gastroenterology. 2006;130:231-64.

Manns MP, McHutchison JG, Gordon SC, *et al.* Peginterferon alfa-2b plus ribavirin compared with interferon alfa-2b plus ribavirin for initial treatment of chronic hepatitis C: a randomised trial. *Lancet.* 2001;358(9286):958-65.

Mariño EL, Alvarez-Rubio L, Miró S, *et al.* Pharmacist intervention in treatment of patients with genotype 1 chronic hepatitis C. *J Manag Care Pharm.* 2009;15(2):147-50.

Rodis JL, Kibbe P. Development of a hepatitis C support group. *Am J Health Syst Pharm.* 2006;63(17):1594-96.

Smith JP, Dong MH, Kaunitz JD. Evaluation of a pharmacist-managed hepatitis C care clinic. Am J Health Syst Pharm. 2007;64(6):632-36.6. Kolor B. Patient education and treatment strategies implemented at a pharmacist-managed hepatitis C virus clinic. *Pharmacotherapy.* 2005;25(9):1230-41.

Snella KA, Sachdev GP. A primer for developing pharmacist-managed clinics in the outpatient setting. *Pharmacotherapy.* 2005;23(9):1153-6

World Health Organisation. Hepatitis C. Fact sheet No. 164, revised October 2000. Available at: http://www.who.int/mediacentre/factsheets/fs164/en/. Accessed February 5, 2009.

Appendix

The Critical Need for Pharmacist Involvement in the Management of Patients with Hepatitis C

LINDA M. SPOONER, PharmD, BCPS, is Associate Professor of Pharmacy Practice, Massachusetts College of Pharmacy and Health Sciences, School of Pharmacy-Worcester/Manchester, Worcester, Massachusetts. *Journal of Managed Care Pharmacy.*

Hepatitis C virus (HCV) infection is a global and national health issue, affecting an estimated 170 million people worldwide and 4 million people in the United States. Approximately 80% of infected individuals will develop chronic HCV infection, which may result in substantial morbidity and mortality due to the development of hepatic fibrosis, liver cirrhosis, and hepato-cellular carcinoma.

Annually, between 8,000-10,000 deaths result from HCV infection in the United States. It has been estimated that direct medical costs secondary to HCV infection will reach $10.7 billion in the United States by the year 2019.

The high cost of HCV drug therapy, close patient follow-up, and laboratory monitoring for virologic response and adverse effects contribute to this staggering figure. Mariño *et al.* present the results of their study assessing the impact of pharmacists in management of patients with chronic HCV infection, specifically genotype 1 infection, in a secondary-care hospital in Catalonia, Spain.

A convenience sample of 50 treatment-naïve patients initiating therapy with once-weekly subcutaneous peginterferon alfa-2b and twice-daily oral ribavirin received consultation from pharmacists throughout the entire course of therapy. Pharmacists provided oral and written disease and drug information, including education about treatment of adverse drug reactions, proper storage of medications, methods of drug administration, and management of missed doses. These visits were provided in tandem with the attending hepatologists at the study site. The authors described an overall sustained virologic response (SVR) of 48%, which is comparable to that observed in other trials of patients with genotype 1 HCV. They noted that this SVR may have been increased by the low rate of early treatment discontinuation in the study. Additionally, the overall mean adherence rate was 85.7%; the adherence rate in the patients achieving SVR was an impressive 95.5%. The authors are commended for focusing their study on the benefits of pharmacist involvement in management of chronic HCV infection. They intervened on patients with genotype 1 virus, a type that is challenging to eradicate due to the lengthy treatment duration required. The study was strengthened by the visual assessment of adherence at each visit using inspection of patients' pill boxes, providing a more accurate assessment of adherence than does patient self-report. The role of the pharmacist is clearly delineated in this study, from the pharmacist's role as an educator to motivator for those patients experiencing an early virologic response at 12 weeks. Along with their face-to-face meetings with patients, the pharmacists' close participation with hepatologists facilitated a multidisciplinary collaboration that enhanced patient care. Similarly, the 24-hour pharmacist support, provided to these patients after hours and on weekends and holidays, was an invaluable addition to the care that they received.

The authors acknowledged that one of the limitations of their study was its lack of a comparison group. Without a control group, it is impossible to quantify the impact that pharmacists had on the SVR in this study. Additionally, this study included only patients with genotype 1 HCV infection. Although this genotype is the most common in the United States (comprising 70%-80% of patients) and in Spain, patients with other genotypes would also likely benefit from pharmacist intervention. Although patients with genotypes 2 and 3 infection typically receive shorter courses of therapy (24 weeks) as compared with genotypes 1 and 4 (48 weeks), the pharmacist can still strongly influence patients with respect to education, adherence, and management of adverse effects. Lastly, this study excluded patients who were co-infected with human immunodeficiency virus (HIV) infection. Since approximately 25%-33% of HIV-positive individuals are co-infected with HCV, a potentially large segment of the HCV-infected population was not considered.

The complicated pharmaco-therapeutic regimens of co-infected subpopulations of patients underscore more clearly the need for pharmacist involvement.

Do Pharmacists Make a Difference in Management of HCV Infection?

A paucity of data are available to illustrate the benefits of pharmacist involvement in HCV management. In 2007, Smith *et al.* published a pilot study that retrospectively evaluated outcomes in a pharmacist-managed HCV clinic at the Los Angeles Department of Veterans Affairs (VA) Health Care System. Overall, 17 of the 27 enrolled patients (63%) achieved a SVR. The authors concluded that their clinic was able to achieve a SVR rate comparable to that of physician-run clinics, while also efficiently providing patient support and education. A major limitation of this study was its lack of a comparison group without pharmacist involvement. Additionally, there may have been bias in the selection of motivated patients for this pilot study, resulting in a higher SVR rate and no patients lost to follow-up. Adherence assessment was not performed. Nevertheless, the study included patients with genotype 1, as well as genotypes

COMMENTARY

The Critical Need for Pharmacist Involvement in the Management of Patients With Hepatitis C 2 and 3 HCV, and provided information about detailed and broad-ranging responsibilities for the pharmacist working in the HCV clinic setting. The only other literature published about the role of the pharmacist in HCV management is descriptive in nature. Kolor described a pharmacist-managed HCV clinic at the VA Long Beach Health Care System, where specially trained pharmacists provided extensive initial and follow-up visits. During the visits, pharmacists independently adjusted doses of drug therapy, ordered laboratory tests to assess virologic response and adverse effects, and referred patients to sub-specialists as needed. This paper did not describe SVR rates or adverse event rates observed inpatients seen in the clinic by pharmacists.

Rodis and Kibbe described an HCV support group developed by a pharmacist and a nurse practitioner in Central Ohio. Although no data were gathered with respect to virologic outcomes, adherence, or adverse effects, the authors noted that they received an increased number of patient referrals to their ambulatory care clinic as a result of their involvement with the support group. Although preliminary and lacking in methodological rigor, these descriptions suggest the potential for pharmacists to play an important part in the management of HCV infection. Pharmacists are in an ideal position to provide care for patients with HCV due to the long duration of therapy, need for close monitoring of adverse effects and laboratory values, and potential dose adjustments required.

It is a natural role for pharmacists to fill, similar to the function that pharmacists have in the management of other chronic disease states, such as diabetes mellitus, hyperlipidemia, and asthma.

Quantifying the benefits of pharmacists in the management of patients with HCV infection will likely permit greater support for their involvement. This important topic area warrants future study using a comparative design in order to assess the costs and benefits of pharmacist involvement.

Why Aren't More Pharmacists Involved in HCV Clinics?

While recognizing the shortage of data quantifying the benefits of pharmacist participation in the management of individuals with chronic HCV infection, one wonders why more pharmacists are not becoming involved in these clinics. Unfortunately, most ambulatory care pharmacists have difficulty allocating time to spend in an additional clinic each week. There may be an overwhelming need for pharmacist management of more prevalent chronic issues such as diabetes mellitus, asthma, and anticoagulation that precludes the ambulatory care pharmacist from diversifying into the HCV arena. Additionally, conflicts between the HCV clinic times and administrative meetings and responsibilities prevent the university-based clinical pharmacist from consistently being involved in the clinic.

Other issues that arise include monetary considerations and awareness of opportunities. Many HCV clinics cannot afford to hire a clinical pharmacist to participate inpatient care. Clinic physicians are often unaware of pharmacists in the area who would be interested in developing a segment of their practice in HCV management. Further, clinical pharmacists may not have considered becoming involved in this area. Ambulatory care pharmacists often assume that clinical pharmacists specializing in infectious diseases will cover HCV clinic management, and vice versa. Many pharmacists are unaware of which practitioners their patients are seeing for management of their HCV infection, since so many different specialists may provide this care, including gastroenterologists, infectious diseases specialists, HIV sub-specialists, and primary care physicians. Although no formal certification or training is required for pharmacists to care for patients with HCV, clinical pharmacists often feel a level of intimidation about the complexity of HCV treatment with respect to medication dosing and adverse effect management. All of these issues contribute to missed opportunities for optimal management of patients with HCV infection. A multidisciplinary approach to the management of this disease will permit further research into the beneficial effects that pharmacists could potentially have on treatment success as well as discovery of avenues for funding. Perhaps an increased awareness of the need for pharmacist participation in HCV clinics can be accomplished with inclusion of pharmacy practice residents in the HCV clinic setting, thereby fostering an early interest in management of this disease. Additionally, pharmacists who manage HIV-positive individuals in the clinic setting are also in an ideal position to become involved in treatment of HCV infection as well, through collaboration with other pharmacists who focus their practices in the ambulatory care arena.

6

Specialised Services of Radiotherapy and Oncology in a Hospital

The clinical practice of Radiotherapy and Medical Oncology, though a recent development in India, is expanding its scope in the curative management of cancer. Radiation Oncology is a highly technology-oriented area and therefore requires both high energy facilities and highly trained manpower for its clinical practice. A better understanding and knowledge of radiotherapy in relation to surgery and recently chemotherapy has brought in radical changes in the concept of Oncology. Also, the development of new radiation sources has given a fillip to the clinical practice of radiotherapy. The perfection in dose measurement and refinement in precision radiation therapy techniques have contributed immensely towards better cure of cancer. The cure largely depends upon the accurate assessment of target volume and precision radiation delivery. The super-voltage cancer radiotherapy has made revolution in the cure of many forms of cancer which were not treatable and curable earlier. Cancer of the uterus and cancer of oral cavity are now curable with high technology radiotherapy in the range of 78-80 per cent, especially when the disease is localised. Similarly, the malignant lymphomas, which were not curable in 1950s and 60s; the Hodgkin's disease and many forms of other cancers, are now treated and cured to the extent of 80-90 per cent in Stages I and II by special techniques of super-voltage radiotherapy. In the case of advanced stages, radiotherapy is used for palliation and comfort. There are very few side effects when the patients are treated by modern techniques with high technology.

In the past, clinical radiotherapy has been weighed down by its inability to provide curative treatment of a large group of patients due to limitations of improved and precise instrumentation (especially high energy radiation sources which include X-ray and electrons), beam direction techniques and better knowledge of radiobiology. The clinical practice of radiotherapy is not developed in private clinics, nursing homes and major private hospitals since this requires special facilities and establishment. Although, radiotherapy has been in practice for more than half a century now, yet it has not achieved the place it deserves in almost all the centres which have radiotherapy facilities. However, the situation is changing now and the attitude of pessimism is subsiding.

It must be recognised that the initial management decision is the most critical component in the treatment of cancer, especially in the application of radiation sources. Therefore, the expertise of trained radiation oncologists (not the general radiologists) should be available when and where the decision is made.

The greatest hindrance perhaps is the unawareness of our planners about the wide applications of radiation sources in the management of cancer, coupled with the non-availability of modern radiation sources.

It is high time that a suitable strategy needs to be developed for the provision of radiotherapy and medical oncology facilities at community level. The facilities of radiotherapy in government institutions are overcrowded and many a time the needy patients wait for longer durations for their term of treatment. The establishment of such facilities would add a new dimension in our cancer control activities. It is very important in a disease like cancer, the sooner the treatment is started, the better, even if it means some extra expenses which are expected well within the reach.

The Centre can be affiliated to a well-established general hospital or may be designed as a free standing centre with close rapport with a good general or community hospital. It is important that necessary working relationship between the referring physician and the surgeon/treatment specialist at the cancer centre can be best achieved in an environment inside a hospital consistent with the modern pattern of medical practice requiring all facilities at one place.

Today, surgery in most of the established general hospitals is well-developed and it requires only augmentation to include the most modern technological developments to equip itself to deal with the complex nature of cancer. Radiotherapy, including chemotherapy, is the one discipline which now needs to be established in free standing cancer centres for quality treatment and better cure. The primary objective of establishing a community cancer centre, based on recent thinking, is to bring to the community the best possible cancer care programme in radiotherapy and chemotherapy. The centre offers many advantages to the community through the concerted efforts of medical and technical manpower coupled with availability of equipments and specialised facilities for modern radiotherapy and/or chemotherapy. The facilities in surgery and pathology and even in radiology are already available in most of the district hospitals and private general hospitals and these can be easily extended to the free-standing community cancer hospitals. Radiotherapy and chemotherapy can be provided to a great majority of patients on an outpatient basis and a large number of patients can be treated on a daily basis without incurring heavy expenditure on inpatient and ward facilities. The supportive facilities like haematology, mainly for blood counts, and biochemistry for tests are the additional requirements in a centre for treatment programme. The CCC with high technology in radiotherapy and chemotherapy is a unique development for health care delivery programme at the district level. One of the most important features of the community cancer centre will be its dedication to and concentration on improving cancer care facilities for the community.

An effective financial planning is an important consideration. The cost of services has to be viewed from the complex nature of treatment facilities for quality control and cancer cure. The programme and facility planning are important in-depth studies for cancer needs of the medical services to be rendered to the community. Long-term financial viability is dependent upon the following factors:

(1) Adequate reimbursement for patient treatment programme,
(2) Community philanthropists and their involvement in the project, and
(3) Special grants from the government and other charitable organisations.

Fund raising and philanthropy are essential elements for the thriving of a community health facility. However, the levels of such facilities vary in each community in a region. To ensure the organisation's ability to meet the patient treatment needs, a good deal of treatment cost should be recouped through patient revenue and charges for the services rendered to them. The objective of this presentation is to suggest a viable financial planning and methodology which may be helpful in establishing a new community cancer treatment centre where high quality treatment facilities are extended to include high technology in radiotherapy and chemotherapy. The main objective for establishment of these centres is to provide high technology which may not be feasible in the usual planning process by the government in view of the limited resources. It is aimed at creating the most modern facilities for early diagnosis and complete treatment for rooting out the disease and enhancing cure. It is also important that a tumour registry programme and epidemiological research facilities may be created in these centres for rendering advice to the community on prophylactic measures. Cancer is a preventable disease and all efforts should be made to improve the general health care delivery programme of cancer patients.

Medical Oncology

The treatment of cancer with single and multiple drug therapy is a newer development and needs establishment in high technology programme along with radiation therapy. In recent years, many new drugs and practice of poly-chemotherapy with multiple drugs have widened the scope for cure in some of the cancer specially when disease is widely disseminated and patients are not suitable for treatment either by surgery and/or radiotherapy. Some of the cancer, especially lymphoma in advanced disseminated stages are now curable almost in the range of 30-50 per cent, a remarkable achievement. Many solid tumours like carcinoma of the breast, ovary (with widespread disease) were not treated in the past but have now become treatable and controllable with development of newer chemotherapy programme. Many childhood cancers which were not treated earlier and have posed challenge in the past are now managed with various combinations of chemotherapy and have become curable in fairly good numbers. The acute leukemia is a special form of blood cancer which was known to be fatal is now managed fairly well with poly-chemotherapy programme. There are many other cancer which are treatable, manageable with chemotherapy and have given a new direction for their control. The practice of medical oncology is a highly specialised branch and also come under high technology area since this requires greatest skill and training. It is important to note that cure in cancer is an important criterion in medicine and this needs development in this establishment along with radiation oncology.

These two forms of treatment-Radiation and Medical Oncology-are also known as non-surgical treatment and are part of high technology development programme in India and many clinics in Western countries. This is a highly technical speciality and needs definite establishment in oncology programme in our community. The following is the special requirement for the Radiation and Medical Oncology set-up:

1. 6-MeV Linear Accelerator Or

Rotational Cobalt-60 unit with 80 cm SSD and electronically controlled consol and collimator.

2. Intra-cavitary and Interstitial Brachytherapy Facilities

This is a specialised highly technical field of radiation therapy where sealed radio-active isotopes are placed in and around the tumour for high dose delivery to the target volume. This is most essential and the only form of treatment for diseases like carcinoma uterus and oral cavity especially the tongue and buccal mucosa. It is important to note that brachytherapy facilities have further developed with after loading systems and have given a new direction since this has reduced considerably the radiation dose to the medical and technical staff. The facilities are not very expensive, however, these require specialised construction work for control of radiation energy. The total cost for a 24 patients' programme is approximately Rs. 5 lacs.

3. The practice of Medical Oncology does not require high expenditure programme

However, this requires in-door bed facilities and day care ward for treatment with multi-drug poly-chemotherapy. The practice certainly requires haematology and other lab. facilities which are to be developed.

4. Medical Ward

A total of 15-20 beds are the total requirement of this oncology programme since majority of the patients are treated as outpatient by radiotherapy and day care ward with chemotherapy. The requirement of the in-door beds are essential for brachytherapy where the patient has to be admitted ranging from 3 to 7 days. The patients who are not mobile and have developed minor and major complications of the disease and/or treatment for their further management, etc.

Two wards with 10 beds each male and female are sufficient for this programme with some facilities for isolation of at least two beds each.

The plan of the total facilities of tele and brachytherapy, day care ward, in-door and ward, outpatient and reception is enclosed.

Manpower

1. *Radiotherapy-One:* Qualification: MD Radiotherapy with a minimum experience of 15-20 years.
2. *Medical Physicist-One:* Non-medical with qualification of M.Sc., DRP (BARC), Bombay with at least 5 years' experience in the field of medical physics with special reference to Radiotherapy.
3. *Medical Technologists-Two* for handling of radiation sources.
4. Clinical haematologist on a part time basis for advice in medical oncology programme.

The Initial Investment and Estimated Annual

Non-Recurring-Capital Investment

(1) The construction for provision of indoor ward, day care ward, reception and waiting room, consultants' rooms, examination room, research lab., and teletherapy facilities (linear accelerator or cobalt as the case may be), the total covered area being approximately 500 sq. ft. (This is a standard requirement for a working set-up as mentioned above and this also includes a super-voltage radiotherapy room which needs special construction. The space needs to be on the ground floor since RCC with 4 ft. wall has to be constructed for high energy therapy equipment).

APPENDIX

MEDICAL EDUCATION IN TODAY'S PERSPECTIVE

Medical education is rightly said to be the mother, which generates trained health manpower for dispensation of an 'effective' and 'efficient' health care delivery system in the country. It is only a 'well nourished' mother, which is capable of giving birth to a full term normal baby. Going by this dictum, until and unless the health of medical education, which incidentally is the mother of effective health care delivery system is maintained, the resultant child in the form of trained health manpower would otherwise be 'malnourished' and also impoverished.

It is in this background, it is required to be appreciated that maintenance of standards of medical education is not just a must, for 'cosmetic' purposes but is mandatory for the purposes of efficient dispensation of the effective health care delivery system, which has a significant bearing on the entire country. This necessitates 'quality incorporations' in medical education in a 'timely' manner, so that it is capable of not only catering to the 'contemporary' requirements, but also is able to address the 'long-term concerns' of 'relevance and consequence'.

The context of medical education needs to be viewed on three important counts namely (1) India being one of the key generators of the trained health manpower, (2) the cost based medical education, and (3) mal-distribution of the trained health manpower resulting in gross inequalities in terms of non-availability of rural health manpower.

It's really a matter of achievement that by virtue of 289 medical colleges with an annual intake of well over 32,000 MBBS seats and with avenues of nearly 13,000 postgraduate seats, India happens to be one of the largest generator of trained health manpower. This estimates that but for the four countries namely Brazil, Russia, India and China, all other countries shall be facing a 'gross deficit' of the trained health manpower, it is inevitable that India will be required to produce doctors who would be able to cater to the global needs. This will mean broadening the scope of medical education, so as to accommodate not just the capacity to cater to the 'national needs' but 'global needs' as well.

The second consideration is significant as it has a social bearing. At one end, it is said that higher education including medical education in the country should be governed by the principles of easy access, equity and affordability. This means that medical education is expected to be available to the eligible talent in the country in terms of merit based 'free and equitable access' and within 'affordable' economical reach. 'Cost-based' medical education turns out to be an antithesis to these otherwise laudable objectives that have a human face. The fact that 'cost-based' medical

Journal of Indian Medical Education, Vol 107, Feb. 2007.

education would be beyond the ambit of the poor who is meritorious, is not just a matter of 'social concern' but is also a big 'human challenge'

The urbanisation blended with commercialisation has resulted in congregation of the trained health manpower in larger urban pockets resultantly the vast rural areas being deprived of medical care and cure in a significant way. Cost-based medical education mandating huge monetary payments ends up in calculating a commercial value system in the minds of the generated doctors, which results in total reluctance for serving the rural poor.

In today's perspective therefore, the inevitable mandate is 'quality-based globally acceptable medical education', which is 'affordable and accessible' to the meritorious and deserving independent of the 'cost polemics'. This calls for serious and diligent application of mind by all concerned, so that an appropriate strategy is carved out which will enable to mitigate the existing malady and create situations which would be capable of catering towards the fulfillment of legitimacy of the expectations of the talented youth of this country and also equitable distribution of trained health manpower to be catering to hitherto unserved areas and poorly privileged population of the country.

KETAN DESAI

Past-National President,
IMA (HQ) and Past President,
Medical Council of India-110002
JIMA, Feb. 2009

7

Management of Mid-life Clinic for Women

For better health of women in mid-life, setting-up a special clinic is essential. This is the period when perimenopausal changes start, menopause occurs and post-menopausal changes set in.

Menopause refers to cessation of mensturation and involves cessation of ovarian activity and involutions/atrophy of female genital organs and the phenomenon is peculiar to human race. The usual age is 45-52 years of age. In most cases the process is gradual, taking several months to years for the menstrual bleeding to come to an end. Simultaneously, the woman becomes coarser in build and appearance and may develop some hairs on face. The waistline is lost and often there is increase in weight. Many women develop psychological changes due to fears of losing youth, feminity, sexual activity and other stressful symptoms in proportion to emotional instability existing before its onset. Common symptoms include depression, nervousness, irritability, lack of concentration, loss of sleep, headaches, giddiness, head noises, loss of appelite or increase a appetite, palpitation, pain in the chest, hot flushes and sweats, painful breasts, pigmentation of skin, increased incidence of blood pressure heart disease, loss of bone density and fractures and several others. Thus, menopause represents change of life and requires management. This can better be achieved in a menopausal clinic, which will inspire more confidence.

Setting up a menopausal clinic

Running a menopausal clinic should involve comprehensive counselling and screening services for climacteric women and such a service should be well organised.

(a) Aims of Menopause Clinic

(i) Provision of information and advice,
(ii) relief of distressing symptoms,
(iii) prevention of osteoporosis,
(iv) Reduction of ischaemic heart disease and strokes,
(v) Screening for breast cancer, uterine and cervical cancers, hypertension, diabetes, hyperlipidaemia and osteoporosis, and
(vi) health education: diet, exercise, anti-smoking, alcohol control, stress management.

(b) Staff Requried for Menopause Clinic

(i) Gynaecologist,
(ii) Staff nurse or assistant trained in dealing with gynecology patients,
(iii) Receptionist to ease the administrative load, and
(iv) Counsellor for patients with mid-life problems including psychosexual difficulties, dealing with genital malignancies, etc.

(c) Requirement of Premises

(i) Room for consultation,
(ii) Examination/treatment room, and
(iii) Waiting area for patients.

(d) Equipment Required

The facility for conducting pap. smear, ultrasonogram, hormone and lipid profile tests and other tests, facility of bone densitometer, etc. have to either exist within the clinic or a good collaborative arrangement is required.

(e) Establishment of Menopause Protocol

This will include:

(i) *Administrative details*—Name, age, address, Tel. No. occupation.
(ii) *Presenting complaints*—To be ticked in the previously mentioned questionnaire. Also enquire about any previous medications taken for the complaints.
(iii) *Gynecological history*—Menstrual history, LMP, parity, current contraception, hysterectomy (and/or) coophorectomy with reasons, smear results.
(iv) *Medical/Surgical history*—DVT, Myocardial infarction, cerebrovascular accident, hypertension, diabetes, breast lump, migraines, jaundice, epilepsy, gastric surgery, gall stones, otosclerosis, thyroid disorders, steroid therapy, etc.

(v) Current medication/allergies.
(vi) *Personal history*—Marital status, employment, smoking, alcohol, diet, exercise, etc.
(vii) *Family history*—Breast cancer, ovarian cancer, uterine cancer, IHD/CVA, osteoporosis.

After taking history and clinical examinations, following tests may be considered:

(a) Full blood count.
(b) Thyroid function tests if features of thyroid disease are present.
(c) Patient with a relevant past history of thrombo-embolism will require a full fibrinolysis.
(d) *Mammogram*—All women aged 50 years or over who have not undergone mammography in the previous 3 years irrespective of whether-patient with history of benign breast lump and or fan-lily history of breast cancer should have HRT or not.
(e) *Hormone profiles*—Plasma FSH and LH levels and E2 levels fluctuate widely during the climacteric and hormone levels are of little value, except in cases of spontaneous premature menopause and also to diagnose ovarian failure in hysterectomized patients.
(f) Pelvic USG is not necessary in the absence of clinical abnormality. USG is required inpatients with a family. history of ovarian cancer whether patient is on HRT or not.
(g) Lipid profile is required inpatients with a strong family history of hyperlipidemia, IHD, hypertension and inpatients who are obese, hypertensive, or smokers.
(h) *Bone density assessment*—where facilities are available, a bone densitometry scan is of particular value for women who, in the absence of climacteric symptoms would take HRT if they were shown to be at a risk of later osteopororosis.

Maintenance of Records

Every patient should have a record card to indicate attendance at the clinic, to document findings, to record details of the treatment and ensure proper follow up.

INVESTIGATIONS

A. A Pap Examination

It is a screening test for cervical cancer. It detects the cancer young and predicts whether one is in a pre-cancerous stage. An abnormal Pap smear could mean that one is in the stage before cancer. If left untreated, this could lead to cervical cancer.

Cervical cancer strikes the cervix—the lower narrow end of the uterus that forms a canal between the uterus and the vagina. It is the fifth leading cause of death from cancer in women. Most cervical cancer deaths occur in women who have never had a Pap smear. Cervical cancer can be prevented. In most cases, if detected early, it can also be cured in 90 percent of the cases. Left untreated, this cancer invades adjacent organs or spreads elsewhere in the body, rendering it difficult to control. The cure rates then drop to 50 per cent or less. All women should undergo Pap smear test, some women are at a higher risk of cervical cancer than others, e.g.

(i) Multiple sex partners or a male partner who has had multiple female partners.
(ii) Genital warts.
(iii) Sexual relations before the age of 18.

Middle aged women should continue with the test at least once every three years.

How it's done?

A Pap exam is a simple procedure in which physician painlessly obtains cells from the surface of cervix, using a special brush or spatula to sample the area where most cancers begin to develop. The cells are placed on a glass slide, which is sent to a laboratory.

If cancerous or pre-cancerous cells are found, the next step is a more thorough examination of the cervix. A Pap test may also detect infections such as bacteria, yeast or viruses.

How Reliable is it?

The accuracy of Pap smear depends on the correct collection, proper staining and accurate interpretation of that specimen in the laboratory. If any of these procedures is inadequate, the diagnostic value of Pap smear could be compromised. In some cases false positive or false negative can occur.

B. Ultrasonogram

This scan is often required to find any structural abnormality in the uterus/ovaris, etc. in a menopausal woman. This is non-invasive, convenient and not expensive. This may be required once in a year.

C. Mammogram

A mammogram is a low-dose X-ray test of a woman's breasts that detects tumours and cysts. It can help differentiate benign tumours from malignant ones. It can detect breast cancer at an early stage. Any abnormality in the breasts will show up as an irregular opaque patch on the resulting image. This procedure has a 92 percent accuracy rate.

Breast self-examinations, along with mammograms and regular examinations by Physician can help detect breast cancer in its early stages.

When a mammogram spots a tumour, a woman is likely to have caught it early, before it has progress to a high-grade growth: When detected clinically, the cancer has usually spread to the lympth nodes. The earlier breast cancer is found, the more likely it is to be treated successfully. It is recommended that women get annual mammograms starting at age-40.

So even if you have had an annual mammogram done for the last decade, you still run a 50-50 chance of being wrongly diagnosed with breast cancer. The tests could include more mammograms, ultrasound scans and biopsies, even if they turn out to be free of cancer. If an abnormality is found, you may need a follow-up appointment. Special mammogram views and/or ultrasound may help clarify findings on the screening mammogram.

D. BMD

Bone Mineral Densitometry is a test that can tell whether or not you have osteoporosis and how likely you are to develop it in the future. Most typically, obteoporosis causes fractures of the spine, hip and wrist. Other bones like the ribs, humerus and pelvis can also be affected. Before bone densitometry was invented, osteoporosis was detected through routine X-rays or a bone biopsy. These methods rarely diagnosed osteoporosis before a fracture had occurred. So, a minimum of 25 per cent of the bone's mass would already have been lost.

Osteoporosis steals more than bone. It's the primary cause of hip fracture, which can lead to permanent disability, loss of independence and, even death. Collapsing spinal vertebrae can produce a stooped posture. Osteoporosis can wreck daily life: The simplest things can cause broken bones—stepping off a car, sneezing, bending to pick up something, even a hug.

Osteoporosis-related fractures occur about four times as often in women than men. Of the individuals who fracture a hip, one-half will be permanently disabled, and almost 20 per cent will require long-term nursing care. Some 20 per cent of the hip fracture victims die within one year, usually from complications like pneumonia or blood clots in the lung related to either the fracture or surgery.

Every woman in her 40s should get a screening, earlier, if she has one or more risk factors for osteoporosis (like a family history). Follow this with a screening about a year after the start of menopause—a time of rapid bone loss. All post-menopausal women must be tested. The most common bone density test in use today is the dual energy X-ray absorptiometry (DXA). A simple, painless, non-invasive procedure. A small X-ray detector scans spine, hips or both. One may be asked to lift legs onto a support to straighten back for the test. The test is safe and does not require any injections.

New technology for measuring bone density is the Heel Ultrasound. This involves immersing foot in a bath of warm water, allowing high frequency sound waves to pass through heel. The test measures the density and quality of the bone in the heel. Another test is the Clinical Bone

Densitometer. This system measures the transmission of high frequency sound waves through the heel but it does not require water.

E. Pelvic Examination

Pelvic examinations are important if one continues to have sex because of the risk of sexually transmitted diseases (STDs). STDs, many of which cause no noticeable symptoms, can increase your risk of cervical cancer and infertility.

A pelvic examination is must if any of the following symptoms are present; irregular periods after first year of menstruation; any unwanted sexual contact or sexual abuse; unusual discharge from vagina; sores or lumps around vagina; itching or burning in genital area; pain in upper thigh, groin or lower abdomen.

Gynaecologist begins by taking blood pressure, weight and pulse. She will ask, when the first day of your last period was. This is also the time to tell her about any problems. Don't keep anything back: Tell her about the timing and frequency of any illness; irregular or painful periods; infections; painful sex. Feel free to discuss weight, hair loss or skin changes, and other issues such as smoking, drinking or emotional or family issues. Gynaecologist will listen to heart and lungs, check breasts for any changes or lumps, and palpate abdominal area for any irregularities. A reliable examination of breasts should take approximately 30 seconds per breast.

A good physician would show how to do a monthly breast self-exam. If one is 35 or older, the physician should also discuss doing a mammogram screening for breast cancer. A manual examination is performed next. Gynaecologist will insert a gloved finger into vagina while palpating lower abdomen to note the size, shape and mobility of uterus, ovaries, cysts, endometriosis and fibroid tumours.

F. Prostate Specific Antigen Test (PSAT)

As a menopausal woman is being examined and investigated, it is pertinent to enquire the urinary history of her husband and investigate him for prostate cancer by PSA test.

A PSA test reveals the level of prostate specific antigen in the blood. There are a number of reasons why a person's PSA could be higher than normal-and prostate cancer could be one of them. An enlarged prostate is an age-related disease. Once thought of as an old man's disease, prostate cancer is now striking more and more men in their 40s, 50s and 60s. Detected early, prostate cancer can be cured. However, in many men, the disease would have spread beyond the prostrate capsule before the cancer is diagnosed. Early enquiry about urinary complaints of a menopausal woman's husband and PSA Test, will provide him early treatment/ prevention against prostate cancer.

G. Other Specific Investigations

Magnetic resonance imaging (MRI) has been advocated in the

diagnosis of endometrial cancer. Similar to ultrasound measurements of endometrial thickness, MRI measurements have a high degree of sensitivity for endometrial carcinoma but lack specificity. MRI may also be used to predict myometrial invasion in established cases of endometrial cancer and is more accurate at this than ultrasound. However, the cost and time required for MRI imaging suggests that it is not a practical method for screening the large number of women with PMB that presently exist.

At present, the management of PMB should be tailored to suit an individual case's clinical merits. No clear evidence for the best method of investigation exists. The International Society for Gynecologic Endoscopy agreed that hysteroscopy could replace dilatation and curettage in the investigation of post-menopausal women with uterine bleeding. It is currently recommended that hysteroscopy and endometrial sampling is the gold standard for diagnosis. This can be performed as an outpatient if suitable facilities are available.

TREATMENT PLAN

Since menopause is caused by cessation of hormonal production in the ovaries, etc., the *sine qua non* of treatment is Hormonal Replacement Therapy (HRT). Administration of one or more hormones, its route and form has been decided by the Gynaecologist as per the need and acceptability of the individual patient. Now several preparations of HRT are available. For the majority of women requiring HRT for the relief of symptoms, it makes no difference which route is chosen and patient preference may be the most important determining factor. In reality, for most women starting HRT, oral tablets will be the best option, but there are some differences in the effects of the various routes which will indicate a specific preference. Preparations of HRT are available for delivery orally, transdermally, by subcutaneous implant or vaginally. In addition, sublingual and intranasal spray options are being evaluated.

A. Oral

Oral oestrogen is the most suitable initial therapy for most women. Now we have a wide range of natural oestrogen preparations containing oestradiol, oestrone, conjugated equine oestrogens and the synthetic steroid tibolone, which has oestrogenic, androgenic and progestogenic activity. The particular merits and main disadvantages of oral administration are summarised below:

Advantages

Easy to take; most people are used to swallowing tablets. Tablets are usually cheaper than other routes of administration, good control due to short half-life, so can be withdrawn quickly, wide choice of preparations available.

Disadvantages

A high dose of oestrogen is required to overcome the extensive metabolism in the intestine and liver before reaching the systemic circulation.

Wide variation in absorption and metabolism during the first pass of intestine and liver.

Alteration of some liver function and protein synthesis. Oral oestradiol is mainly converted to oestrone.

Higher incidence of minor side effects than with other routes, requires daily dosage. All tablets contain lactose.

B. Transdermal Oestrogen

Oestrogen is absorbed well through skin and subcutaneous fat, as well as vaginal epithelium, nasal and sublingual mucosa. The main advantage of all these routes of administration is that metabolism in the intestine and liver is avoided. Pure oestradiol can, therefore, be administered directly into the systemic circulation causing a predominant rise in plasma oestradiol concentration, and an oestradioloestrone ratio similar to that found in premenopausal women. Therefore, transdermal should be preferable to oral oestradiol.

Advantages	Disadvantages
Lower dose pure oestradiol	Skin reactions
Avoids intestine and liver metabolism	More expensive than tablets
Physiological oestradiol oestrone ratio	Not well tolerated in warm climates
Reduces serum triglyceride	Variable absorption
Few side effects	

An alternative transdermal administration is by application ofa gel containing oestradiol. This has been available for some years. It is a hydro-alcoholic gel containing 0.06% w/w 17B-oestradiol. A measured dose of 0.75 mg oestradiol is dispensed and the usual recommended starting dose is two measures daily applied to arms or legs. This route of administration allows the woman a feeling of greater control over her therapy, and is gradually becoming more popular.

C. Implants

Pellets of crystalloid oestradiol have been available for subcutaneous implant for a long time. However, despite a long history and many advantages of this route of administration, it is not widely used. Insertion of the pellets requires a minor surgical procedure which may be one reason for limited popularity, though it is easy, takes only 3-4 min. and is safe. Pellets of oestradiol are available in 25, 50 and 100 mg doses. The 50 mg dose is most commonly used for post-menopausal oestrogen replacement, and given at 6 monthly intervals produces a circulating level of approximately 400 pmol/1 at one year. For the prevention of osteoporosis, a level of at least 300 pmol/l is required and higher levels may achieve greater replacement of bone.

In some cases there is a need to take additional progestogen or Testosterone in a 100 mg pellet, particularly if they are troubled by headaches, loss of energy, depression and especially loss of libido. This is usually given at the same time as oestradiol. The need to add progestogen to regimens of HRT for women with a uteruses protect the endometrium is well established and accepted.

D. Vaginal Oestrogen

For older women in particular who are troubled by symptoms related to urogenital ageing, local oestrogen therapy is often more appropriate, but these problems are not well recognised or treated. Local oestrogen administration will provide relief, but is often given for too short a time to have an adequate response. Systemic therapy does not always produce an improvement in vaginal symptoms, and for women with symptoms of systemic and local oestrogen deficiency, a combination of systemic and vaginal oestrogen may be necessary initially, until the vaginal epithelium has responded. For the older woman who does not wish to experience the effects of systemic oestrogen, the use of a natural oestrogen vaginal preparation can avoid significant systemic absorption. There are several creams and pessaries and a vaginal tablet. A soft 5 cm diameter ring, Estring, releases oestradiol locally over 3 months, and is more user-friendly.

All routes of administration of HRT are beneficial. For most women the oral route will be the simple, cheapest and most suitable for initial therapy. Future developments of intra-uterine devices releasing progestogen, vaginal rings and the oral selective oestrogen receptor modulators (SERMs) will further increase the options so that very few women will not be able to find some suitable therapy. With life expectancy increasing, the need to improve compliance into old age will be even greater so that longevity can be matched by good quality of life as well.

E. Role for Progestogens

Progestogens are effective in preventing endometrial hyperplasia and carcinoma in women on oestrogen replacement and so have been proposed and in some cases used to treat/prevent endometrial lesions in women on tamoxifen therapy.

F. Hysterectomy Cases

In those cases, where menopause is induced suddenly by surgical removal of life run and ovaries, sudden symptoms of menopause plus depression are induced. Here HRT has to be given and psychological symptoms have also to be looked into. The therapeutic effect of hysterectomy include both the cure of physical symptoms and improvement of resultant depression. Inpatients with pre-existing psychiatric illness, depression is unlikely to settle after hysterectomy and in those with over-anxious neurotic personality, the emotional stress of surgery may precipitate depression. Ovarian failure is the more plausible cause of depression, but it is often overlooked and remains untreated after hysterectomy. With appropriate case selection, psychiatric evaluation and adequate preoperative counselling many causes of post-hysterectomy depression may be prevented. The practice of regular endocrinological monitoring after hysterectomy to detect the need for oestrogen replacement and a near routine replacement of combined oestrogen and testosterone replacement after bilateral oophorectomy should also be adopted to avoid post-hysterectomy depression.

G. The Future

The possibility now exists to prevent and treat osteoporosis, breast cancer, cardiovascular and probably central nervous system diseases without incurring other health risks. Molecular mimicry will enable the development of drugs with only the moiety that engages and activates precise and specific receptors without side effects in non-target tissues. If, for example, the cardioprotective effect of oestrogen is localised to a part of the molecule distinct from the part that exerts its sexual role, then selective modulation may enable a designer oestrogen extend its cardioprotective benefits to men without fear of emasculating them HRT as we know it today consists of arbitrary doses of oestradiol and occasionally, token testosterone supplements. But the sex steroid precursors produced cyclically in variable but balanced quantities by the ovary may exert as yet unrecognised metabolic functions by activating DNA sequences other than the ERE as exemplified by 17-episterol. The recognition and exploitation of these putative genes and their functions will 'fine tune' our concept and application of HRT.

8

Rehabilitation Centre: Essential in Every Hospital

Rehabilitation is a medical service to patient that is designed to prepare the patient for useful, productive and happy living in his community. No matter, how serious or disabled is the patient, must be regarded from the first day of his illness as one who will some day return to a normal and satisfactory mode of living. To bring him back to the normal state, rehabilitation must be started from the day of his admission in the hospital. Rehabilitation is a specialisation in medicine. It is an integral part of medical care. The world is recording increasing rate of accidents, metabolic diseases, neo-plastic diseases, cardiovascular diseases and neuromuscular diseases day-by-day. The average life expectancy age has been increased and side by side chronic illnesses also becoming high. Psychiatric problems, social problems, vocational problems requires long-term continuous care. Increasing population, urbanisation, industrialisation and migration, demands more hospital beds. Whereas at present the bed population ratio is only 0.4 bed to 1000 population. Dr. Mudaliar Committee had recommended 1 bed per 1000 population in 1959-61. Inspite of the advancement made in the field of medicine, the required bed number is still inadequate. The allocation of finance for health sector is megre, but we need to give primary rehabilitative services either in O.P.D. or in established rehabilitation centres.

According to WHO Tech. Series No. 419 (1969) on Medical rehabilitation the expert committee recommended to create rehabilitation centres in regional and intermediate hospitals, and pilot medical rehabilitation centres should be established in coordination with social and educational services. In order to promote education in rehabilitation, faculties of medicine should create provision of rehabilitation medicine and establish schools for allied health and rehabilitation personnel.

Rehabilitation has various connotations. Occupational therapy and physiotherapy are used sometimes in place of rehabilitation. But, they are not one at the same. According to World Health Organisation rehabilitation, "As applied to disability. This is the combined and co-ordinated use of medical, social, educational and vocational measures for training or retraining the individual to the highest possible level of functional ability." Physiotherapy and occupational therapy also included in medical care and they are different from rehabilitation. However, department of physiotherapy, occupational therapy and rehabilitation arc parts of the hospital. Physiotherapy deals with physical treatment by means of a course of exercises, cold or hot message, water bath, light treatment and electrical message. The major purposes of physiotherapy is relief of pain, prevention and correction of disability, to restore strength and vigour, mobility and co-ordination. It includes various tests to identify muscular and nerve defects joint movements and functional disabilities. Whereas occupational therapy is medically directed treatment of the physically or mentally disabled by means of constructive activities designed and adopted by a professionally qualified occupational therapist to promote the restoration of useful function.

Physical Facilities

Rehabilitation department should be located in ground floor attached near outpatient department. Many patients can get treatment from outpatient department and go back home. But many of the patients may require round the clock care inpatient ward. The department should be spacious with all required equipment and supplies. For each of therapy, should be a separate cubicle or rooms. Such as cubicle for diathermy, radiant heat, active-therapy, message, water treatment, active exercise room, passive exercise room, health education room, and room to teach daily living for parapligic patients to live without aid.

Apart from the cubicle, there should be facilities for open air grounds, gymnasium and swimming pool.

Offices are very essential for planning, discussing and keeping records. Therefore, there should be offices for Director, Office Superintendent, Physiotherapists, occupational therapist, nursing superintendent, speech therapist, psychotherapist, etc. In addition to the above, there should be provision for record officer, store room and sanitary annexes.

Team Approach

Rehabilitation department of hospital must adopt a team approach inpatient care, which should utilize the specialised skills of physician, physical therapist, occupational therapist, social worker, speech and hearing therapist, nurse, vocational counsellor, psychologist and prosthetic specialist.

Administration

The Director of Physical Medicine shall be the incharge of the department. He should possess specialisation in physical medicine. He will be able to practice full time of his speciality. He should be authorised for admission and discharge of patients. He will supervise the safety of the department and ensure safe care to all patients. He will assess plan, co-ordinate and implement all programmes related to rehabilitation. He proposes staff and budget for the department.

Follow-up Clinics

In order to have easy reach of skilled ease, there should be followup clinics in the town or city. Once they have treated from the centre, for further care if needed can get guidance from follow-up clinics. This saves the time of the community and reduces hospital rush. But it should be well-planned and co-ordinated.

Follow-up Visits

Sometimes if follow-up clinics are not available, facilities for follow-up visit from the rehabilitation centre to be facilitated. Adequate staff with transport facilities may be the additional requirement.

References

Rusk, Howard A., *Rehabilitation Medicine,* St. Louis, The C.V. Mosby and Co., 1971.

W.H.O., *Hospital Planning and Administration,* Geneva, W.H.O., 1966.

W.H.O., W.H.O. Expert Committee on *Medical Rehabilitation,* Tech. Series No. 419, 1969, Geneva, W.R.O., 1969.

9

Physiotherapy in a Hospital: Immense Scope

Physiotherapy is a fairly recent medical profession with an immense scope for profound study and exploration. Although, when it was initiated into the medical field, it had diploma to offer which, however, in due course of time, has been extended to comprehensive course of one and a half year. For further exhaustive study courses like MPT, Ph.D. and specific specialisation's various areas of physiotherapy have been established.

The physiotherapy can be defined as a branch of health, which deals with the management of various body disorders through scientific application of physical agents to promote optimum health and function. It aims to identify, prevent, correct or alleviate acute or prolonged movement dysfunction of anatomic or physiologic origin through physical measures. The physical agents utilised are heat, cold, light, electricity, water, exercises and manipulation.

The Indian Association of Physiotherapists have defined Physiotherapy as the means of Modern Scientific Physiotherapeutic system of medicine. This includes examination, treatment, advice and instruction to any person preparatory to or for the purpose of or in connection with Movement dysfunction, bodily malfunction, and physical disorder/ disability. It also includes healing pain from injury, disease, Physical and mental conditions using physical agents, activities and devices including Exercises, Mobilisation, Manipulation and Electrotherapy for diagnosis, prevention and treatment.

Aspects of Physiotherapy

The varied aspects of physiotherapy which includes prevention at all the three levels that is Primary, Secondary and Tertiary. As far as curative aspect is concerned it includes manual, mechanical and electrotherapy treatments to cure the patients. It covers the promotive aspect by providing ample scope for higher studies and immense area for research too. To rehabilitate the physically disabled this field helps the disabled to adapt to the new jobs with least mental trauma.

There are three treatment modalities for all the diseases-medical, surgical, physical. Physiotherapy falls in the third category. Disabilities and related problems of physical dysfunction are as old as humanity. But the present day science of physiotherapy had its origin after World War II, when a large number of soldiers and civilians suffered from many types of injuries resulting into amputation deformities and backbone injuries causing paralysis of limbs. These disabled patients required a long-term management to enable them to become physically efficient enough to come back to main stream of social life. The restoration of physical strength, freedom of joint movement could be achieved/for these patients by careful assessment of their abilities and need of skilled persons only. Thus, the science of physiotherapy grasped the ground and therefore has made a rapid progress to occupy an important place in health care profession.

Physiotherapy role is spread over practically the medical spectrum, sprain, neurological disorders, chest, heart diseases, muscle and bone treated by medical practitioners, who refer them for further physical therapy to physiotherapist. Undoubtedly, it is one of the most important rehabilitation services of our times. Physiotherapy is a dynamic health care profession and is an integral part of the health care system. The physiotherapy is applicable to all phases of health care, prevention of ill effects, restoration of function and rehabilitation.

The Main Aims of Physiotherapy

The following points broadly signify the main aims of physiotherapy:

1. To relieve pain and inflammation.
2. To promote healing.
3. To maintain and increase the mobility of joints.
4. To maintain and increase the strength, power, endurance and volume of muscles.
5. To maintain and improve posture.
6. To maintain and improve neuromuscular co-ordination.
7. To maintain and improve vital capacity (Respiratory function).
8. To make patient ambulatory and last but not the least is to.
9. Make patient independent to perform activities of daily living.

The medicines have their limitations and many a times have an adverse effect. The problems of joint mobilizing and joint strengthening a weak muscle, improving neuromuscular co-ordination, restoring the respiratory control, etc. cannot be dealt by the prescription of medicines. It requires an active direct and skillful management by physical agents. The physiotherapy is neither supplementary nor complementary to medicine surgery but an essential need of the patient and appropriate remedy for his problems. The remarkable feature about physiotherapy is that it has no side effects. Moreover, besides lending physical stability and fitness to the patients, it also helps them to readapt to their social environment harmoniously and congenially.

Widening Horizons of Physiotherapy

In earlier years after World War II, the role of physiotherapy was mostly confined to orthopedics patients but slowly in these years, the science established its identity and found its effectiveness in restoration of physical disability. The physical agents were viewed more critically and researchers carried on, that led to advent of a wide range of sophisticated electrotherapeutics modalities. The physiotherapy moved out of orthopedic area to neurological area where a large number of patients suffered from chronic physical problems. The physiotherapy has also proved not only effective but also essential. Its role in orthopedic surgery was already established but it was realised that preoperative and post-operative physiotherapy enabled patient to be quickly back to his pre-disease state. Physiotherapy can prevent many serious complications involved in an operation and in the patients requiring long-term bed rest. The respiratory function can be adequately maintained and improved by physiotherapy.

Physiotherapists are employed not just in ortho and rehabilitation departments but also in neurology, ICU, cardio thoracic, plastic surgery, ante-natal and prenatal sectors. Another area of work is that of sports. There are times when even a physiotherapist cannot do much about it, it is here that his role becomes doubly important. The permanently disabled and handicapped are all gently taught how to innate humanity accept their bodily dysfunctions and how to live inspite of them. It is the physiotherapist which makes him a massiah for his patients, which is why it is a career successfully pursued by the chosen few.[1]

More and more people will need physical therapy as medical advances save the lives of larger proportion of new born with severe birth defects. Growth will result from advances in medical technology that permit the treatment of disabling conditions of the past, for example, the development of hip and knee replacements for those with arthritis needed specific regime of exercises which only physiotherapy could meet.

Burgeoning of Physiotherapy

According to the W.H.O., one therapist is needed for every 10,000 people but in India there are only 5,000 qualified physiotherapists, meaning a shortage of 95,000 to meet our population needs. In countries like U.S.A. and Australia, no patient is discharged before going through the hands of the therapists, but in India the importance to the therapy is yet to be realised.

A. Role of Physiotherapists in Primary Care

Physiotherapists have a major role to play in the provision of the primary care. As a clinician involved in the examination in the evaluation, diagnosis, prognosis, intervention and prevention and prognosis, intervention and prevention of musculoskeletal and neuromuscular disorders, physical therapists are well positioned to provide those services as the members of the primary care team.

B. Role in the Secondary and Tertiary Care

They play major roles in the secondary and tertiary care. Patients with musculoskeletal, neuromuscular cardiopulmonary, or integument conditions frequently were initially treated by another health care practitioner and then referred to the physical therapist for the secondary care.

Tertiary care is provided by the physical therapists is highly specialised, complex and technology-based setting (e.g. heart and lung transplant units, burns unit) or when supplying specialised service (e.g. to patients with spinal cord lesions or closed-head trauma) in the response to requests for consultation that are made by other health care practitioners.[2]

Electrotherapy

Electrotherapy is the branch of physiotherapy that deals with treatment through the various machines. These are:

Ultrasound Therapy

Ultrasound Therapy is any vibration at a frequency above the sound range several different frequencies are used in for Physiotherapy treatment. This treatment is given after soft tissue injuries, as the mechanical effect helps to remove traumatic exudate and reduces the danger of adhesion formation. Accelerated protein synthesis stimulates the rate of repair of damaged tissues. Analgesia produced by the ultrasound allows early use of the part. The frequency used for the therapeutic purposes is 1-3MHz.

Short Wave Diathermy, Microwave Diathermy. The frequency used is 27.12 MHz in case of S.W.D. and 2457 MHz in case of M.W.D. S.W.D is used to accelerate the resolution of chronic inflammation, relieve pain and reduce muscle spasm. M.W.D are Electromagnetic radiations which are absorbed by the body which provokes ionic movement, rotation of dipoles and electron orbit distortion to produce heat and ultimately relieve pain.

Hot Rays

Hot Rays are given with the help of different kinds of infra red lamps. These are absorbed by the skin and produce heat.

Wax Therapy

The wax transmits energy to the tissues by giving up energy as it solidifies. Thus, it provides effective low temperature heating of the part.

Ultra Violet Rays

Ultra Violet Rays are used to heal the ulcer and cure the infection at the wound.

Nurve and Muscle Stimulator

Nerve and Muscle Stimulator is used for re-education of muscle action. Training new muscle action and to maintain muscular viability in nerve injuries too it is used.

Mechanical Therapy

Mechanical Therapy, which uses mechanical equipment to help the patient do recovery exercises and tractions for neck and back are given generally when the pain radiates to the arms or legs. The traction can be either mechanical, electrical or computerized one.

Exercise Therapy

The therapeutic exercises may be defined as scientific application of body movements designed specifically to maintain or to restore the normal function to the diseased or injured tissues. The word exercise is derived from the word "Ex.", which means "out" and "Arc" component, which means, "to lock", so exercise means to free or unlock.

Hippocrates (460 B.C.), the famous Greek physician and the father of medicine, recognized, the importance for strengthening muscles and improving mental attitude.

The aims of exercise therapy are:

1. To promote activity and to minimize the effects of inactivity.
2. To regain normal range of joint movement without delay.

Manual therapy are exercise done by the therapist to help patients to alleviate the pain to mobilize and strengthen the part according to the requirement. Hydrotherapy is a part of exercise therapy as a whole the body is immersed in water and the major therapeutic effect is due to exercise in the water in the pool. Whirlpools are stainless-steel tanks of various sizes. The smaller ones accommodate one limb. It refers to the Turbulence produced by electric pump, which mixes air and water into the jet stream. The agitated water stimulates the skin surface mechanically.

Chest Physiotherapy

Chest Physiotherapy is gaining a lot of importance as mortality and morbidity of the patient depends on the lung function, therefore chest physiotherapy has become an integral part of intensive care unit, post-operative care and for long-term bedridden patients. The aims of chest physiotherapy are:

1. To prevent airway obstruction and accumulation of secretions that interfere with the normal respiration.

2. To reduce the energy cost during respiration than breathing retraining.
3. To maintain/improve chest mobility.
4. To improve cough effectiveness.

Various problems in the field of physiotherapy

1. As there is growing popularity of this profession; among the students, it is important that the things should be organised in the right manner, before there is chaos.
2. Physical therapy predicted to increase rapidly through 2005. A growing vulnerability people are too chronic and debilitating conditions especially among elderly people, which imply more demand of therapeutic services.
3. Baby boomers are also entering the prime age of heart attacks and strokes, which will increase the demand for cardiac and physical rehabilitation.
4. The growing interest in health promotion should also increase the demand for physical therapy services. More employers are now evaluating work sites, developing exercise programme, teaching in safe work habit to employees in the hope of reducing injuries.
5. Every Sports too would employ a therapist to keep his team fit.

A physiotherapy department at P.G.I. is one of the best departments in India. The following lines give the description of the physiotherapy services at P.G.I. Physiotherapy services at P.G.I. were added in the year 1965 and over a period it improved from 1 therapist to 13 therapists with the most modern equipments.

The posts in the department are as follows:

1. Consultant
2. Suptd
3. 3 Senior physiotheraphists
4. 4 physiotherapists and 6 junior physiotherapists

The organogram of the existing hierarchy in the department. The department is divided into two sub-departments:

1. One for the indoor patients in the main PGI building. The indoor patients are the patients requiring consultation and treatment in various wards, which includes intensive care unit orthopedics surgery and wards. 6 therapists are posted in the different wards.
2. Other is for the outdoor patients which in the PGI campus in the New O.P.D. block and 7 therapists are posted in the O.P.D.

Functioning of the Department

1. These duties changes every year, O.P.D. consists of two units, i.e. unit 1 and unit 2.
2. Each unit has 4 therapists.
3. Each unit has 3 O.P.D. days to see the new patients and the other three days are non-O.P.D. days where therapist is busy treating his long cases.

On an average 225 patients attend the department daily. These physiotherapy services are available on all days including the gazzetted holidays where again staff is called on rotation. During the last 4 years the department is running a 4 and years degree course in physiotherapy. The course started in year 1995 Sept. with 10 students and at present there are 50 students in all. Various interdepartmental C.M.E. programmes and research projects are carried out. Special hand clinic and lymphoedema clinic are run in the department.

Table 9.1 shows number of patients in last four years.

TABLE 9.1

New Patients	1993-94	1994-95	1995-96	1997-98
	5198	5626	5050	4904
Revisits	21331	22729	20351	28916

Table 9.1 shows the numerical value of the patients visiting the Physiotherapy department as new patients and revisits are the patients corning to undertake physiotherapy treatment in the years 1993 to 1998.

P.G.I. has made an incredible progress in all the departments, with each passing year. Physiotherapy department too, has been propitiously refurbished. Apart from a dedicated and committed staff, latest equipments ~oo have been installed that would enhance the physiotherapeutic treatment.

Stupendous success can be achieved in the physiotherapy dept once the provision for Hydrotherapy unit is fully functional, this will lead to new pinnacle of standards of P.F.I.

NOTES AND REFERENCES

1 "Physiotherapy—Dimensions of the Field", *The Physiotherapy Voice*, June 94, No. 1.

2 Who are Physical Therapists, and what do they do?, *Physical Therapy*, Nov. 1997, Vol. 77, No. 11.

References

Dilip Pate, Geetha Bharithan, Sarla V. Bhatt, "Changing Concept of Physiotherapy", *Journal of Indian Association of Physiotherapist,* Dec. 1996, 1, 1, 39-41.

Dr. Dinesh, Physiotherapy 1995, *Physiotherapy Voice,* July 1995, 5.

Life After 200 Years—Reader's Digest.

N.S. Yadav, "Development of Physiotherapy in India", *Journal of Pediatric Surgery in Developing Countries,* Sept. 1993, 1.1.

Tarun Behl: "Physical Therapy", *The Daily Tribune,* Sept. 28, 1997, p. 2.

"What types of interventions do Physical therapist provide?" *Physical Therapy,* Nov. 1997, Vol. 77, No. 1.

10

Hospital Library Services: Great Resource

Man is a social animal. He grows, develops and responds to the social environment. He is exposed to knowledge explosion in the process of socialisation. He needs to prepare himself to meet the explosion. He wants to communicate his thoughts and experiences through generation to generation. Thus, the idea of library organisation originates from the concept of collecting the thoughts, ideas and experiences of human beings preserved for use by the present and future generations. According to Dr. CM. White, "Library has been perfected as the principal vehicle for carrying forward and making available the intellectual resources that need to be accumulated for use, this statement means for one thing that formal education that all level can be conducted more effectively with well-equipped librarians."

According to Pierce Butler, library is a social organisation—a necessary unit in the social fabric effectively planned and utilised for transmitting the accumulated experiences of society to individual members of the society through the instrumentality of books and other graphic accounting, and holistic materials—maps, charts, phonorecords, microfilms, etc. (See appendix attached to this chapter)

Dr. S.R. Ranganathan describes: "Libraries should become multipurpose social institutions to assemble, organise, preserve socialize, and serve all expressed thoughts embodied in manuscripts, books and periodicals." An organised and up-to-date library can play a vital role in hospital field.

Medical and nursing profession is advancing day-by-day at par with other professions. The quality of health care services and patient care depends upon the preparation, knowledge, attitude and professional competencies of doctors and nurses. They should keep about with changing needs of society and equipPed with up-to-date knowledge. In-service education, and quality library may meet the required need of the professionals. See Appendix attached to this chapter for more on Libraries as a source of knowledge and information.

Aims of Establishing Hospital Library

1. To identify, collect and stock educational materials for hospital staff including doctors, nurses and paramedical professionals.
2. To organise stock of collected educational materials which will enable the readers to utilise the library to the maximum.
3. To communicate the staff/readers about the new arrival of educational literature in library.
4. To co-ordinate with intra- and inter-departmental agencies.
5. To facilitate hospital research work.

Types of Library in Teaching Hospital

1. General nursing library (if nursing school is attached).
2. Departmental or Ward library composed of permanent and borrowed books.
3. Medical library.
4. Integrated library which is used by doctors, nurses, pharmacists, etc.

Physical Facilities of a Hospital Library

(a) Location

Library should be located in a calm and quite place away from outpatient department and emergency units. It should be located at the centre of the hospital so that all wards staff have accessibility to it. It should be well-ventilated, well-lighted and have one entrance. It should be air-conditioned or normal temperature is maintained by cooling or heating system according to the weather.

(b) Spacing and Accommodation

While planning for library, room for its expansion must be considered. The staffing pattern in hospitals varies, and the area of library room depends upon the number of readers available at a time in the library. It should be large enough to stock library books, periodicals, and other educational literature.

Area—depends upon the number of readers it cater. Minimum—150 sq. ft.

Office of the librarian—105 sq. ft.

Reading magazine, journal, etc., space area—336 sq. ft., Reading room—18 sq. ft. per reader.

Space for display rack, shelves, catalogue cabinets, bulletin boards, etc.

Tables and Chairs for readers.

Store room for stocking hard wares and softwares.

Organisation of Library

To obtain the maximum success of library, the following conditions are to be fulfilled:

(a) There should be a library committee to advise the proceedings.
(b) There should be a librarian and library staff.
(c) There should be policies to govern it.
(d) There should be a budget.

(a) Library Committee

The library committee services as an advisory body to the librarian and forms a link between the librarian and the professional staff. It is desirable to have representation from medical, nursing and other paramedicals in library committee. The functions of library committee shall be the following:

1. To define the job description of librarian and library staff.
2. Establishing objectives, philosophy, policies and rules and regulations for library administration.
3. Advise on selection and purchase of periodicals and text books.
4. Preparation of library budget.
5. Compilation of statistics on the use of library.
6. Recording and reporting on committee meetings.
7. Encouraging for library research.

(b) Librarian

There should be a full time librarian for the management of library. The library needs a person who has graduation in library sciences and he has knowledge in medical, health, biological and social sciences. The functions of librarian shall be:

1. Maintaining library stock.
2. Available in library.
3. Maintains books and journal on the accessibility of readers.
4. Maintains accession register.
5. Classify and catalogue all books.
6. Selects, purchase and keeps book/journal according to the advice of library committee.
7. Makes library rules and regulations with library committee members.
8. Participates in orientation of library.

9. Makes inventory of the library and helps in physical verification.
10. Maintains records and reports.
11. Maintains library up-to-date with proper mending and binding.

(c) Library Policies

Librarian and library committee shall formulate policies for library. That will define and clarify the following aspects:

1. Membership subscription or free of cost privilege for the readers.
2. If there is no membership subscription system, whether any deposit money should be collected from members, if so, what and when it should be refunded.
3. Who shall be responsible for purchase, stock, inventory and maintenance?
4. The book/journal which may be borrowed.
5. The period for which the book/journal may be borrowed.
6. How many books shall be issued to a member?
7. Hours at which the library will open and close.
8. What is the hour for issuing and returning?
9. Policies for loan.
10. Policies for charging fine.
11. Policies for loss of books.

Library Collection, Arrangement and Maintenance of Material

The library should equip with books, periodical, audio-visual aids and other selected materials which has scope in medical and nursing education. It should provide a wide variety of periodicals concerned with nursing and medical subjects, biological, physical, social and behavioural sciences. It should include dictionaries, audio-visual aids like charts, model, maps, slides, film strips, film rolls, posters, flannel graph, etc.

Book Selection

For effective services to the readers, the library committee will assign a library purchase committee which should be headed by a Chairman and include members, all professors of various departments, nursing and pharmacy departments. According to the fund available, the quality should be maintained by purchasing latest edition in less number and with a variety of new books/journals. If available few amount should be kept for developing cultural! social taste for social magazines, fictions, etc.

Requisition

Author, title, place of publication, publisher, date, price and number of copies desired should be worked out, on which the signature of Head of the Department should be obtained. That is the requisition form. On arrival of order, the order slip is received by the librarian, verified and the bills are sent to the business office for payment.

Library Records

1. Accession Register

This gives a detail information of the books received:

(a) Accession number.
(b) Author.
(c) Title and edition.
(d) Publisher.
(e) Price.
(f) Date of receipt.
(g) Date of withdrawal from stock.
(h) Source.

2. Kardex

It is a quick reference to obtain a reference material.

3. Book Labelling

Ownership stamp, spine label and date label is mentioned in each book.

4. Arrangement of Books

Books should be placed in open shelves to permit and easy use at all times. This should be arranged according to the classification system adopted. Pamphlets and other materials may be placed in special cabinets, current journals may be placed in magazine rack. Always the materials should be placed in such manner that the readers should not waste their time.

5. Classification

A professional library usually arranges books according to subject classification. For a hospital library Dewey Decimal number classification will be helpful than other classifications. For example:

000—General, 100—natural science, 200—social science, 300—nurses and nursing, 490—medicines, 500—hospital economy, 600—Food, nutrition and dietetics, 700—public health, 800—philosophy, psychology and religion, 900—general culture. Each division is again sub-divided into ten sub-divisions.

Another scheme of classification by mixed notation of Alphabets and numerals introduced by Miss. J. Williamson, Librarian, School of Nursing, University College Hospital, London, can also be useful, for example

A—History of Medicine, B—Anatomy, C—Physiology, 0—Microbiology, E—Nutrition, F—Pharmacology, G—Basic Nursing, H—Medicine, J—Surgery, K—Ear, Nose, Throat, L—Ophthalmology, MGynaecology, N—Obstetrics, P—Paediatrics, Q—Geriatrics, R—Psychiatry, S-Psychology, T—Educational Theory.

When the classification is made, the book should be placed in the shelf allotted. Whatever classification is it may be, it should be easily adaptable to all phases of medicine and nursing.

Cataloguing

In order to maintain cataloguing, a uniform system is essential.

Before circulating the library materials, the following points to be kept in mind:

1. It should be checked with bill or order.
2. Enter into the stock books-source, date of receipt, cost, total, etc.
3. Cut any uncut pages.
4. Emboss the stamp with mark of ownership on page edge, on sides of each cover, and on set pages throughout the book.
5. Write the accession number and date in front or back of the title page of the book.
6. Classify and place them in shelves.
7. New should be opened carefully to prevent tear.
8. Books should get enough space in shelves to avoid overcrowding.
9. Protect the edges of the books while shelving.
10. Regular dusting and cleanliness is essential for its preservation.
11. Books damaged or torned should be sent for mending
12. Books/journals or periodicals should be sent for binding as and when needed.
13. Immediate binding is required when any book is badly loosened.

Issue Procedures

There are two methods of discharging books:

I. Browne System

In this method, two cards are required—one card is given to student on which the loan books are entered (Borrowers Card)—other card is kept at the back of each book in a small envelope.

2. Register System

In this title of the book, author of the book, accession number, name of the person, date of issue and date of return is written. Person who borrows the book has to sign in the register with date. This method is useful for hospital library.

Records and Reports

Records are very essential to know about the utility of the library. The budget is prepared on that account. A daily record of attendance is very useful. The report is prepared by the librarian and send it to the Administrator monthly/quarterly or so. It is valuable for research purpose.

Evaluation of Library

Library services should be evaluated by the staff and library committee annually. A suitable proforma should be prepared on the basis of criteria developed by the committee.

Mukherjee and Others, Library Organisation and Administration, Calcutta, World Press Private Ltd., First Edition, 1972.

Philomina, G., "The Nursing College Library", NJI, Vol. XXXVII, No. 6, Qune, 1986, pp. 151-53.

APPENDIX

KNOWLEDGE AND INFORMATION MANAGEMENT IN LIBRARIES

N.SUBRAMANIAN

1. INTRODUCTION

This is the era of knowledge and information explosion. The unprecedented growth of knowledge and information has impacted all organisations including the libraries. The conventional functions of libraries are collect, process, disseminate, store and retrieve information to provide better **services** to the end users. In the digital environment, the role of libraries is changing to provide the competitive advantage for its users. The success of **library** and information centre depends upon their ability to utilize information knowledge of its staff to serve the user community. The ICT has played a significant role in this dynamics which has not only made access across the globe easier, but has facilitated integration of thought processes, synergy in working methods and places, team learning and in enhancing organisational transparency. With the development of IT and its applications in libraries, the concept of document **management** has been changed to information **management** and again, the entire scenario of information **management** has started its change to knowledge **management**.

2. KNOWLEDGE

Knowledge is an intellectual capital when people out of creation, add value to information. It is generated. Knowledge is classified and modified. It may be indexing. It is shared. Sharing of knowledge is a core element of knowledge **management**. IT has provided with number of possible solutions for sharing via e-mail, intranet, etc. Davanport (1998) defined knowledge as follows: Knowledge is fluid framed experiences, values, contextual information as expert insights that provides a framework for evaluation and incorporating new experiences of information.

Daniel Bell defines knowledge as a set of organised statements of facts or ideas, presenting a reasoned judgment or an experimental result, which is transmitted to others through some communication medium in some systematic form.

3. INFORMATION

Marc Porat states that "Information is data that has been organised and communicated." Stehen Abram sees the process for knowledge creation and use as a continuum where data transforms into information, information transforms into knowledge and knowledge drives and undergoing behavior and decision making. Information is visible, independent from action and decision, different informat after processing, physical product, independent from existing environment, easily transferable and duplicate. Knowledge is invisible, closely related to action and decision, different in thought after processing, spiritual product, identified with existing environment, transferable through learning and not duplicate.

4. TYPES OF KNOWLEDGE

Knowledge is classified into three types:

1. Explicit knowledge
2. Tacit knowledge
3. Cultural knowledge

Explicit knowledge

It is formal and easy to communicate to others. It is the knowledge of rationality. That is, policies, rules, specifications and formulae. It is also known as declarative knowledge.

Tacit knowledge

It is complex form of knowledge. It has two dimensions namely technical and cognitive. This is personal knowledge, which is in human mind and difficult to formalize and also difficult to communicate.

Cultural knowledge

B.B. Chand describes the cultural knowledge as knowledge which includes assumptions and beliefs. It is used to understand, describe and explain the reality as well as conventions. It is also useful to form the framework among organisational members, recognize the new information and evaluate alternative interpretations and actions.

5. KNOWLEDGE MANAGEMENT

Knowledge **management** is generally understood to mean the sharing of knowledge inside or outside of an organisation. Knowledge sharing has been greatly facilitated by modern computer based technology. There is no agreed definition of Knowledge **Management**, even among practitioners. The term is used loosely to refer to a broad collection of organisational practices and approaches related to generating, capturing, and disseminating know-how and other content relevant to the organisation's business. Knowledge is no just an explicit tangible "thing", like information, but information combined with experience, context, interpretation and reflection. Knowledge involves the full person, integrating the elements of both thinking and feeling. Knowledge **management** is the process of creating, capturing and using knowledge to enhance organisational performance. It is most frequently associated with two types of activities:

- to document and appropriate individual's knowledge, and
- to disseminate it through such venues as a company vide database.

- Knowledge **management** is a method of gathering information and making it available to others process of systematically and actively managing and leveraging the stores of knowledge in an organisation process of transforming information and intellectual assets into enduring values
- a system or framework for managing the organisational processes that create, store and distribute knowledge as defined by its collective data. Jennifer Rowlay stated, "Knowledge **management** is concerned with the exploitation of an organisation.... Organisations that succeed in knowledge **management** are likely to view knowledge as an asset and to develop organisational norms and values, which support the creation and sharing knowledge."

Galagan proposed the following knowledge **management** processes:

- Generating new knowledge
- Accessing knowledge from external sources
- Representing knowledge in documents, databases and so on
- embedding knowledge in processes, products or **services**
- transferring existing knowledge
- using accessible knowledge indecision-making
- facilitating knowledge through culture and incentives
- measuring the value of knowledge assets and the impact of knowledge

Knowledge management in library and information centers

Business world is changing in the new knowledge economy and in the digital age, libraries of all types are undergoing drastic changes also. The new role of libraries in the 21st century needs to be as a learning and knowledge center for their users. As a learning organisation, libraries should provide a strong leadership in knowledge **management**. Unlike the business organisation, the learning organisation should sharing of knowledge with others outside. Libraries should improve their knowledge **management** in all of the key areas of **library services**.

The exponential growth in human knowledge in a variety of formats, libraries need to develop their resources, access and sharing strategies from printed to electronic and digital resources. Restricted by limited funding, technology, staff and space, libraries must carefully analyze the needs of their users and seek to develop cooperative acquisition plans to meet the needs of users.

Libraries should be developed and maintained an integrated online public access catalogue (OPAC) with both internal and external resources as well as printed and other formats of knowledge. Useful websites and knowledge sources should be regularly searched and selected from the internet and included in OPACs. A system for the reviewing and,updating of these resources should be performed. Going beyond explicit knowledge, libraries should also develop to capture all that tacit knowledge that is of importance to their users, their organisations, and to the internal operations of libraries. The website of each **library** should serve as a "portal" for all sources of relevant knowledge and information whether explicit or tacit,whether on site or remote and in all formats.

In the current digital and networked knowledge age, the size of information sources on the web is growing exponentially. No one really knows exactly how many web pages are on the internet, because new web pages are added every second. Universities and research organisations are knowledge reservoirs. These highly valued intellectual assets, regardless of whether they are explicit or tacit, should be inventoried, archived, indexed, frequently updated and made accessible in digital form, Libraries should use the new approach to capture web information by cooperative efforts such as Dublin core metadata and the cooperative online resources catalogue (CORC).

Other new methods such as data mining, text mining, content **management**, search engines, spidering programmes, natural language searching, linguistic analysis, semantic networks, knowledge extraction, concept of yellow pages, and such technologies in information visualisation as two dimensional or three dimensional knowledge mapping, etc., have been a part of recent developments in knowledge **management** systems.

6. RESOURCES SHARING AND NETWORKING

Traditionally, libraries have a long practice of resource sharing and networking. These have been greatly expanded by the rapid development of computer, telecommunication networking and digital technologies.

The sources of the cooperative work and resources sharing of OCLC (Online Computer **Library** Center) and Ohio LINK (Ohio **Library** and Information Network) in US, is the best examples in resource sharing and networking with the result of the full cooperation and participation of all member libraries without selfishness. Large and major libraries must take the lead in such an Endeavour.

7. CHARACTERISTICS OF KNOWLEDGE MANAGEMENT IN LIBRARIES

The role of KM in Libraries will become more and more important along with the development of knowledge economy. It is a new **management** mode. The following superiority and characteristics are incomparable with conventional **management**.

1. Information technology is a tool for KM
2. Human resource **management** in KM
3. User **Services** in KM

Information technology is a tool for KM

To facilitate the implementation of knowledge **management**, a well-defined and operational knowledge **management** system should be in place. Latest information technology should be used in the libraries. In this regard, the **library** director/librarian should consider himself as the chief knowledge officer of the entire organisation and should work together with the chief information officer, heads of the planning department, the computer and information technology center, the human resource **management** department, the finance department, etc., to design and develop such a system. Such knowledge **management** system should be built on the existing computer and information technology infrastructure including upgraded intranet, extranet, internet and available software programmes to facilitate the capture, analysis, organisation, storage and sharing of internal and external information resources for effective knowledge exchange among users, resource persons (faculty, researchers, subject experts, etc.), publishers, government agencies, business and industries and other organisations via multiple channels. In recent years, many of the newly developed information technology for databases and information/document **management** can be utilised in knowledge **management** such as data warehousing, data mining, text mining, etc.

Human resource management in KM

The most important resource in the knowledge economy system is the talents who grasp knowledge. The talent competition has become the focus of market competition in the knowledge economy era. In the knowledge economy era, the libraries will attach importance to vocational training and lifelong education of **library** staff to raise their scientific knowledge level and ability of acquiring and innovative knowledge. They also will respect the human value, guide and bring into play wisdom potentialities of **library** staffs. It is an important way for raising work efficiency of **library** staff. An all round improvement of **library** staff's quality and positioning of the human value will become important objectives of knowledge **management** in **Library** and Information centers. The **library** staff members of Universities and research committees should be inventoried, indexed regularly and be made searchable and accessible through electronic databases created and maintained by libraries. The expertise should be appreciated with appropriate rewards and incentives. As a learning organisation, libraries should allocate annual funding to provide continuing education and staff training to all staff members. Knowledge must be renewed and expanded to prevent it from becoming stagnant.

Libraries should also encourage the transfer of knowledge and experience from experienced staff to new staff members. A mentoring system should be in place to help new comers to learn from experienced **library** staff. Informal seminars, discussion sessions for staff can interact and exchange "lessons learned" "best practices" and other experiences should be scheduled at regular intervals and at convenient times sit and chat rooms can be created through intranet libraries should be attending to favorable working conditions and environment, which will contribute to better staff retention.

User services in KM

The utmost goal of knowledge **management** is to provide users with a variety of quality **services** in order to improve the communication, use and creation of knowledge. Information about each user can be obtained by analyzing the records of user registration, surveys, circulation and inter **library** loan, frequently asked reference questions and the use of e-journals and digital resources, etc. User satisfaction and needs should be collected through periodical user's surveys. The findings should be used for the planning and redesign of the existing **library services**.

Some of the manual **services** of the **library** such as "new publication alert" and "dissemination of information" should be done automatically by employing the "push technology" with great efficiency and convenience. Each **library** user can also set-up his virtual "my **library**/portal" for new information /resources provided by the **library**.

8. TECHNOLOGIES FOR KNOWLEDGE MANAGEMENT

Library and information centers should be developed/modified based on the perfect environment for new media applications. Due to impact of globalisation, economic competition and revolution of ICT, the libraries are under going tremendous change its environment. ICT tools and techniques, knowledge **management** systems, internet, web resources, digital libraries have made a significant change in the existing **library** systems and **services**. It is a major challenge for the **library** professionals. Knowledge acquisition is the starting point ot knowledge **management** in Libraries. The application of IT, enlarges the scope of knowledge acquisition, rises knowledge acquition, speed and reduces knowledge acquisition cost. It is impossible to accomplish such important tasks by using man's brain only in the modern society in which the knowledge changes with each passing day. It will be possible to link closely knowledge sources and knowledge workers by computer networks, thus constructing knowledge networks in libraries based on realisation of single point informationalisation.

Data-wise technologies developed the following list of technologies for the knowledge **management**:

- Intranet within an organisation
- Document **management** systems
- Information retrieval systems
- Relational and object databases
- Electronic publishing
- Groupware and work flow systems
- Push technologies
- Help desk applications
- Brain storming applications
- Data warehousing and data mining

9. CONCLUSION

KM is an emerging field, much tooted or hyped since late 1990s. Due to the complicated nature of knowledge and its **management**, it is often difficult to estimate or demonstrate the value of the Knowledge **Management**. In the business world, knowledge **management** has been regarded as strategically important for organisations to gain a competitive advantage over their competitions, to add value their products, to win greater satisfaction from their customers.

In the **library** world, there is a lesson to be learned from the business world.

For any **library** to succeed in implementing knowledge **management** will require a strong leadership and vision from the top administration. Information Technology and systems can provide effective support in implementing knowledge **management**. Libraries should work together with Information Technology Professionals and others to develop the appropriate knowledge **management** systems. Libraries, with limited budget and human resources, should utilize the current **management** structure and technology to implement KM, either bottom-up or top-down. With an effort, KM will help to increase libraries operational efficiency and later to the ever increasing needs of our clientele.

References

Dearstyne, B.W. (2000). Greeting and shaping the future: Information professionals as strategists and leaders. *Information Outlook.* Aug 2000.

Denning, S. (2001). The Strategy of Knowledge. http://www.stevedenning.com/stategy_knowledge-sharing.html

Kantor, R.M.(2001). Evolve!: Succeeding in the Digital culture of tomorrow, New Haven, Harvard Business school press.

Peacock, J and Middleton, M (1999). Mixed mode education: Implication for **library** user **services**. *New Library World.* 100(1146) 11-19pp.

Shanhong, Tang(2000). Knowledge **Management** in Libraries in the 21st Century. In the 66 IFLA Council and General Conference, held at Jerusalem, Israel, 13-18 Aug 2000.

Stratigos, A. (2001). Knowledge **management** meets future information users. Online, Jan. 2001.

Wag Yunbua(1999). Knowledge Economy and the development of the **Library**. **Library** work and Research. 1999 (6) 17-19pp.

Index